D1379924

Evidence-based
Obstetric Anesthesia

To my wife Janice and our sons Zvi, Moshe and Yoni – SHH

To Bill, Matthew and Mark – MJD

Evidence-based Obstetric Anesthesia

Edited by

Stephen H. Halpern

Director of Obstetrical Anaesthesia
Sunnybrook and Women's College Health Sciences Centre
University of Toronto
Toronto
Ontario
Canada

M. Joanne Douglas

Clinical Professor
Department of Anaesthesia
University of British Columbia and British Columbia's Women's Hospital
Vancouver
British Columbia
Canada

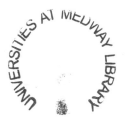

 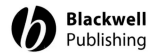

Blackwell Publishing, Inc., 350 Main Street, Malden, Massachusetts 02148-5020, USA
Blackwell Publishing Ltd, 9600 Garsington Road, Oxford OX4 2DQ, UK
Blackwell Publishing Asia Pty Ltd, 550 Swanston Street, Carlton, Victoria 3053, Australia

First published 2005

Library of Congress Cataloging-in-Publication Data

Evidence-based obstetric anesthesia / edited by Stephen H. Halpern, M.
Joanne Douglas.
    p. ; cm.
  Includes bibliographical references and index.
  ISBN-13: 978-0-7279-1734-8
  ISBN-10: 0-7279-1734-X
  1. Anesthesia in obstetrics.   2. Evidence-based medicine.
  [DNLM: 1. Anesthesia, Obstetrical.   2. Evidence-Based Medicine.
I. Halpern, Stephen H.   II. Douglas, M. Joanne.

  RG732.E975 2005
  617.9′682—dc22

                                        2004028825

ISBN-13: 978-0-7279-1734-8
ISBN-10: 0-7279-1734-X

A catalogue record for this title is available from the British Library

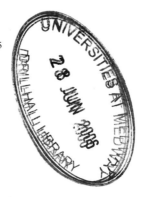

Set in 9.5/12pt by Graphicraft Limited, Hong Kong
Printed and bound in India by Replika Press Pvt. Ltd

Commissioning Editor: Mary Banks
Project Manager: Alice Nelson
Development Editor: Nick Morgan
Production Controller: Kate Charman

For further information on Blackwell Publishing, visit our website:
http://www.blackwellpublishing.com

The publisher's policy is to use permanent paper from mills that operate a sustainable
forestry policy, and which has been manufactured from pulp processed using acid-free
and elementary chlorine-free practices. Furthermore, the publisher ensures that the text
paper and cover board used have met acceptable environmental accreditation standards.

Contents

Contents

Contributors

Pamela Angle MD, FRCP(C)

Assistant Professor, Dept of Anaesthesia, Sunnybrook and Women's College Health Sciences Centre, University of Toronto, 76 Grenville St, Toronto, Ontario M5S 1B2, Canada

Terrance W. Breen MD

Dept of Anesthesiology, Duke University Medical Center 3094, Durham, NC 27710, USA

Michelle Chochinov MD, FRCP(C)

Dept of Anaesthesia, Sunnybrook and Women's College Health Sciences Centre, University of Toronto, 2075 Bayview Ave, Toronto, Ontario M4N 3M5, Canada

Peter T-L. Choi MD, MSc, FRCP(C)

Assistant Professor, Dept of Anaesthesia, University of British Columbia, 910 West Tenth Ave, Vancouver, British Columbia V5Z 4E3, Canada

M. Joanne Douglas MD, FRCP(C)

Clinical Professor, Dept of Anaesthesia, Faculty of Medicine, University of British Columbia and British Columbia's Women's Hospital, 4500 Oak St, Vancouver, British Columbia V6H 3N1, Canada

Yehuda Ginosar BSc, MB BS

Lecturer in Anesthesiology, Hebrew University Medical School, Jerusalem, Israel, and Senior Anesthesiologist, Dept of Anesthesiology and Critical Care Medicine, Hadassah Hebrew University Medical Center, POB 12000, Jerusalem 91120, Israel

Eric Goldszmidt MD, FRCP(C)

Dept of Anaesthesia, Mount Sinai Hospital and University of Toronto, 600 University Ave, Toronto, Ontario M5G 1X5, Canada

Stephen H. Halpern MD, MSc, FRCP(C)

Director of Obstetrical Anaesthesia, Sunnybrook and Women's College Health Sciences Centre, University of Toronto, 76 Grenville St, Toronto, Ontario M5S 1B2, Canada

Darren Hart RM

Research Midwife, Dept of Obstetrics and Gynaecology, Guy's and St Thomas' Hospital, London SE1 7EH, UK

Kamal Hussain MB BS, FFARSCI

Obstetric Anaesthesia Fellow, Dept of Anaesthesia, Sunnybrook and Women's College Health Sciences Centre, University of Toronto, 76 Grenville St, Toronto, Ontario M5S 1B2, Canada

Jean E. Kronberg PhD, MD, FRCP(C)

Associate Professor, Dept of Anaesthesia, University of Toronto and Active Staff, Sunnybrook and Women's College Health Sciences Centre, University of Toronto, 76 Grenville St, Toronto, Ontario M5S 1B2, Canada

Barbara L. Leighton MD

Dept of Anesthesiology, Washington University, Campus Box 8054, 660 S. Euclid Ave, St Louis, MO 63110-1093, USA

Stefan Lucas MD

University of Rochester, School of Medicine and Dentistry, Dept of Anesthesiology, 601 Elmwood Avenue, Rochester, NY 14642, USA

Chahé Mardirosoff MD

Service d'Anesthésie et Réanimation, Polyclinique de Savoie, 8, rue F. David, 74100 Annemasse, France

Pamela J. Morgan MD, CCFP, FRCP(C)

Associate Professor, Staff Anaesthesiologist, Sunnybrook and Women's College Health Sciences Centre, University of Toronto, 76 Grenville St, Toronto, Ontario M5S 1B2, Canada

Geraldine O'Sullivan MD, FRCA

Dept of Anaesthetics, Guy's and St Thomas' Hospital, London SE1 7EH, UK

Niall L. Purdie MB ChB, FFARCSI

Dept of Anaesthesia, Sunnybrook and Women's College Health Sciences Centre, University of Toronto, 76 Grenville St, Toronto, Ontario M5S 1B2, Canada

Ian F. Russell MB ChB, FRCA

Honorary Senior Lecturer, Academic Dept of Obstetrics and Gynaecology, Hull University, and Consultant Anaesthetist, Dept of Anaesthesia, Hull Royal Infirmary, Anlaby Road, Hull HU3 2JZ, UK

Andrew Shennan MD, MRCOG

Senior Lecturer in Obstetrics and Gynaecology, Dept of Obstetrics and Gynaecology, Guy's and St Thomas' Hospital, London SE1 7EH, UK

Margaret Srebrnjak BSc, MD, FRCP(C)

Dept of Anaesthesia, Sunnybrook and Women's College Health Sciences Centre, University of Toronto, 76 Grenville St, Toronto, Ontario M5S 1B2, Canada

Dorothy E.A. Thompson MB ChB, FRCP(C)

Honorary Staff, Dept of Anaesthesia, Sunnybrook and Women's College Health Sciences Centre, University of Toronto, 76 Grenville St, Toronto, Ontario M5S 1B2, Canada

Martin R. Tramèr MD, DPhil

Consultant Anesthetist, Division of Anesthesiology, Geneva University Hospitals, CH-1211 Geneva, Switzerland

Martin van der Vyver MB ChB, MMed(Anes), FCA(SA)

Sunnybrook and Women's College Health Sciences Centre, University of Toronto, 76 Grenville St, Toronto, Ontario M5S 1B2, Canada

Carolyn F. Weiniger MB ChB

Dept of Anesthesia, Hadassah University Hospital, POB 12000, Jerusalem 91120, Israel

William Wight MB BS, FRCA

Consultant Anaesthetist, Dept of Anaesthesia, Royal Victoria Infirmary, Newcastle upon Tyne NE1 4LP, UK

Preface

Since the introduction of anesthesia to obstetric practice by James Young Simpson in 1847, there have been controversies concerning its use. In addition to the larger issue of any medical intervention during normal childbirth, the lay public and medical community have struggled with the balance between the benefits and the risks of analgesia and anesthesia to the mother and fetus during labor and delivery. These controversies persist despite numerous advances in our knowledge about the physiology and pharmacology related to pregnancy and childbirth.

Compared to other fields in medicine, many of the issues in obstetric anesthesia can be difficult to study. This is because the obstetric anesthesiologist often sees the patient for the first time under emotionally and physically stressful circumstances. While some of the early animal studies were helpful in delineating the physiology of pregnancy, this information was accepted as dogma and applied, sometimes inappropriately, to humans. Even the results of some of the older human studies were more likely to reflect the biases of the researchers than the "truth." Many of these early studies have not been repeated but a growing body of high quality research in the field of obstetric anesthesia has been published in the last 20 years.

The purpose of this book is to identify and synthesize the strongest research in obstetric anesthesia in order to promote best practice. There are many areas that will not be found in this volume because of the absence of sound research on the subject. Most of the topics were chosen because they were of interest to clinicians and/or there was extensive, rigorous research on the subject matter. Perhaps in the future, as more research becomes available, other topics will be added.

The contributors were asked to write each chapter in the form of a systematic review. Rather than providing a general discussion, each chapter was designed to answer one or more discrete clinical questions. The basis of each chapter is an extensive literature review for each topic for the best evidence. In an effort to reduce bias, most of the information presented comes from randomized controlled trials or high-quality cohort studies. This type of data does not exist for topics that deal with rare events such as maternal mortality, aspiration pneumonitis and epidural hematoma. The contributors of chapters on these topics relied on data from national surveys and other databases for some of the information.

The contributors then summarized the data. In most cases this was done qualitatively through the extensive use of data tables. In some cases, a formal meta-analysis could be performed. Finally, each contributor interpreted the existing data to answer the clinical questions originally posed. Thus, the information on each topic is meant to be complete, accurate and accessible to clinicians. In some areas, there are obvious gaps in our knowledge and these are highlighted.

The book is divided into three main sections. The first deals with analgesia for labor, which is probably the most controversial area related to obstetric anesthesia. This includes chapters about informed consent, new techniques (patient-controlled epidural analgesia, combined spinal epidural analgesia), new drugs (ropivacaine, levobupivacaine) and controversies about equipment (epidural catheters). The efficacy of nitrous oxide is discussed in light of information that has rarely been presented previously. Finally, there is a brief, but thorough, examination of the use of TENS for labor analgesia.

The second section – Anesthesia for cesarean section – contains two chapters on the prevention and treatment of hypotension associated with spinal anesthesia. One discusses which fluids are best, the other which vasopressor. Following these chapters is a discussion on the treatment of postoperative pain and the side-effects resulting from that treatment. Finally, the assumption that "regional anesthesia is good and general anesthesia is bad" is discussed in some detail.

The third and final section – Complications of obstetric anesthesia – contains a number of controversial topics. Should the parturient with a low platelet count be offered epidural analgesia? Does epidural analgesia cause long-term back pain? Is the airway of the parturient really different from non-pregnant patients? Other topics presented in this section include the issue of postdural puncture headache in the parturient and analgesia for external cephalic version.

This book is intended for the use of all clinicians who practice obstetric anesthesia. Trainees at all levels can benefit both from the content and the approach to clinical problems. Rather than taking the words of their mentors at face value, we would encourage them to ask "how do you know that?" or seek the best evidence themselves.

As more research is being performed and published the conclusions drawn from this current literature review may change. Hopefully, this book will stimulate further research leading to a clearer understanding as to the role of obstetric anesthesia in pregnancy and childbirth.

We would like to take this opportunity to thank the contributors to the book for doing such a thorough job researching their topics and presenting it in a manner that, hopefully, clinicians and students will find useful.

SHH
MJD

Acknowledgments

We would like to thank the Hebrew University, Jerusalem, Israel for providing a Joels Visiting Professorship in the Department of Anesthesiology and Critical Care Medicine to Dr Halpern and Sunnybrook and Women's College Health Sciences Centre, Toronto, Canada for providing his sabbatical support.

We would also like to thank British Columbia's Women's Hospital and Health Centre for their support of Dr Douglas.

PART 1
Analgesia for normal labor

CHAPTER 1

Consent for obstetric analgesia and anesthesia

M. Joanne Douglas

Background

Informed consent is based on the ethical principle of autonomy and has several components. The requirements for informed consent are that:

1 it must be given voluntarily;
2 the patient must have the capacity (ability) to understand the information that is presented;
3 the consent must be specific to the person doing the procedure and to the procedure;
4 the risks and benefits of the procedure must be explained and understood; and
5 all questions must be answered.

In addition, the individual should have time to consider the information that is presented, although for the woman in pain that often is a short interval.[1]

The obstetric anesthesiologist often faces a dilemma in obtaining informed consent for neuraxial analgesia/anesthesia in the laboring parturient. Many anesthesiologists consider it impossible to obtain informed consent from a woman who is in pain, and in particular if she has received an opioid, such as meperidine.[2–4] Some women prepare birth plans prior to labor indicating that they do not want an epidural under any circumstances. This presents an ethical dilemma if these women change their minds when confronted with the pain of labor and request an epidural.[1] It can be argued that they prepared their birth plan without full knowledge as to the degree of pain that they might encounter. The anesthesiologist faced with a birth plan that states "no epidural" is concerned that the woman in pain is not fully competent to provide informed consent to the epidural.[5,6] Scott[7] discussed this dilemma in her editorial where she considered it "unethical to withhold pain relief" to a woman in pain because she had previously written a birth plan stating that she did not wish for an epidural.

It is useful to review the literature for studies that explore obtaining informed consent in the laboring parturient, the information to be provided and the most effective way to present that information.

Methods: literature search

Studies included in this review were cohort studies or surveys dealing with the issue of informed consent for labor epidural analgesia. The outcomes of interest were whether women postpartum could recall the risks that were included in the informed consent,[8,9] whether written or oral information was more effective in the consent process,[10,11] and the information women wanted to know prior to giving consent for epidural analgesia.[11–13]

A computer search of the MEDLINE® and EMBASE® databases covering the time period 1980–August 1, 2003 was performed using the key words: [consent], [informed consent], [analgesia], [obstetrics], [obstetric anesthesia/anaesthesia], [labor/labour analgesia], [labor/labour analgesia, epidural] and [ethics]. The search was limited to human studies that were published in English and full text was available from the University of Toronto. The bibliographies of articles that were retrieved were searched for additional references and those articles reviewed. Some studies from the general anesthesia literature were reviewed to contrast the experience of laboring women with that of the general surgical population.[14–17]

Results

Seven studies were found using the above search strategy.[8–13,18] One was a randomized trial,[10] the remainder were prospective surveys or retrospective assessments. No study was excluded (Table 1.1). The total number

Table 1.1 Characteristics of studies.

Authors	Study type & country	Population	Number of subjects	Time data collected	Main outcome	Comments
Swann et al.[8]	Survey, Australia	Nulliparas	40	36–48 h postpartum	Recall of risk comparing women who attended epidural antenatal class	Lack of randomization to antenatal classes, no description of population, no consistent provider of information pre-epidural
Affleck et al.[9]	Survey, USA	Mixed parity	101	< 24 h postpartum	Recall of risk	Heterogeneous population, 7 had only mild pain
Gerancher et al.[10]	Randomized survey, USA	Mixed parity	113/group	5–7 months postpartum	Recall risk: verbal vs verbal + written information	Population not described, 73% followed up, no measure baseline knowledge
White et al.[11]	Audit before and after intervention, UK	Mixed parity	100/group	1 day postpartum	Recall risk: verbal vs verbal + written information	25–30% previous epidural, interviewers not blinded, interview of groups separated by time
Pattee et al.[12]	Survey, Canada	Mixed parity	60	1–2 months postpartum	What complications parturients want to know, did pain influence ability to give consent	Systematic sampling, retrospective, lack generalizability, 86% postgraduate education, 35% previous epidural, 64% received opioids pre-epidural, variability in time of survey < 4 h–8 weeks
Jackson et al.[13]	Prospective survey, Canada	Mixed parity	60	Pre-epidural	What parturients want to know, understand risk	25% previous epidural, 75% postgraduate education, 46% opioids presurvey, epidural only given after survey completed
Beilin et al.[18]	Survey, USA	Mixed parity	320	24 h postpartum	Knowledge and concerns re. epidural	Vaginal delivery + cesarean section included

of participants included in the seven studies was 981 parturients.

Overall, the evidence provided in the studies is not strong (Table 1.1). In many there was no full description of the individuals surveyed in the population (e.g. educational status), although most described the number of multiparas and nulliparas. There was no indication as to how the number of women surveyed was determined and most of the surveys were conducted at varying time periods following delivery.

Other design issues lead to difficulties in interpreting the results. For example, if the woman cannot recall risks during a postpartum interview or questionnaire, this does not exclude the possibility that she understood the risks at the time of consent. Therefore, a survey that relies on the recall of risk may be meaningless. A woman's postpartum assessment as to her competency at the time of the consent may be influenced by the outcome of the labor (healthy or ill baby, vaginal or operative delivery, postpartum pain from an episiotomy or tear). Yet none of the surveys stratified for the obstetric outcome. The woman's response to a survey might be biased if she did not want an epidural but agreed to it because of the severity of her pain. Similarly, it is difficult to rely on responses to questionnaires or interviews that women

Consent for obstetric analgesia and anesthesia

Table 1.2 Risks discussed by Affleck et al.[9]

Infection
Bleeding
Nerve damage
Urinary retention
High spinal block
Block failure
Nausea and vomiting
Respiratory depression
Pruritus
Intravenous injection (with cardiovascular collapse)
Postdural puncture headache
Local anesthetic toxicity (potential seizure)
Hypotension

completed before being given analgesia because her answers might have been influenced by her desire to obtain analgesia as rapidly as possible.

In addition to the problems listed above, other characteristics of the studies make interpretation difficult. Some of the surveys combine the results of mixed populations of parturients (multiparas who had received an epidural with a previous pregnancy and nulliparas). It may be difficult to generalize the results to parturients of different ethnic and educational backgrounds when the majority of participants were well educated. Many of the surveys were small, leading to a lack of precision in the findings. Finally, and possibly most importantly, none of the studies describe a rigorous process to determine whether or not their questionnaires produce reliable and valid results.

Postpartum recall of risks

In an effort to determine the effectiveness of the consent process, Swan and Borshoff[8] assessed postpartum recall of epidural risk explanation in 40 laboring women who had an epidural. Prior to insertion of the epidural, a brief, detailed explanation of the risks of the procedure was given focusing on backache, postdural puncture headache (PDPH) and "more serious" complications. "More serious complications" were explained in general terms. Women were then surveyed 36–48 h postpartum for recall and a comparison was made as to recall of risk between those who had the antenatal education classes offered at their hospital and those who had not.

Sixty-five percent had attended antenatal classes but only 40% attended the session on epidural analgesia.

All 40 women recalled having an epidural but only 67% recalled that risks were discussed. Recall of all three areas of risk (PDPH, backache, serious complications) was higher in the group that had received antenatal education; median score 2.31 (maximum 3) vs 0.92. Those who had received epidural antenatal information had significantly better recall of each specific risk.

Affleck et al.[9] administered a standardized oral discussion of anesthetic risks to 101 laboring women prior to epidural catheter insertion (Table 1.2). The women could discuss any concerns. Postpartum (< 24 h after consent) they were surveyed and asked to:

1 verbalize any risks they could recall; and
2 identify the risks they could recall from a printed list of eight risks, five of which were real and three were false. Descriptive analysis was used.

All women recalled the informed consent discussion and insertion of the epidural. Patients recalled an average of 2.0 ± 1.3 risks with 13% recalling no risks, 22% one risk, 29% two risks and 25% three risks. When only one risk was recalled the most commonly recalled risk was PDPH (64%). The five true risks were identified by more than 50% of the women. In contrast to Swan's study there was no difference in risk recall between those who attended prenatal classes and those who did not.

Is recall of risk better when written information is provided?

Two studies examined the best way to present information prior to epidural analgesia. Gerancher et al.[10] enrolled 113 consecutive laboring women during the daytime over a 1-month period. All women had a structured preanesthetic interview by one of the investigators. This interview was carried out prior to administration of any form of labor analgesia, including parenteral medications. The interview included questions regarding the woman's medical condition and a verbal presentation of anesthetic options, risks and procedures (total time 10 min). A written 10-point check list was used to ensure that all topics were covered.

The women were randomly assigned to receive the interview as documented above (verbal group) or the same interview plus a written informed consent form containing the same information (verbal + written group). The "informed consent" form was simultaneously reviewed by the investigator and signed by the woman, and the investigator and women in this group received a copy of the consent form. The verbal group did not review, receive or sign a similar consent form. The women were contacted 5–7 months later at which time 10 objective questions (five true risk questions, two false risk questions and three situational questions) were asked to assess their degree of recall.

Eighty-two of the original 113 women (72.5%) were contacted postpartum; 44 in the verbal + written group and 38 in the verbal only group. Seventy-five percent in the verbal + written group and 78% in the verbal only group had received epidural analgesia. Median recall scores were 80 (70–90) in the verbal only group and 90 (80–100) in the verbal + written group ($P <$ 0.01). Seventy-six responded that written consent would help them remember the different options, risks and procedures. Six (one verbal + written, five verbal only) considered it unhelpful and four of the six felt that written consent would be alarming. Two of these four (both verbal group) felt they were unable to give informed consent.

White et al.[11] performed an audit prior to (control group) and following adoption of the use of an epidural written information card (subject group) which was prepared following consultation with antenatal and postnatal women, midwives and anesthesiologists. This information card was given to the subject group to read prior to a verbal discussion of the risks involved with epidural analgesia. Both groups had structured interviews on the first postpartum day to discover what the women understood when they gave consent. Eleven questions about epidurals were asked, mainly focusing on potential complications.

Two hundred women participated: 100 in the pre-written information group (control) and 100 in the post-written information group. There was a statistically significant improvement ($P < 0.05$) in the number of correct answers to eight of the 11 questions when the information card was used.

What do women want to know?

In the past many anesthesiologists felt that it was unrealistic to expect the laboring woman to cope with information regarding epidural complications when she was having pain. As an essential ingredient of informed consent is providing information regarding the risks and benefits of the proposed procedure, one must ask the question "How much does the patient want to know?" Two studies addressed this issue.

Pattee et al.[12] surveyed 60 women during the first 2 months postpartum. One month of every 3 months was chosen for systematic sampling and eligible women were those who received epidural analgesia for an uncomplicated vaginal delivery. Approximately 50% of the women were interviewed by survey in hospital and those who were discharged early, at home via telephone call. All of the interviewers were trained by the first author. Questions were either categorical (yes/no) or scored on a 0–10 scale. The questions covered demographics as well as epidural complications that were included in the discussion prior to obtaining consent.

Sixty-five percent of the women responded that it was their first epidural. Sixty-four percent of the parturients had received opioids prior to the epidural but they were as satisfied with the consent process as were the women (34%) who had not had opioids. Women wanted all epidural complications disclosed as they considered them important. If a major complication such as death or paralysis had a risk of more than 1 : 10,000, 66% would not have an epidural. Women did not feel that distress, even though they had considerable pain (8.8/10), interfered with their ability to give consent nor did it affect their comprehension of the information provided (3.0/10). Useful information regarding the epidural came from the anesthesiologist (40%) or from prenatal courses (38%). All patients felt that information with respect to epidural anesthesia should be provided well before labor began (9.4/10).

Jackson et al.[13] prospectively surveyed 60 laboring women between May 1 and October 1, 1999. A single individual interviewed each woman immediately after the request for an epidural was made. All surveys were completed during the daytime and all women requesting an epidural were considered eligible. In addition to brief demographic data, a visual analog score (VAS) was completed regarding pain, anxiety and desire to have an epidural. The goals of the study were to determine what the laboring woman wanted to know before consenting to epidural analgesia and if she felt that she could understand the risks. The survey then gave a list of possible epidural complications and asked the importance of each (Table 1.3). This was followed by a series of questions (Table 1.4).

Table 1.3 Possible epidural complications discussed by Jackson et al.[13]

1 Headache
2 Backache
3 Infection around the spine
4 Temporary low blood pressure
5 Inability to urinate
6 Spinal anesthesia (temporary total body paralysis)
7 Convulsions
8 Death or permanent paralysis
9 Effects on baby
10 Prolongation of labor
11 Inability to walk during labor

Table 1.4 Questions asked by Jackson et al.[13]

1 Level of risk considered significant
2 Where they had obtained epidural information
3 Level of agreement as to whether pain/anxiety affected their ability to understand the information given
4 Whether a relative or friend would be helpful in their decision
5 Whether they felt pressure to have an epidural
6 Whether they had received a "painkiller" in labor prior to the epidural

Four women could not complete the survey: three because of labor pain and one because of the birth of her baby. Four patients did not understand what was meant by the "level of risk considered significant." Most of the women (75%) had some college or university education and 25% had epidural analgesia for a previous labor. Eighty percent realized that epidurals were not risk free and knew of alternatives and 46% had received an opioid earlier in labor. All had a high degree of pain (7.5/10) and anxiety (7.2/10) and the median length of labor prior to the request was 6 h (SD 14 h, range 1–76 h). All wanted to hear about all potential epidural complications but felt that knowing the complications would not stop them from having an epidural. They considered headache, confinement to bed and prolongation of labor as less important side-effects while seizure, death or paralysis and effects on the baby were of greater importance. Of interest, 52% of women did not want to know the incidence of the complications. The women in this survey felt less able to understand the information because of pain and anxiety (4.9/10) than those in the study by Pattee et al.[12]

Beilin et al.[18] wanted to know whether pregnant women want to have an interview with an anesthesiologist before the start of labor. On postpartum day 1, a 17-item questionnaire was given to 407 consecutive women who had given birth either vaginally or by cesarean section. The questionnaire took 10–15 min to complete. Three hundred and twenty women completed the questionnaire (79%). Fifteen percent (26) of 174 women felt that they did not receive sufficient information and 11 of these felt that the pain of labor interfered with their ability to concentrate.

Consent for anesthesia in other contexts

Overall, there are few studies involving consent for epidural analgesia for labor. However, the results from these few studies are similar to those in the general surgical population. Clark et al.[19] studied the risk information retained before and after either a verbal or verbal + written consent process in consecutive non-obstetric inpatients. Surprisingly, the verbal only group retained more information about anesthetic risk than did the verbal + written group. In contrast, Garden et al.[14] found that full disclosure of risks in 45 patients about to undergo cardiac surgery significantly increased knowledge about anesthesia. Provision of written information did not increase the level of anxiety.

There have been several studies looking at what the non-obstetric patient wants to know prior to anesthesia for surgery.[14–17] Most found that patients under the age of 50 years wanted to know more about potential complications than those over 50 years.[17] Patients in these studies wanted the opportunity to meet their anesthesiologist preoperatively and discuss their anesthetic. The studies by Pattee et al.[12] and Jackson et al.[13] also found that laboring women wanted to have all complications discussed but were reluctant to know the incidence. Because of the education level of the women in Jackson's study the results may not be applicable to all laboring women.

Although a majority of patients wish to know about complications, a survey of Canadian anesthesiologists, published in 1985, found that 48% of anesthesiologists identified at least one complication that they never discussed with their patients.[20] This complication was considered very important by the anesthesiologist. Twenty-one percent of anesthesiologists identified four or more such complications that they did not discuss.

At the same time 74% felt that their patients were seldom or never adequately informed prior to labor and over 80% felt that it was the anesthesiologist's responsibility to educate the women. It would be interesting to repeat this study today to see if the results would be similar.

Current anesthesia practice

Is a separate written consent necessary to document that informed consent has been obtained? In Canada, a written consent form does not necessarily indicate that an informed consent was obtained.[4] In the UK, the majority of obstetric anesthesiologists obtain verbal, rather than written, consent for epidural analgesia.[3] In a survey with a return rate of 60%, more American anesthesiologists indicated that they obtain separate written consent for obstetric anesthesia (for labor and cesarean section). This is in contrast to UK anesthesiologists (47% vs 22%).[21] Written consent for epidural analgesia for labor was obtained by 33% of American and 11% of UK anesthesiologists, even if the woman was judged to be mentally impaired by pain or analgesic drugs. More risks and benefits of epidural analgesia are discussed by American anesthesiologists. Royal College of Anaesthetists' tutors in Great Britain and Northern Ireland were surveyed with respect to their practice in providing information and obtaining consent.[22] There was a 77% response rate. Sixty-two percent of departments provided information on obstetric analgesia and anesthesia and 80% stated that it was possible for a woman to discuss anesthetic techniques with an anesthesiologist.

Conclusions

What can we learn from these studies? First, many laboring women want to know the risks that are involved with an epidural before they give consent. Second, knowledge of the risks does not appear to deter women from consenting to the procedure. Third, provision of written information increases the chance that a woman may recall the complications that are associated with an epidural in the postpartum period. Lastly, the studies by Pattee et al.[12] and Jackson et al.[13] found that most women wanted all of the risks associated with epidural analgesia explained prior to insertion of an epidural and that these women felt that neither pain nor previous opioid altered their ability

to understand those risks. However, there still is a low rate of recall of the informed consent discussion. It is important to realize that failure to recall risk does not indicate that the informed consent process was inadequate or that the woman did not comprehend the information given at the time of the consent. It simply indicates that after a period of time the patient could not remember the information that was provided.

All of the studies are limited by small numbers, heterogeneous populations, dependency on recall of a discussion that took place when the woman was in pain and generalizability of the studies to all women requesting epidural analgesia during labor. Information provided prior to labor will allow women to make a more informed choice.

How do we deal with the woman who has a birth plan that states "no epidural" but then asks for an epidural during labor? Many anesthesiologists would withhold epidural analgesia for fear of legal repercussions. The literature does not deal directly with this issue other than in letters to the editor. Just as one can give consent, one can also change one's mind when confronted with the pain of labor. Ideally, the anesthesiologist will have seen the woman in early labor or prior to labor to ensure that she has all of the facts, understands the possible complications, has adequate time to consider her decision and is not being influenced by her caregivers, her partner or others in her room. However, if suddenly faced with a woman who had a birth plan and who has now changed her mind because of severe pain, I would insert an epidural after a discussion with the woman. I agree with Scott who stated: "It is unethical, I would maintain, to withhold pain relief from a greatly distressed woman, actually begging for an epidural, solely because of a statement written in her Birth Plan at a time of 'not knowing', which states 'I do not wish to have an epidural in labor'."[7] The only possible legal ramification may arise if a woman's birth plan states that: "Even if I change my mind when confronted with labor pain I am not to have an epidural." Known as the Ulysses directive, it may be ethically sound to administer an epidural but legally it could be interpreted as a battery.[1,23] Many anesthesiologists would argue that the woman who has written a Ulysses directive has capacity and can change her mind. Under these circumstances they would administer an epidural.[5,6] Whether an epidural is administered or not, it is important to see these women postpartum and have a frank discussion about the issues surrounding the decision. Some women, who had indicated that they did not want an epidural and who then change their mind and receive an epidural, may feel that they have failed in that they were unable to cope with labor pain. A postpartum discussion may allay their anxiety and ensure that any questions they may have are addressed.

References

1 Brooks H, Sullivan WJ. The importance of patient autonomy at birth. *Int J Obstet Anesth* 2002;**11**:196–203.

2 Knapp RM. Legal view of informed consent for anesthesia during labor. *Anesthesiology* 1990;**72**:211.

3 Bogod D. Obstetric anaesthesia and medical negligence. *Clin Risk* 2002;**8**:243–5.

4 Smedstad KG, Beilby W. Informed consent for epidural analgesia in labour. *Can J Anesth* 2000;**47**:1055–9.

5 Roberts J. Consent issues in obstetric anaesthesia. *Anaesthesia* 2002;**57**:1232–3.

6 Meek T. A response to "Consent issues in obstetric anaesthesia". *Anaesthesia* 2003;**58**:405–6.

7 Scott WE. Ethics in obstetric anaesthesia. *Anaesthesia* 1996;**51**:717–8.

8 Swan HD, Borshoff DC. Informed consent – recall of risk information following epidural analgesia in labour. *Anaesth Intensive Care* 1994;**22**:139–41.

9 Affleck PJ, Waisel DB, Cusick JM, Van Decar T. Recall of risks following labor epidural analgesia. *J Clin Anesth* 1998;**10**:141–4.

10 Gerancher JC, Grice SC, Dewan DM, Eisenach J. An evaluation of informed consent prior to epidural analgesia for labor and delivery. *Int J Obstet Anesth* 2000;**9**:168–73.

11 White LA, Gorton P, Wee MYK, Mandal N. Written information about epidural analgesia for women in labour: did it improve knowledge? *Int J Obstet Anesth* 2003;**12**:93–7.

12 Pattee C, Ballantyne M, Milne B. Epidural analgesia for labour and delivery: informed consent issues. *Can J Anaesth* 1997;**44**:918–23.

13 Jackson A, Henry R, Avery N, VanDenKerkhof E, Milne B. Informed consent for labour epidurals: what labouring women want to know. *Can J Anesth* 2000;**47**:1068–73.

14 Garden AL, Merry AF, Holland RL, Petrie KJ. Anaesthesia information – what patients want to know. *Anaesth Intens Care* 1996;**24**:594–8.

15 Farnill D, Inglis S. Patients' desire for information about anaesthesia: Australian attitudes. *Anaesthesia* 1993;**48**:162–4.

16 Moores A, Pace NA. The information requested by patients prior to giving consent to anaesthesia. *Anaesthesia* 2003;**58**:703–7.

17 Lonsdale M, Hutchison GL. Patients' desire for information about anaesthesia. Scottish and Canadian attitudes. *Anaesthesia* 1991;**46**:410–2.

18 Beilin Y, Rosenblatt MA, Bodian CA, Lagmay-Aroesty MM, Bernstein HH. Information and concerns about obstetric anesthesia: a survey of 320 obstetric patients. *Int J Obstet Anesth* 1996;**5**:145–51.

19 Clark SK, Leighton BL, Seltzer JL. A risk-specific anesthesia consent form may hinder the informed consent process. *J Clin Anesth* 1991;**3**:11–3.

20 Slusarenko P, Noble WH. Epidural anaesthesia: concerns regarding informed consent. *Can Anaesth Soc J* 1985;**32**:681–2.

21 Bush DJ. A comparison of informed consent for obstetric anaesthesia in the USA and the UK. *Int J Obstet Anesth* 1995;**4**:1–6.

22 Watkins EJ, Milligan LJ, O'Beirne HA. Information and consent for anaesthesia: a postal survey of current practice in Great Britain. *Anaesthesia* 2001;**56**:879–82.

23 Walton S. Birth plans and the falacy of the Ulysses directive. *Int J Obstet Anesth* 2003;**12**:138–9.

CHAPTER 2

Epidural analgesia and the progress of labor

Barbara L. Leighton & Stephen H. Halpern

Introduction

Epidural analgesia effectively relieves labor pain and is often chosen by parturients because of the known efficacy of the technique. However, some authors express concern about potential side-effects of epidural analgesia on the progress of labor, the fetus and the newborn. Recently, it has been stated that: "Nulliparous women should be told that they are less likely to have a spontaneous vaginal delivery, that they are more likely to have an instrumental vaginal delivery, and that their labor is likely to be longer"[1] should they choose to request epidural analgesia. Whether or not this is true has been a subject of debate for many years and unfortunately, the matter is difficult to resolve. In other fields of medicine, it is often possible to design a randomized controlled trial to test various hypotheses. In this case, there are severe constraints on the types of clinical trials that can be performed.

In this chapter we review the various types of study architecture that can be used to determine the effect of epidural types of analgesia on the progress of labor. Each type of study has its strengths and weaknesses. We then systematically review the available data concerning the effect of epidural analgesia on the cesarean section rate, operative vaginal delivery rate and duration of labor. This review is an update of a previously published systematic review and the details of the search strategy are published elsewhere.[2] The last literature search was completed on April 15, 2004.

Study designs

Three types of studies have been reported to measure the effect of epidural analgesia on the incidence of cesarean and instrumented vaginal delivery: cohort observational studies (prospective and retrospective); randomized controlled trials in which epidural analgesia is compared to parenteral analgesia (often opioids); and observational studies in which a prospective cohort is compared with a retrospective cohort after an epidural service has been instituted ("before and after" studies). Each of these study designs has advantages and disadvantages. For ethical reasons, there have been no placebo-controlled randomized trials.

Observational studies

Compared with other study designs, observational studies are inexpensive and investigators can rapidly obtain data on a large number of patients. These studies have shown a strong association between epidural analgesia and the incidence of cesarean section.[3] This association was present even when multivariate statistics were used in an attempt to control confounding variables.[4] The authors of these studies concluded that epidurals probably *caused* the negative outcomes, and one group suggested that these data be routinely discussed with patients in order to help them make an informed decision.[5] However, women who have a more painful latent phase of labor are more likely to have a dysfunctional labor leading to requests for more analgesia and more obstetric interventions.[6,7] Increased pain and prolonged latent phase are also the reasons many patients choose to have epidural analgesia. Therefore, increased pain may be a marker for poor obstetric outcome, and these patients are more likely to request epidural analgesia.

In many observational studies, there is clear evidence that patients who request epidural analgesia are at higher risk for obstetric intervention because

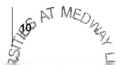

of multiple demographic factors. For example, in one study in which the population was of mixed parity, there were significantly more nulliparous patients in the epidural group.[8] Commonly, other demographics are unbalanced. Lieberman et al.[4] performed a retrospective analysis of data obtained from nulliparous, low-risk patients who had enrolled in another trial. Patients were allowed to choose their method of analgesia. In this trial, there was more than a fourfold increase in the risk of cesarean section in patients who received epidural analgesia (17% vs 4%, $P < 0.05$). However, important demographics, such as maternal height and weight, fetal weight, progress of labor before epidural analgesia, rate of progress before labor analgesia and maternal race were statistically different between treatment groups and favored women who did not receive epidural analgesia. Although the authors attempted to adjust for baseline characteristics in their analysis, this was not possible because of the large number of known and unknown differences in demographics. Further examples of unbalanced demographics can be found by examining studies in which women choose their own analgesia, whether the data are collected prospectively or retrospectively (see reference 1 for a complete listing of these studies to the year 2002). The data from observational studies are therefore not reliable and will not be considered further.

Randomized contolled trials

In many clinical scenarios, randomized controlled trials are considered to be the most rigorous evidence available to determine effects of treatment. In this case, randomized controlled trials are particularly difficult to perform because of the clear superiority of the analgesia in the epidural group compared with, for example, parenteral opioids. It is not possible to blind these studies. Because there is some subjectivity in deciding the need for and timing of cesarean or instrumented vaginal delivery for dystocia, knowledge of the patient treatment group by caregivers could introduce bias. A second concern is that women with a definite desire for or against epidural analgesia do not enroll in these trials. A large proportion of women make this decision before the onset of labor, eliminating many parturients from study participation. This may reduce the generalizability of the results to the general obstetric population. Finally, patients may not follow their

group assignment. If they are randomized too early, they may not require any analgesia and may refuse group assignment. This problem can be reduced by assigning the group when the patient requests analgesia. Later, if the analgesia is inadequate, the patient may choose to "cross over" and receive the alternate treatment. Usually this occurs when the patient has not been assigned to the epidural group. If enough patients change groups, the randomization may be threatened.

In spite of these difficulties, random allocation to epidural versus parenteral opioid labor analgesia was reported in 15 studies enrolling 4619 healthy patients.[9–23] In addition, 1223 patients in a single study were randomized to receive either parenteral meperidine or subarachnoid analgesia followed by a continuous epidural infusion (CSE).[24] Finally, there were 854 pre-eclamptic patients in two studies.[25,26] Additional data on one of the studies[19] have become available in a review article.[27]

As shown in Table 2.1, the studies have been performed in the USA, Canada, Scandinavia, Great Britain and India. All of the studies that were available in full manuscript form were rated for quality of reporting, based on the Jadad scale[28] (see Appendix for a full description of the scale). Normally, this three-item scale has a maximum score of 5 points (2 for appropriate randomization, 2 for blinding and 1 for accounting for all the enrolled patients). Because of the obvious differences in the effectiveness of the analgesia, none of the studies were blinded. Therefore the maximum quality score available is 3. As shown in Table 2.1, most of the patients were enrolled in high-quality studies. A heterogeneous population of patients was studied, although most were healthy nulliparous patients in spontaneous labor. As can be seen from Table 2.1, multiparous and hypertensive patients are also represented.

Because blinding is impossible, other strategies are required to reduce caregiver bias in the results. For this reason, it is important that the protocols for the use of oxytocin to augment labor and indications for operative delivery be written and monitored for compliance. The protocol for each included study is shown in Table 2.2. Eleven of the studies reported the existence of a protocol for the management of labor[9–11,14,15,19,21,22,24,26,29] and three reported a protocol for operative delivery.[11,22,24]

Table 2.1 Study characteristics.

Reference and year	Country of origin	Quality score	Population Nulliparous : multiparous	Induced labor included	Comments
Healthy parturients					
Robinson* 1980	UK	1	58 : 0	Unknown	
Robinson* 1980	UK	1	0 : 35	Unknown	
Philipsen[†] 1989, 1990	Denmark	3	104 : 7	Yes	
Thorp 1993	USA	3	93 : 0	No	The trial was stopped early for "ethical" reasons
Ramin 1995	USA	2	693 : 637[‡] 484 : 385[§]	No	Parity and cervical dilation at request for analgesia were unbalanced between groups. Intent to treat data available from reference 27
Clark 1998	USA	3	318 : 0	No	Both intent to treat and protocol compliant data were presented
Muir 1996	Canada	Not rated	50 : 0	No	Abstract
Sharma 1997	USA	3	386 : 329	No	
Nikkola 1997	Finland	2	20 : 0	Unknown	Primary outcome was the effect of analgesia on the neonate
Bofill 1997	USA	3	100 : 0	No	The trial was stopped early because of slow recruitment
Gambling 1998	USA	3	650 : 573	No	CSE + continuous infusion. Analyzed as intent to treat and protocol compliant
Loughnan 2000	UK	3	614 : 0	Unknown	
Howell 2001	UK	3	369 : 0	Yes	Primary outcome was back pain
Sharma 2002	USA	3	459 : 0	No	
Jain 2003	India	3	123 : 0	No	3 groups Group 1= epidural Group 2 = IM meperidine Group 3 = IM tramadol
Halpern 2004	Canada	3	242 : 0	No	Multicentered trial
Hypertensive parturients					
Lucas 2001	USA	3	525 : 213	Yes	Admitted with the diagnosis of pre-eclampsia. Enrolled when analgesia requested
Head 2002	USA	3	75 : 116	Yes	Admitted with the diagnosis of severe pre-eclampsia but no contraindications to epidural analgesia

* This manuscript contained data for nulliparous and multiparous patients which were analyzed separately. Therefore they are presented as two studies.

[†] Data from this cohort of patients was presented in two manuscripts.

[‡] Total number of enrolled patients; used to calculate the cesarean delivery incidence by intent-to-treat.

[§] Number of protocol-compliant patients; used for all other maternal and neonatal outcomes in this study.[27]

CSE, combined spinal epidural; IM, intramuscular.

Table 2.2 Analgesic protocol, epidural analgesia.

Study	Labor protocol	Criteria for operative intervention	Analgesic protocol, parenteral analgesia	Analgesic protocol, epidural	Crossover rate
Normal parturients					
Robinson 1980 (both studies)	Not stated	Not stated	Meperidine 150 mg + perphenazine 5 mg IM q 4 h as requested by the patient supplemented by 50% N_2O and methoxyflurane 0.35% as requested by the patient	Bupivacaine 0.5% 5–10 mL bolus doses as needed, no infusion	None reported
Philipsen 1989	Not stated	Not stated	Meperidine 75 mg IM as requested by the patient supplemented by N_2O 50% as requested by the patient	Test dose 1% lidocaine with epinephrine. Bolus doses of 0.375% bupivacaine, no infusion. No top-ups in second stage. N_2O 50% as requested by the patient	None reported
Thorp 1993	Electronic fetal monitoring for all patients. No elective instrumented vaginal deliveries. Dystocia diagnosed only after "documentation of adequate labor" by internal uterine pressure monitor. Fetal distress diagnosed by persistent ominous fetal heart rate tracing or scalp pH	Not stated	Meperidine 75 mg + promethazine 25 mg IV q 90 min as needed	0.25% bupivacaine bolus, bupivacaine 0.125% infusion adjusted to maintain a T10 level. Infusions were continued through second stage of labor if adequate progress was made	1/48 patients assigned to the epidural group did not receive an epidural. 1/45 patients assigned to the parenteral opioid group also received an epidural
Ramin 1995	Protocol in labor floor manual. Early amniotomy, intrauterine pressure catheter, electronic fetal monitoring, oxytocin, no elective forceps	Criteria for low forceps, not for cesarean section	Meperidine 50 mg IV q 4 h as requested by the patient + promethazine 25 mg with the first dose. Epidural if inadequate pain relief	Bupivacaine 0.25% bolus, bupivacaine, 0.125% with 2 µg/mL fentanyl infusion to maintain a T8 level	103/666 in the parenteral opioid group also received an epidural 232/664 randomized to receive an epidural received no medication

Continued

Table 2.2 (*continued*)

Study	Labor protocol	Criteria for operative intervention	Analgesic protocol, parenteral analgesia	Analgesic protocol, epidural	Crossover rate
Muir 1996	"Strict" definitions for diagnosis and management of labor	Not stated	IV patient-controlled analgesia meperidine 1 mg/kg loading dose	Bupivacaine 0.125% + epinephrine + meperidine bolus, bupivacaine 0.125% + epinephrine + meperidine patient-controlled epidural analgesia	11/22 in the parenteral opioid group also received an epidural
Clark 1997	"Active management of labor"	"Obstetrical reasons"	IV meperidine 50–75 mg q 90 min as needed	Lidocaine 1% test dose, bupivacaine 0.25%/50 μg fentanyl bolus, bupivacaine 0.125%/fentanyl 1 μg/mL infusion, adjusted to maintain a T10 level	84/162 in the parenteral opioid group also received an epidural group 5/156 in the epidural group received IV opioids (no epidural) 4 received no medication
Nikkola 1997	Not stated	Not stated	IV patient-controlled analgesia fentanyl, stopped in 2nd stage	Bupivacaine 0.5% 6 mL followed by 4 mL boluses as requested by the patient, no infusion, epidural "not routinely given" in 2nd stage	4/10 in the parenteral opioid group also received an epidural
Sharma 1997	Protocol in labor floor manual. Early amniotomy, electronic fetal monitoring, oxytocin, no elective forceps	Criteria for low forceps, not for cesarean section	Meperidine 50 mg plus promethazine 25 mg followed by meperidine IV PCA	Bupivacaine 0.25% bolus, infusion bupivacaine 0.125% with 2 μg/mL fentanyl to maintain a T10 level	Of 358 women assigned to the meperidine group, 93 did not receive any medication and 5 received an epidural after receiving meperidine. Of 357 women assigned to the epidural group, 115 received no medication and 8 received only parenteral opioids
Bofill 1997	Active management of labor. Criteria for oxytocin augmentation	Cesarean section decision made by a perinatologist blinded to patients analgesia assignment. 50/100 patients had instrumented vaginal deliveries for "resident training"	Butorphanol 1–2 mg IV every 1–2 h as needed	Bupivacaine 0.25%/fentanyl 50–100 μg bolus, infusion of bupivacaine 0.125% and fentanyl 1.5 μg/mL	2/49 in the epidural group received no medication. 12/51 in the parenteral opioid group received opioid plus an epidural

Study					
Loughnan 2000	Active management of labor	Decision to do an operative delivery was made by midwifery and medical staff not involved with the study	Meperidine IM q 2 h as requested by the patient to a maximum of 300 mg	Bupivacaine 0.25% 10–15 mL followed by bupivacaine 0.125% at 10–15 mL/h until the 2nd stage	Of the 304 women who were randomized to epidural, 244 received an epidural, 13 received meperidine and an epidural, 47 received either meperidine or Entonox®. Of the 310 women randomized to meperidine, 132 received meperidine, 89 received an epidural, 86 received an epidural and meperidine, and 3 received Entonox®
Howell 2001	Not stated	Not stated	Meperidine 50–100 mg repeated "according to midwifery practice"	Bupivacaine 0.25% 10 mL initially, bolus doses of 5–10 mL bupivacaine 0.25% as requested by the patient	61 of 184 women in the epidural group did not receive an epidural 52 of 185 women in the non-epidural group received an epidural
Sharma 2002	Written protocol	Written protocol	Meperidine via IV PCA	Bupivacaine 0.25% with fentanyl; bupivacaine 0.06%/fentanyl 2 µg/mL patient-controlled epidural and 5 mL/h background infusion	In the IV meperidine group 207/233 followed the protocol. Of the 26 violations, 14 received an epidural In the epidural group 214/226 followed the protocol
Jain 2003	Not stated	Not stated	2 groups: meperidine 1 mg/kg q 4 h IM or tramadol 1 mg/kg	Bupivacaine 10 mL of 0.15% with 30 µg fentanyl. Top-ups with 0.15% bupivacaine with 15 µg fentanyl or a continuous infusion of bupivacaine 0.1% with 1 µg fentanyl per mL at 10 mL/h	None were allowed
Halpern 2004	Labor managed by protocol	Predefined. Monitoring committee for protocol violations	Intravenous patient-controlled analgesia using fentanyl	Epidural patient-controlled 0.08% bupivacaine with 1.67 µg/mL fentanyl	51 of 118 women in the IV PCA group received an epidural. 3/124 in the PCEA group received a non-protocol epidural because of failure of analgesia

Continued

Table 2.2 (*continued*)

Study	Labor protocol	Criteria for operative intervention	Analgesic protocol, parenteral analgesia	Analgesic protocol, epidural	Crossover rate
Combined spinal epidural technique (normal parturients)					
Gambling 1998	Written protocol	Written protocol – elective forceps were not permitted	Intravenous meperidine and promethazine by request to a maximum of 400 mg meperidine/4 h	CSE with 10 μg sufentanil followed by 8 mL of 0.25% bupivacaine. Then 0.125% bupivacaine with 2 μg/mL fentanyl at 8–10 mL/h	In the IV meperidine group 352/607 followed the protocol. Of the 255 that did not, 102 received a CSE and 42 declined analgesia. In the CSE group, 400/616 followed the protocol. Of the 216 that did not, 82 received meperidine and 52 declined analgesia
Pre-eclampsia					
Lucas 2001	? – Written protocol for pre-eclampsia management	Not stated	IV meperidine and promethazine followed by IV PCA	Epidural initiated with incremental doses of 0.25% bupivacaine followed by 0.125% bupivacaine with 2 μg/mL fentanyl as a continuous infusion	Of the 366 women in the meperidine group, 340 followed the protocol. Of the 26 that did not, none received an epidural.Of the 372 women assigned to the epidural group, 51 did not follow the protocol. Of these none received meperidine but 7 did not receive any analgesia
Head 2002	Not stated	Not stated	IV meperidine 50–75 mg as needed	Bupivacaine 0.25% in incremental doses followed by bupivacaine 0.125% with 2 μg/mL fentanyl at 10 mL/h	One patient in the meperidine group received an epidural

CSE, combined spinal epidural; IM, intramuscular; IV, intravenous; PCA, patient-controlled analgesia; PCEA, patient-controlled epidural analgesia.

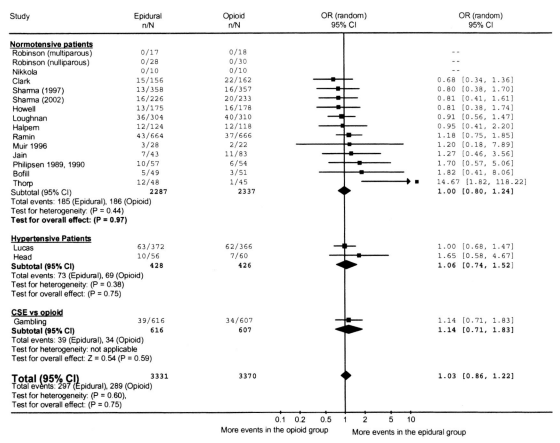

Study	Epidural n/N	Opioid n/N	OR (random) 95% CI	OR (random) 95% CI
Normotensive patients				
Robinson (multiparous)	0/17	0/18		--
Robinson (nulliparous)	0/28	0/30		--
Nikkola	0/10	0/10		--
Clark	15/156	22/162		0.68 [0.34, 1.36]
Sharma (1997)	13/358	16/357		0.80 [0.38, 1.70]
Sharma (2002)	16/226	20/233		0.81 [0.41, 1.61]
Howell	13/175	16/178		0.81 [0.38, 1.74]
Loughnan	36/304	40/310		0.91 [0.56, 1.47]
Halpern	12/124	12/118		0.95 [0.41, 2.20]
Ramin	43/664	37/666		1.18 [0.75, 1.85]
Muir 1996	3/28	2/22		1.20 [0.18, 7.89]
Jain	7/43	11/83		1.27 [0.46, 3.56]
Philipsen 1989, 1990	10/57	6/54		1.70 [0.57, 5.06]
Bofill	5/49	3/51		1.82 [0.41, 8.06]
Thorp	12/48	1/45		14.67 [1.82, 118.22]
Subtotal (95% CI)	2287	2337		1.00 [0.80, 1.24]
Total events: 185 (Epidural), 186 (Opioid)				
Test for heterogeneity: (P = 0.44)				
Test for overall effect: (P = 0.97)				
Hypertensive Patients				
Lucas	63/372	62/366		1.00 [0.68, 1.47]
Head	10/56	7/60		1.65 [0.58, 4.67]
Subtotal (95% CI)	428	426		1.06 [0.74, 1.52]
Total events: 73 (Epidural), 69 (Opioid)				
Test for heterogeneity: (P = 0.38)				
Test for overall effect: (P = 0.75)				
CSE vs opioid				
Gambling	39/616	34/607		1.14 [0.71, 1.83]
Subtotal (95% CI)	616	607		1.14 [0.71, 1.83]
Total events: 39 (Epidural), 34 (Opioid)				
Test for heterogeneity: not applicable				
Test for overall effect: Z = 0.54 (P = 0.59)				
Total (95% CI)	3331	3370		1.03 [0.86, 1.22]
Total events: 297 (Epidural), 289 (Opioid)				
Test for heterogeneity: (P = 0.60),				
Test for overall effect: (P = 0.75)				

0.1 0.2 0.5 1 2 5 10

More events in the opioid group   More events in the epidural group

Fig. 2.1 Cesarean section rate. The number of patients who had a cesarean section, the odds ratio (OR) and 95% confidence interval (CI) (random effects model) are shown for each study. The size of the box is proportional to the weight of the study in the meta-analysis. The scale is logarithmic. For studies with no cesarean sections, the OR could not be calculated.

Only one study reported monitoring of the protocol.[11] Of interest, one investigator reported that many patients in the epidural group had a forceps delivery for resident training purposes,[9] illustrating how the method of analgesia may influence obstetric decisions. The protocol for the delivery of epidural analgesia was variable and represented the differences in practice settings. Compliance to the analgesic protocol was highly variable and depended on the patient population and the method of analgesia used for the non-epidural group (Table 2.2).

The clinical trials were sufficiently similar to perform a meta-analysis on the incidence of cesarean section (Fig. 2.1). There was no statistically significant heterogeneity between studies although one of the studies reported very different results than all the others. This study was remarkable because it was stopped early for "ethical reasons" after the incidence of cesarean section was found to be significantly higher in the epidural group than in the opioid control group.[23] In this study, incidence of cesarean section in the control group was much lower (2%) and that of the epidural group (25%) much higher than the historical norm (15%) for that institution. Of note, this was the only study that reported a statistical difference between groups. As shown in Fig. 2.1, the odds ratio was 1.03 (95% confidence interval [CI] 0.86–1.22, $P = 0.75$). The absolute risk difference between groups was 0% (95% CI −1.0–2.0%, $P = 0.69$). There was a subgroup of seven studies and a total of approximately 2300 patients in which less than 10% of patients did not adhere to the analgesia protocol.[13,17,18,21–23,25,26] In

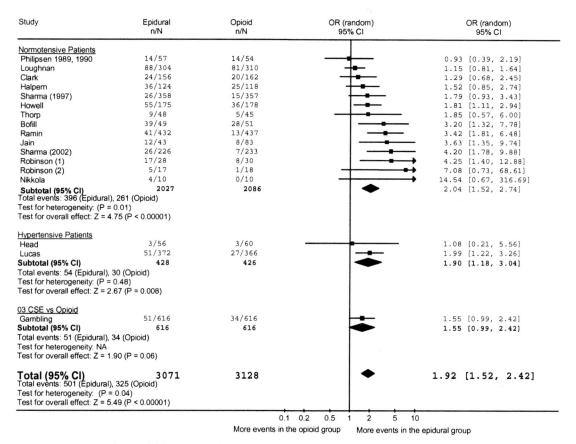

Fig. 2.2 Instrumental vaginal delivery rate. The number of patients who had an instrumental vaginal delivery, the odds ratio (OR) and 95% confidence interval (CI) (random effects model) are shown for each study. The scale is logarithmic. The size of the box is proportional to the weight of the study in the meta-analysis.

this subgroup, there was also no significant difference in the cesarean section rate. The odds ratio was 1.15 (95% CI 0.76–1.67, P = 0.48).

Of interest, the incidence of instrumental vaginal delivery (vacuum extraction + forceps) was higher in the epidural group. The odds ratio was 1.9 (95% CI 1.5–2.4, P < 0.001) (Fig. 2.2). These studies are heterogeneous, likely because of the different clinical criteria used in each study for the use of forceps. These criteria ranged from strict written protocols (see Table 2.2) to a clear preference for forceps deliveries when the patient had epidural analgesia.[9] However, of the 16 studies that report this outcome, 15 report an increased incidence associated with epidural analgesia (Fig. 2.2). Eight of these were statistically significant.

The duration of the first stage of labor was reported in nine randomized controlled trials (eight full manuscripts)[9,10,12–14,20,22,23] comprised of approximately 2200 patients. There was no difference in the duration of the first stage of labor, with a weighted mean difference of approximately 24 min (95% CI 4–54 min, P = 0.09). There was significant heterogeneity in this outcome because of the different populations studied (nulliparous, multiparous and mixed parity) and differences among studies in defining the beginning and end of the first stage of labor.

The duration of the second stage of labor was reported in 11 studies[9–14,17,18,20,22,23] comprised of approximately 2550 patients. Epidural analgesia prolonged the second stage of labor by approximately 16 min (95% CI 10–23 min, P < 0.0001). Again, there was

Table 2.3 Randomized controlled trials comparing low-concentration to high-concentration local anesthetic.

Study	Quality score	Population (parity)	Low dose		High dose		Comments
			N	Protocol	N	Protocol	
Collis 1995	2	Mixed	98	CSE with B 2.5 mg + F 25 µg Intermittent boluses of B 0.1% + F 2 µg/ mL 10–15 mL	99	Epidural B 0.25% 10 mL Intermittent bolus B 0.25%, 6–10 mL	No blinding 5 CSE did not receive CSE, rather B via epidural catheter
COMET 2001	3	Nulliparous	666	**1** CSE with B 2.5 mg + F 25 µg **2** Epidural B 0.1% + F 2 µg/mL 15 mL Both followed by continuous infusion of B 0.1% + F 2 µg/mL 10 mL/h	388	Lidocaine 2% 3 mL via epidural + B 0.25% 10 mL Intermittent boluses of 0.25% B 10 mL	No blinding. Study repeated (COMET 2 reported here) because of faulty randomization. 3 groups comparison. 2 low-dose groups (CSE and epidural) vs 1 high-dose group (epidural B 0.25%)
James 1998	5	?	40	Epidural 15 mL B 0.1% + F 50 µg followed by intermittent bolus B 0.1% + F 30 mL	40	15 mL B 0.25% followed by intermittent boluses of B 0.25% 10 mL	Sample size based on visual analog scores averaged over the labor. 5 in the low dose and 2 in the high dose withdrawn from the primary outcome but mode of delivery was described for all patients
Nageotte 1997	2	Nulliparous	505	CSE 10 µg S followed by 0.0625% B + 2 µg/ mL F at 12 mL/h	253	Epidural 0.25% 11 mL + 50 µg F followed by 0.125% B + 2 µg/ml F at 10 mL/h	3-group comparison. Low dose divided into ambulation and no ambulation. Not blinded. Primary outcome not identified

B, bupivacaine; CSE, combined spinal epidural; F, fentanyl; S, sufentanil.

significant heterogeneity in the outcome – however, in all studies the second stage of labor was prolonged in the epidural group. This prolongation was statistically significant in six of the studies.[11–14,22,23]

Additional evidence concerning the outcome of labor comes from randomized controlled trials that compare low-dose to high-dose epidural analgesia. The argument that epidural analgesia causes an excess number of obstetric interventions (cesarean section or instrumental vaginal delivery) is strengthened if a dose–response relationship can be shown. For this reason, Angle et al.[30] retrieved all randomized controlled trials that compared low-concentration to high-concentration epidural labor analgesia that reported obstetric outcomes. They defined "high concentration" as bupivacaine concentration 0.125% or more and "low concentration" as less than 0.125% bupivacaine. The addition of epidural opioid was

allowed in both groups to enhance analgesia. They found four randomized controlled trials comprised of approximately 2000 patients that met these criteria.[31–34] The study characteristics of these studies are shown in Table 2.3. In these studies, high-concentration epidural analgesia resulted in a reduction in the rate of spontaneous vaginal delivery. The odds ratio was 1.32 (95% CI 1.1–1.6, $P = 0.003$). The incidence of cesarean section was slightly lower in the high-dose group (odds ratio 0.9, 95% CI 0.6–1.4, $P = 0.63$). However, the incidence of instrumental delivery was higher (odds ratio 1.31, 95% CI 0.9–1.8, $P = 0.12$).

An additional study by Reynolds et al.[35] supports the finding that high-concentration epidural analgesia leads to an increase in obstetric interventions. This study is a summary of five separate reports, comparing low-concentration (0.0625% bupivacaine) with high-concentration (0.125% bupivacaine) epidural infusions

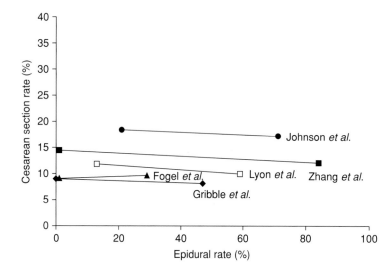

Fig. 2.3 Epidural rate versus cesarean section rate in institutions that introduced (or disbanded) an epidural service on demand. Data from published studies (see text).

at one institution. However, the loading dose was not controlled and all patients received 0.25% bupivacaine if analgesia was inadequate. While the study did not meet the criteria of the meta-analysis above, it does support the conclusions. Patients in the high-concentration group were less likely to experience a spontaneous vaginal delivery than those who received a low concentration. Logistic regression showed that there was a statistically significant increase in the incidence of obstetric intervention as the dose of bupivacaine (in milligrams) increased.

Before and after studies

In an attempt to avoid some of the problems encountered in randomized controlled trials, some investigators have studied institutions that had no epidural analgesia service for labor and then, over a brief period of time, introduced epidural analgesia into practice. While many factors can threaten the validity of this design (such as changes in practice or personnel over the study period), when compared with randomized controlled trials there are some advantages. This approach eliminates the problem of patients choosing epidural analgesia when assigned to another treatment group because epidural analgesia was not available. Similarly, these studies (provided the data are collected in a comprehensive and reliable manner) are more generalizable to the full population because the patients have not "chosen" to be studied. Since 1990, there have been five published studies that have done

this.[36–40] As can be seen in Fig. 2.3, there was no appreciable change in the cesarean section rate, even with a large incremental change in the epidural rate. Further, a recent meta-analysis of published and unpublished data showed that there was no increase in the incidence of operative vaginal delivery[41] after the epidural service was instituted.

Conclusions

Since 1980, there have been numerous studies performed to determine whether epidural analgesia interferes with labor, resulting in an increased need for obstetric interventions. Because of the nature of the question, no single study design is capable of giving "the answer." Observational studies that allow the patient to choose her mode of analgesia are inappropriate because many of the risk factors for cesarean section cause pain, resulting in requests for epidural analgesia.

Currently, the best evidence comes from randomized controlled trials that compare epidural to non-epidural analgesia. When combined, these studies clearly indicate that epidural analgesia does not result in an increase in the cesarean section rate. This is supported by the failure of randomized controlled trials comparing low-concentration with high-concentration local anesthetics to demonstrate a dose–response. Further support comes from before and after studies, showing no change in the rate of cesarean section in institutions that suddenly institute an epidural service.

Epidural analgesia may cause an increase in the operative vaginal delivery rate. These data are consistently shown in the randomized controlled trials comparing epidural with non-epidural analgesia. There may be many reasons for the association. First, the second stage of labor is prolonged. This may lead obstetricians to perform an operative vaginal delivery in order to shorten this stage of labor. Second, the analgesia provided by epidural analgesia may change the behavior of caregivers by reducing their concern for pain caused by operative vaginal delivery. However, this is may not be true in all cases because the increased operative delivery rate also occurred in studies that had written protocols for the management of the second stage of labor. Finally, it may be possible to reduce the incidence of obstetric interventions by reducing the dose of local anesthetic to the minimum amount required to provide analgesia. Further work to determine the best way of doing this is required.

References

1 Lieberman E, O'Donoghue C. Unintended effects of epidural analgesia during labor: a systematic review. *Am J Obstet Gynecol* 2002;**186**:S31–S68.

2 Halpern SH, Leighton BL, Ohlsson A, Barrett JF, Rice A. Effect of epidural vs parenteral opioid analgesia on the progress of labor: a meta-analysis. *JAMA* 1998;**280**:2105–10.

3 Morton SC, Williams MS, Keeler EB, Gambone JC, Kahn KL. Effect of epidural analgesia for labor on the cesarean delivery rate. *Obstet Gynecol* 1994;**83**:1045–52.

4 Lieberman E, Lang JM, Cohen A, D'Agostino RJ, Datta S, Frigoletto FD Jr. Association of epidural analgesia with cesarean delivery in nulliparas. *Obstet Gynecol* 1996;**88**:993–1000.

5 Goldberg AB, Cohen BA, Lieberman E. Nulliparas' preferences for epidural analgesia: their effects on actual use in labor. *Birth* 1999;**26**:139–43.

6 Hess PE, Pratt SD, Soni AK, Sarna MC, Oriol NE. An association between severe labor pain and cesarean delivery. *Anesth Analg* 2000;**90**:881–6.

7 Wuitchik M, Bakal D, Lipshitz J. The clinical significance of pain and cognitive activity in latent labor. *Obstet Gynecol* 1989;**73**:35–42.

8 Niehaus LS, Chaska BW, Nesse RE. The effects of epidural anesthesia on type of delivery. *J Am Board Fam Pract* 1988;**1**:238–44.

9 Bofill JA, Vincent RD, Ross EL. Nulliparous active labor, epidural analgesia, and cesarean delivery for dystocia. *Am J Obstet Gynecol* 1997;**177**:1465–70.

10 Clark A, Carr D, Loyd G, Cook V, Spinnato J. The influence of epidural analgesia on cesarean delivery rates: a randomized, prospective clinical trial. *Am J Obstet Gynecol* 1998;**179**:1527–33.

11 Halpern SH, Muir HA, Breen TW, *et al.* Multicenter randomized controlled trial comparing patient-controlled epidural with intravenous analgesia for pain relief in labor. *Anesth Analg* 2004;**99**:1532–8.

12 Howell CJ, Kidd C, Roberts W, *et al.* A randomised controlled trial of epidural compared with non-epidural analgesia in labor. *Br J Obstet Gynaecol* 2001;**108**:27–33.

13 Jain S, Arya VK, Gopalan S, Jain V. Analgesic efficacy of intramuscular opioids versus epidural analgesia in labor. *Int J Gynaecol Obstet* 2003;**83**:19–27.

14 Loughnan BA, Carli F, Romney M, Doré CJ, Gordon H. Randomized controlled comparison of epidural bupivacaine versus pethidine for analgesia in labor. *Br J Anaesth* 2000;**84**:715–9.

15 Muir HA, Shukla R, Liston R, Writer D. Randomized trial of labor analgesia: a pilot study to compare patient-controlled intravenous analgesia with patient-controlled epidural analgesia to determine if analgesic method affects delivery outcome. *Can J Anaesth* 1996;**43**:A60.

16 Nikkola EM, Ekblad UU, Kero PO, Alihanka JM, Salonen MAO. Intravenous PCA in labor. *Can J Anaesth* 1997; **44**:1248–55.

17 Philipsen T, Jensen N-H. Epidural block or parenteral pethidine as analgesic in labor: a randomized study concerning progress in labor and instrumental deliveries. *Eur J Obstet Gynecol Reprod Biol* 1989;**30**:27–33.

18 Philipsen T, Jensen N-H. Maternal opinion about analgesia in labor and delivery: a comparison of epidural blockade and intramuscular pethidine. *Eur J Obstet Gynecol Reprod Biol* 1990;**34**:205–10.

19 Ramin SM, Gambling DR, Lucas MJ, Sharma SK, Sidawi JE, Leveno KJ. Randomized trial of epidural versus intravenous analgesia during labor. *Obstet Gynecol* 1995;**86**:783–9.

20 Robinson JO, Rosen M, Evans JM, Revill SI, David H, Rees GA. Maternal opinion about analgesia for labor: a controlled trial between epidural block and intramuscular pethidine. *Anaesthesia* 1980;**35**:1173–81.

21 Sharma SK, Sidawi JE, Ramin SM, Lucas MJ, Leveno KJ, Cunningham FG. Cesarean delivery: a randomized trial of epidural versus patient-controlled meperidine analgesia during labor. *Anesthesiology* 1997;**87**:487–94.

22 Sharma SK, Alexander JM, Messick G, *et al.* Cesarean delivery: a randomized trial of epidural analgesia versus intravenous meperidine analgesia during labor in nulliparous women. *Anesthesiology* 2002;**96**:546–51.

23 Thorp JA, Hu DH, Albin RM, *et al.* The effect of intrapartum epidural analgesia on nulliparous labor: a randomized, controlled, prospective trial. *Am J Obstet Gynecol* 1993; **169**:851–8.

24 Gambling DR, Sharma SK, Ramin SM, *et al.* A randomized study of combined spinal–epidural analgesia versus intravenous meperidine during labor: impact on cesarean delivery rate. *Anesthesiology* 1998;**89**:1336–44.

25 Head BB, Owen J, Vincent RD, Shih G, Chestnut DH, Hauth JC. A randomized trial of intrapartum analgesia in women with severe pre-eclampsia. *Obstet Gynecol* 2002; **99**:452–7.

26 Lucas MJ, Sharma SK, McIntire DD, *et al.* A randomized trial of labor analgesia in women with pregnancy-induced hypertension. *Am J Obstet Gynecol* 2001;**185**:970–5.

27 Sharma SK, Leveno KJ. Update: epidural analgesia does not increase cesarean births. *Curr Anesthesiol Rep* 2000; **2**:18–24.

28 Jadad AR, Moore RA, Carroll D, *et al.* Assessing the quality of reports of randomized clinical trials: is blinding necessary? *Control Clin Trials* 1996;**17**:1–12.

29 Thorp JA, Parisi VM, Boylan PC, Johnston DA. The effect of continuous epidural analgesia on cesarean section for dystocia in nulliparous women. *Am J Obstet Gynecol* 1989;**161**:670–5.

30 Angle P, Halpern S, Morgan A. Effect of low dose mobile versus high dose epidural techniques on the progress of labor: a meta-analysis. *Anesthesiology* 2002;**96**(suppl 1): P-52.

31 Collis RE, Davies DWL, Aveling W. Randomised comparison of combined spinal–epidural and standard epidural analgesia in labor. *Lancet* 1995;**345**:1413–6.

32 Comparative Obstetric Mobile Epidural Trial (COMET) Study Group UK. Effect of low-dose mobile versus traditional epidural techniques on mode of delivery: a randomized trial. *Lancet* 2001;**358**:19–23.

33 James KS, McGrady E, Quasim I, Patrick A. Comparison of epidural bolus administration of 0.25% bupivacaine and 0.1% bupivacaine with 0.0002% fentanyl for analgesia during labor. *Br J Anaesth* 1998;**81**:507–10.

34 Nageotte MP, Larson D, Rumney PJ, Sidhu M, Hollenbach K. Epidural analgesia compared with combined spinal–epidural analgesia during labor in nulliparous women. *N Engl J Med* 1997;**337**:1715–9.

35 Reynolds F, Russell R, Porter J, Smeeton N. Does the use of low dose bupivacaine/opioid epidural infusion increase the normal delivery rate? *Int J Obstet Anesth* 2003;**12**:156–63.

36 Fogel ST, Shyken JM, Leighton BL, Mormol JS, Smeltzer JS. Epidural labor analgesia and the incidence of cesarean delivery for dystocia. *Anesth Analg* 1998;**87**:119–23.

37 Gribble RK, Meier PR. Effect of epidural analgesia on the primary cesarean rate. *Obstet Gynecol* 1991;**78**:231–4.

38 Johnson S, Rosenfeld JA. The effect of epidural analgesia on the length of labor. *J Fam Pract* 1995;**40**:244–7.

39 Lyon DS, Knuckles G, Whitaker E, Salgado S. The effect of instituting an elective labor epidural program on the operative delivery rate. *Obstet Gynecol* 1997;**90**:135–41.

40 Zhang J, Yancey MK, Klebanoff MA, Schwarz J, Schweitzer D. Does epidural analgesia prolong labor and increase risk of cesarean delivery? A natural experiment. *Am J Obstet Gynecol* 2001;**185**:128–34.

41 Segal S, Su M, Gilbert P. The effect of a rapid change in availability of epidural analgesia on the cesarean delivery rate: a meta-analysis. *Am J Obstet Gynecol* 2000;**183**:974–8.

CHAPTER 3

Maintenance of epidural analgesia for labor – continuous infusion or patient controlled

Stephen H. Halpern

Introduction

The early use of epidural labor analgesia consisted primarily of a single dose of local anesthetic through the needle near the end of the second stage of labor. This type of analgesia was quite limited because of the short duration of pain relief compared with the total time of labor. In an effort to prolong analgesia, large doses of local anesthetic were often given, resulting in maternal hypotension, significant risk of local anesthetic toxicity, severe motor block of the lower extremities and a reduction in the parturient's ability to push effectively. If the local anesthetic wore off before the birth of the baby, the whole procedure of epidural placement needed to be repeated.

In the mid 1970s, epidural catheters came into common use. In the 1980s, it became possible to offer the parturient low concentrations of local anesthetic, with or without an opioid such as fentanyl or sufentanil, as a continuous epidural infusion (CEI). This avoided a number of problems associated with clinician-administered intermittent bolus techniques such as uneven analgesia and potential local anesthetic toxicity. However, many patients still required local anesthetic boluses from the clinician, and some had an unacceptably dense motor block of the lower extremities.

In 1988, Gambling *et al.*[1] described patient-controlled epidural analgesia (PCEA) for labor pain. This technique allowed the patient to match the dose of analgesia to the pain as the labor progressed. It also allowed for patient variability in dose requirements. Other research supports the concept that patient satisfaction may be increased by allowing her to have an increased amount of control over the labor and delivery process, including pain control.[2]

PCEA has some potential disadvantages compared with CEI. The delivery system, including the pump and disposable items, is more expensive. In addition, it takes more time to set up the equipment and explain it to the patient. Some patients may not wish to control their analgesia because of fatigue and some may prefer to leave it to the "professionals."

The purpose of this chapter is to compare the methods commonly used for maintaining labor analgesia. PCEA without a background infusion has been extensively compared with CEI. In addition, there are a number of studies that examine the addition of a background infusion to PCEA. While the technique of intermittent clinician-administered bolus continues to be practiced and is useful, it will not be considered further here. The results of studies that investigate this modality yield results that are specific to the setting of the study. For example, the time between patient requesting analgesia and obtaining it is dependent on the availability of an anesthesiologist or the ability of the midwife or nurse to administer top-ups. This is different for different units and may vary over time in the same unit, depending on concurrent clinical demands at the time of request.

PCEA versus CEI

This section is an update of a recent meta-analysis.[3] The last search of MEDLINE®, EMBASE® and Science Citation Index® for randomized controlled trials that compare PCEA with CEI was completed in January 2004. Full manuscripts were rated for quality of reporting using the Jadad scale[4] (see Appendix for a description of the scale). The main outcomes of interest included the number of patients who required non-scheduled clinician bolus doses (top-ups), the incidence of motor block, patient satisfaction and obstetric outcomes. In addition, some of the studies reported neonatal outcomes. Patients in the PCEA group had no background infusion and the analgesic solutions were identical in each group. There were 10 separate trials, resulting in 11 manuscripts. These are summarized in Table 3.1 in order of Jadad score[5–15]. There were seven investigations that used bupivacaine and three that used ropivacaine in concentrations of 0.1–0.2%. Many of the studies were small but one study contained more than 100 patients.[12] Some were not blinded.[5,6,8,12,13,15] None specifically mentioned that assignment was concealed before enrollment. Because of the similarity among studies in design, it was appropriate to combine the outcomes of these studies in a meta-analysis. However, there was significant heterogeneity in some of the outcomes. These were identified and are discussed below.

There was a significant decrease in the requirement for clinician top-ups in patients who received PCEA compared with CEI (Fig. 3.1). This was highly statistically significant (Table 3.2). As Fig. 3.1 shows, three of the seven studies that reported this outcome had a statistically significant reduction in clinician top-ups, and the other four reported a trend in the same direction. The use of PCEA would result in a 19% decrease in the number of patients who require clinician top-ups (95% confidence interval [CI] 9–29%). This yields a "number needed to treat" (NNT) of 5.2 (95% CI 3.4–11).

Patients received less local anesthetic in the PCEA group. In one study, the difference approached 50%.[9] While the pooled difference was statistically significant, there was also significant heterogeneity in the result (Table 3.2). This can be explained by differences in the concentration and dosages of drugs and by the use of different drugs and additives. Finally, heterogeneity may result from the study of different populations of patients (nulliparous versus mixed parity). Of note, while the results are heterogeneous, the direction of change is consistent among the studies. Therefore, it is clear that the use of PCEA can reduce the amount of drug used, although the magnitude of the reduction depends on the factors identified above.

None of the studies reported a statistically significant difference between groups in pain scores during the first stage of labor. One study reported significantly better pain relief in the second stage of labor[6] in patients who received PCEA. While others reported increasing pain scores over time, none specifically reported these scores during the second stage of labor.

Because epidural analgesia can be achieved using a relatively low dose of local anesthetic, none of the studies reported toxicity. However, the increased doses found in the CEI groups resulted in an increased incidence of maternal motor block (Table 3.2, Fig. 3.2). Dense motor block was reported infrequently. In one study, patients experienced a dense motor block (but not complete) during 20% of measurements throughout labor. The incidence was the same in both groups.[8] Two studies reported patients with a dense motor block (Bromage score = 2).[9,10] For most of the study period, none of the patients in the PCEA group in either study had high degrees of motor block, while one or two patients in the CEI group did. This difference was not statistically significant, possibly because of the small sample size of both studies.

While differences in the incidence of motor block could be demonstrated between groups, there was no difference in maternal satisfaction scores. This may be primarily because the satisfaction scores were very high in both groups. It should be noted that maternal satisfaction was not the primary outcome of any of the studies and that the actual measurement was not made with a tool with proven reliability or validity. On a theoretical basis, PCEA may be associated with an increase in maternal satisfaction. Increased maternal freedom for intrapartum decision-making has been associated with an increase in satisfaction[2] and therefore it might be reasonable to expect this aspect to extend to labor analgesia in some women.

None of the other maternal or neonatal outcomes were different between groups (Table 3.2). Important outcomes such as the incidence of cesarean delivery and instrumental vaginal deliveries were measured in all studies and were similar. PCEA did not significantly change the length of the second stage of labor, indicating that patients are able to adequately judge the amount of analgesia required for the expulsion phase. The incidence of neonatal depression in both groups was similar and very low.

The equipment used for the delivery of both PCEA and CEI appears to be reliable. Only two studies explicitly report failure of equipment[8,13] and the incidence in both studies was less than 10%. One study

Table 3.1 PCEA versus continuous infusion. Study characteristics.

Study	Quality score	No. of patients PCEA/CEI	PCEA group treatment	CEI group treatment	Population	Comments
Smedvig 2001[14]	4	27/29	R 0.1% F 2 µg/mL Bolus 5 mL Lockout 10 min, max 25 mL/h	R 0.1% F 2 µg/mL 8 mL/h	Nulliparous	
Curry 1994[7]	4	30/30	B 0.125% Bolus 6 mL Lockout 20 min, no max	B 0.125% 10 mL/h	Mixed parity	Breech presentations were allowed to deliver vaginally
Gambling 1993[11]	4	55/13	B 0.125% F 2.5 µg/mL E 1 : 400,000 Bolus 2–6 mL Lockout 10–30 min	B 0.125% F 2.5 µg/mL E 1 : 400,000 8 mL/h	Nulliparous	4 different bolus doses for PCEA were studied and compared with CEI
Ferrante 1991[9]	3	20/20	B 0.125% F 2 µg/mL Bolus 3 mL Lockout 10 min, no max	B 0.125% F 2 µg/mL 12 mL/h	Mixed parity	
Ferrante 1994[16]	3	15/15	B 0.125% F 2 µg/mL Bolus 3 mL Lockout 10 min, no max	B 0.125% F 2 µg/mL 12 mL/h	Mixed parity	Two other groups with continuous background infusion were included in this study
Boutros 1999[5]	2	48/50	B 0.125% S 0.5 µg/mL Bolus 5 mL Lockout 10 min, max 50 mL/4 h	B 0.125% S 0.5 µg/mL at 8–14 mL/h	Mixed parity	The investigators included a third group of patients that received intermittent boluses
Eriksson 2003[8]	2	40/40	R 0.1% S 0.5 µg/mL Bolus 4 mL Lockout 20 min, no limit	R 0.1% S 0.5 µg/mL 6 mL/h	Mixed parity	Data from 2 institutions. 17 patients were excluded, 8 because of rapid delivery, 8 because of technical pump problems, and 1 because of pre-existing exclusion criteria. The primary outcome (drug dose) was the basis of a power analysis. Randomization was performed using an urn with 80 tickets, 40 per group
Collis 1999[6]	1	44/46	B 0.1% F 2 µg/mL Bolus 10 mL Lockout 30 min, no max	B 0.1% F 2 µg/mL 10 mL/h	Nulliparous	Initiated with combined, spinal epidural. A group that received intermittent boluses from midwives was included
Purdie 1992[12]	1	75/84	B 0.25% Bolus 3 mL	B 0.125% 10 mL/h	Nulliparous	Data on the same population of parturients divided between the two manuscripts
Tan 1994[15]			Lockout 5 min, max 4 boluses/h			
Sia 1999[13]	1	20/20	R 0.2% Lockout 15 min, max 150 mL/h	R 0.2% 8 mL/h	Nulliparous	

B, bupivacaine; CEI, continuous epidural infusion; E, epinephrine; F, fentanyl; PCEA, patient-controlled epidural analgesia; R, ropivacaine; S, sufentanil.

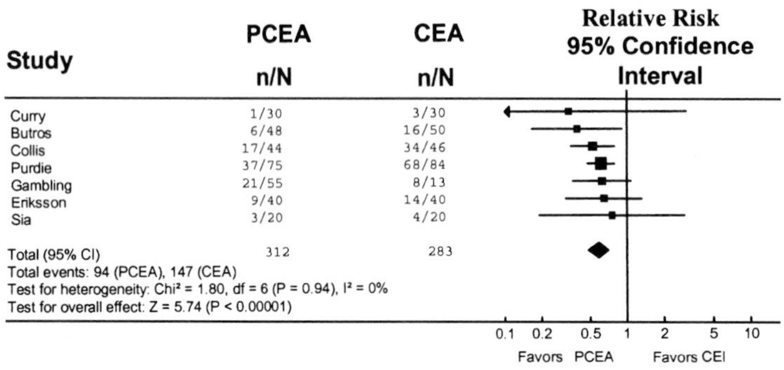

Fig. 3.1 Number of patients who required unscheduled clinician top-ups (n) and the total number of patients in each study (N) is shown. The relative risk and 95% confidence intervals are illustrated for each study on a logarithmic scale. The boxes represent the relative contribution of each study to the pooled estimate. The diamond represents the pooled relative risk. A relative risk of less than 1.0 favors the PCEA group. CEI, continuous epidural infusion; PCEA, patient-controlled epidural analgesia.

Table 3.2 PCEA versus CEI: outcomes.

Outcome	No. of studies (reference)	PCEA N or n/N	CEI N or n/N	WMD or RR (95% CI)	P value	Heterogeneity
Number of patients requiring clinician top-ups	7[5–8,11–13]	94/312	147/283	0.58 (0.48–0.07)	< 0.0001	NS
Mean dose of local anesthetic (mg/h)	9[5–9,11,13,14,16]	297	261	−3.6 (−5.0 to −2.1)	< 0.00001	< 0.001
Motor block: number of patients with motor weakness	5[5,6,8,11,13]	39/204	56/164	0.35 (0.20–0.59)	0.0001	NS
Maternal satisfaction: VAS scores	3[5–7]	119	124	0.06 (−3.9 to 0.52)	0.8	NS
Mode of delivery: cesarean section	10[5–9,11–14,16]	50/373	55/347	0.82 (0.57–1.17)	0.27	NS
Mode of delivery: instrumental deliveries	10[5–9,11–14,16]	112/373	108/347	0.98 (0.8–1.2)	0.85	NS
Length of first stage (min)	2[9,16]	35	35	21 (−38 to 80)	0.5	NS
Length of second stage (min)	4[9,12,13,16]	115	117	−10 (−22 to 0.8)	0.07	NS
Apgar < 7 at 1 min	7[5,6,8,9,11,13,16]	28/241	14/204	1.58 (0.83–3.0)	0.16	NS
Apgar < 7 at 5 min	7[5,6,8,9,11,13,16]	5/241	1/204	2.7 (0.50–14)	0.25	NS
Hypotension	6[8,9,11–13,16]	4/234	3/192	1.42 (0.33–6.2)	0.60	NS

CEI, Continuous epidural infusion; CI, confidence interval; NS, not statistically significant; PCEA, patient-controlled epidural analgesia; RR, risk ratio; VAS, visual analog score; WMD, weighed mean difference.

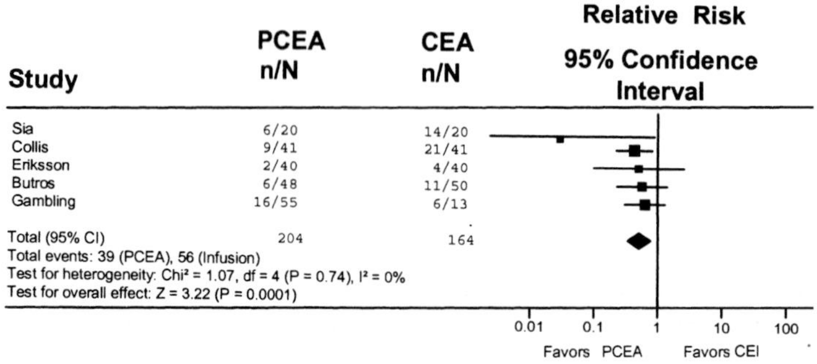

Fig. 3.2 Number of patients that had a motor block (n) and the total number of patients in each study (N) is shown. The relative risk and 95% confidence intervals are illustrated for each study on a logarithmic scale. The boxes represent the relative contribution of each study to the pooled estimate. The diamond represents the pooled relative risk. A relative risk of less than 1.0 favors the PCEA group. CEI, continuous epidural infusion; PCEA, patient-controlled epidural analgesia.

excluded a patient because she was unable to follow the instructions to operate the PCEA device.[10]

PCEA and CEI appear to be equally safe. The incidence of hypotension is low and similar between groups (Table 3.2). None of the studies reported excessively high sensory levels.

The addition of continuous infusion to PCEA

The addition of a background infusion to patient-controlled analgesia may further reduce the need for clinician interventions and may result in better maternal satisfaction. However, this may come at the expense of an increase in drug dose, motor block and interference with the progress of labor. There

have been five randomized controlled trials that have compared PCEA with PCEA with a continuous background infusion. Three of these are available as full manuscripts;[16–18] the information from two are only available as abstracts.[19–21] The details of these studies are shown in Table 3.3.

The three published studies were small and 0.125% bupivacaine, with or without additives, was used. Each employed small volumes for the patient-controlled boluses. In addition, the background infusion varied from 3 to 6 mL. Under these circumstances it is not surprising that the continuous infusion appeared to make very little difference in the main outcomes studied.

In a larger study, Campbell et al.[19,20] reported a comparison of ropivacaine 0.08% with 2 µg/mL of

Table 3.3 PCEA versus PCEA + continuous infusion: study characteristics.

Reference and year	Quality score	No. of patients PCEA/ PCEA + CEI	PCEA group treatment	PCEA + CEI group treatment	Population	Comments
Ferrante 1994[16]	3	15/30	B 0.125% Bolus 3 mL Lockout 10 min	2 groups 3 mL/h (N = 15) and 6 mL/h (N = 15)	Mixed	An additional study group had continuous infusion alone (N = 15)
Petry 2000[18]	2	37/37	B 0.125% S 0.75 µg/mL E = 1 : 800,000 Bolus 3 mL Lockout 12 min	Addition of 3 mL/h	Mixed	
Davin 1994[21]	Abstract	29 parturients (total)	B 0.125% S 1 µg/mL Bolus 5 mL Lockout 15 min	Addition of 5 mL/h	?	"Both groups achieved high quality analgesia with few and moderate side-effects." No quantitative data available
Paech 1992[17]	3	25/25	B 0.125% F 3 µg/mL Bolus 4 mL Lockout 15 min	Addition of 4 mL/h	Mixed	More than 90% of parturients in each group were satisfied with pain relief
Campbell 2004[19]	Abstract	141/144	R 0.8% F 2 µg/mL Bolus 5 mL Lockout 10 min	Addition of 10 mL/h	Nulliparous induced	Additional information is available in a second abstract (see below)
Campbell 2004[20]	Abstract	104/107	R 0.8% F 2 µg/mL Bolus 5 mL Lockout 10 min	Addition of 10 mL/h	Nulliparous induced	Subset of the patients above that did not have a cesarean delivery

B, bupivacaine; CEI, continuous epidural infusion; E, epinephrine; F, fentanyl; PCEA, patient-controlled epidural analgesia; R, ropivacaine; S, sufentanil.

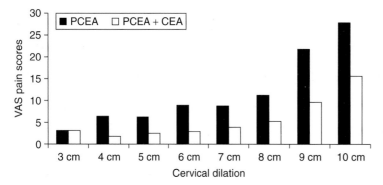

Fig. 3.3 PCEA versus PCEA + continuous infusion. Data from Campbell *et al.*[19] Visual analog score (VAS) pain scores (vertical) versus cervical dilation (horizontal) are shown. The VAS scores are significantly higher for all cervical dilations in the PCEA group. CEA, controlled epidural analgesia; PCEA, patient-controlled epidural analgesia.

fentanyl with and without a 10 mL/h background infusion. This study, reported as two abstracts, was designed to have sufficient power to detect differences in obstetric outcomes as well as outcomes relating to pain relief. Although there were no differences in the obstetric outcomes,[20] there was a statistically significant difference in the number patients who received clinician top-ups (41% vs 27%, $P = 0.03$), and better pain relief in both the first and second stages of labor in the group that received the background infusion (Fig. 3.3).[19] However, there was also a significantly higher volume of local anesthetic used in the PCEA + CEI group. There was no difference in the incidence of motor block (< 4%) or ability to ambulate (85%) between groups (Campbell, personal communication, December 2004).

Conclusions

Both PCEA and CEI provide excellent analgesia for labor. PCEA has a number of clear advantages compared with CEI. These include a reduction in the need for clinician top-ups, a reduction in the amount of drug needed and a reduction in the incidence of motor block. While there was no demonstrable difference in patient satisfaction, this may be because of very high maternal satisfaction with epidural analgesia, regardless of the mode of maintenance, or because there were deficiencies in the tool used for measurement. There is no difference in any obstetric or neonatal outcomes. Both modalities appear to be reliable and safe.

It is difficult to determine whether or not the addition of CEI to PCEA provides additional benefit. Published studies are too small to demonstrate any dif-

ferences. One large study, available only as an abstract, showed that the addition of CEI to PCEA provided better pain relief with fewer clinician top-ups when compared with PCEA alone. There was no difference in any of the obstetric outcomes. From these limited data, it appears that there may be some advantages to the addition of a continuous background infusion. Confirmation of this impression is required before the addition of CEI to PCEA can be recommended.

References

1 Gambling DR, Yu P, Cole C, McMorland GH, Palmer L. A comparative study of patient-controlled epidural analgesia (PCEA) and continuous infusion epidural analgesia (CIEA) during labour. *Can J Anaesth* 1988;**35**:249–54.

2 Hodnett ED. Pain and women's satisfaction with the experience of childbirth: a systematic review. *Am J Obstet Gynecol* 2002;**186**:S160–72.

3 van der Vyver M, Halpern S, Joseph G. Patient-controlled epidural analgesia versus continuous infusion for labour analgesia: a meta-analysis. *Br J Anaesth* 2002;**89**:459–65.

4 Jadad AR, Moore RA, Carroll D, *et al.* Assessing the quality of reports of randomized clinical trials: is blinding necessary? *Control Clin Trials* 1996;**17**:1–12.

5 Boutros A, Blary S, Bronchard R, Bonnet F. Comparison of intermittent epidural bolus, continuous epidural infusion and patient-controlled epidural analgesia during labor. *Int J Obstet Anesth* 1999;**8**:236–41.

6 Collis RE, Plaat FS, Morgan BM. Comparison of midwife top-ups, continuous infusion and patient-controlled epidural analgesia for maintaining mobility after a low-dose combined spinal–epidural. *Br J Anaesth* 1999;**82**:233–6.

7 Curry PD, Pacsoo C, Heap DG. Patient-controlled epidural analgesia in obstetric anaesthetic practice. *Pain* 1994;**57**:125–7.

8 Eriksson SL, Gentels C, Olofsson CH. PCEA compared to continuous epidural infusion in an ultra-low-dose regimen for labor pain relief: a randomized study. *Acta Anaesthesiol Scand* 2003;**47**:1085–90.

9 Ferrante FM, Lu L, Jamison SB, Datta S. Patient-controlled epidural analgesia: demand dosing. *Anesth Analg* 1991;**73**: 547–52.

10 Ferrante FM, Barber MJ, Segal M, Hughes NJ, Datta S. 0.0625% bupivacaine with 0.0002% fentanyl via patient-controlled epidural analgesia for pain of labor and delivery. *Clin J Pain* 1995;**11**:121–6.

11 Gambling DR, Huber CJ, Berkowitz J, *et al*. Patient-controlled epidural analgesia in labour: varying bolus dose and lockout interval. *Can J Anaesth* 1993;**40**:211–7.

12 Purdie J, Reid J, Thorburn J, Asbury AJ. Continuous extra-dural analgesia: comparison of midwife top-ups, continuous infusions and patient controlled administration. *Br J Anaesth* 1992;**68**:580–4.

13 Sia AT, Chong JL. Epidural 0.2% ropivacaine for labour anal-gesia: parturient-controlled or continuous infusion? *Anaesth Intensive Care* 1999;**27**:154–8.

14 Smedvig JP, Soreide E, Gjessing L. Ropivacaine 1 mg/mL, plus fentanyl 2 µg/mL for epidural analgesia during labour: is mode of administration important? *Acta Anaesthesiol Scand* 2001;**45**:595–9.

15 Tan S, Reid J, Thorburn J. Extradural analgesia in labour: complications of three techniques of administration. *Br J Anaesth* 1994;**73**:619–23.

16 Ferrante FM, Rosinia FA, Gordon C, Datta S. The role of continuous background infusions in patient-controlled epidural analgesia for labor and delivery. *Anesth Analg* 1994; **79**:80–4.

17 Paech MJ. Patient-controlled epidural analgesia in labour: is a continuous infusion of benefit? *Anaesth Intensive Care* 1992;**20**:15–20.

18 Petry J, Vertcauteren M, van Mol I, van Houwe P, Adriaensen HA. Epidural PCA with bupivacaine 0.125%, sufentanil 0.75 µg/mL and epinephrine 1/800,000 for labor analgesia: is a background infusion beneficial? *Acta Anaesthesiol Belg* 2000;**51**:163–6.

19 Campbell DC, Breen TW, Halpern S, Muir H, Nunn R. Determination of the efficacy of PCEA alone compared to PCEA + CIEA using ambulatory labor analgesics. *Anesthesiology* 2004;**100**:Suppl A11.

20 Campbell DC, Breen TW, Halpern S, Muir H, Nunn R. Randomized controlled trial comparing PCEA vs PCEA + CIEA on labor outcome using ambulatory analgesics. *Anesthesiology* 2004;**100**:Suppl A20.

21 Davin C, Brichant JF, Falieres X, Lamy M, Hans P. Patient-controlled epidural analgesia during labor: pure demand dos-ing or continuous infusion plus demand dosing? *Anesthesiology* 1994;**81**:A1161.

CHAPTER 4

The use of transcutaneous electrical nerve stimulation for labor pain

Carolyn F. Weiniger

Introduction

The drugless therapies available for labor range from the ancient (massage, oils and acupuncture) to the modern (intracutaneous saline injections and transcutaneous electrical nerve stimulation [TENS]). There are numerous potential advantages to the use of drugless therapies compared with conventional pain relief. Most are easy to administer. Maternal side-effects such as nausea, vomiting, altered sensorium and pruritus can be avoided. Similarly, placental passage of drugs and their effect on the fetus and newborn can be reduced. For these reasons, many women would prefer to avoid or reduce the amount of medication administered during labor and delivery. Many women would also prefer to avoid side-effects from spinal and epidural analgesia, such as postdural puncture headache and motor weakness of the lower extremities.

Transcutaneous electrical nerve stimulation has been used for labor for more than 25 years.[1] Most commonly, electrodes are placed over the T10–L1 dermatomes bilaterally, 1.5–3 cm lateral to the spinous processes of the back to provide analgesia for the first stage of labor. A second set of electrodes is placed over the S2–S4 dermatomes for the second stage of labor. Often a single machine has the capacity to activate all four electrodes simultaneously ("dual channel"). Less commonly, electrodes have been placed cranially or suprapubically. The amount of current can be changed by the woman as labor progresses, giving her a sense of control over the pain of labor. In theory, TENS provides analgesia either by blocking pain impulses to the brain by stimulating A-fiber transmission, or by increasing the local release of β-endorphins.[2] While TENS shares the advantages of other drugless therapies, there are some disadvantages to its use. The TENS machine itself is expensive to purchase and therefore some patients prefer to rent the unit for use during labor and delivery. There are additional costs associated with the disposable electrodes and batteries. Transcutaneous electrical nerve stimulation is incompatible with other drugless therapies such as hot water baths. Finally, some clinicians feel that it is important to train the woman to use TENS before she is in labor.

Although it is unclear whether or not TENS provides labor analgesia, it is an extremely popular mode of analgesia.[3] This chapter reviews the clinical trials that studied the use of TENS in labor to determine its effectiveness. MEDLINE®, EMBASE®, Science Citation Index® and Cochrane Controlled Trials Register databases were searched from the inception of the databases until March 2004 using the following words as text, and key words: [Transcutaneous electrical nerve stimulation], [TENS], [labo(u)r] and [pregnancy]. The bibliographies of the retrieved articles were hand searched in order to identify additional reports. The search was restricted to published randomized controlled trials (RCTs) or quasi-RCTs, written in English. Non-randomized studies, abstracts, case series and case reports were excluded. Further, we eliminated clinical trials that did not place the leads on the back. Each randomized study was rated for quality using the Jadad scale[4] (see Appendix for a full description of the scale). Studies with a quality score of 3 or more were considered to be high quality.

There were 12 studies, presented in 11 manuscripts, that met the inclusion criteria.[2,5–14] Of these one had a randomized and quasi-randomized (alternate assignment by time of admission) component.[6] In one additional study all patients were assigned to group using alphabetical (quasi-randomization) assignment.[7] In total, there were 598 women in the control group and 570 in the TENS group. Seven of the 12 studies were of high quality. The methodological details, quality and main results are presented in Table 4.1.

In all studies, a commercially available TENS machine that allowed the patient to change the settings as labor progressed was provided to the study group during early active labor. Only three papers describe any patient training or who did the training.[2,11,15] One paper specifically chose patients without prior instruction.[12] All studies described the TENS electrodes as placed on the lower back, using the dual electrode system. In six of the studies, the control group received a "sham" TENS in an attempt to blind the patient and caregivers to treatment group[2,11–15] and in three they received "usual care"[5,7,9] without an attempt at blinding. One study contained three groups – TENS, inactive control and usual care,[10] and one study contained an inhaled nitrous oxide control.[6] Finally, one study contained two treatment groups (TENS and intradermal sterile water) that were compared with an unblinded "usual care" group.[9] Only three of the studies reported a sample size calculation.[11,12,14]

Study findings

Analgesia

Pain scores
Seven studies reported differences in pain scores between the TENS group and control. This was measured on pain scale (0–4),[15] a visual analog scale for pain,[2,9,12] a pain relief scale (4 or 5 points "complete or good" to "none").[5,7,11] These pain scores were measured at various times during the first and second stages of labor. Only one study showed a statistically significant improvement in pain scores[5] (Table 4.1). Of note, one study found that the control group had less pain at 7 cm dilation compared with the TENS group.[7]

Requests for other medications
Patients in all studies were allowed to request additional medications. None of the studies reported any difference in the amount of medications requested. One study noted an increase in the requests for analgesia in the TENS group (23/100 vs 14/100) although the difference was not statistically significant.[7]

The primary outcome of one of the studies was the amount of meperidine used during labor.[2] In addition to TENS or sham TENS, each patient received patient controlled intravenous analgesia with meperidine. There was no difference between groups in the number of milligrams of meperidine, the number of requests for medication or the number of successful requests.

Tsen et al. superimposed TENS or sham TENS on epidural analgesia with 0.25% bupivacaine[14] or spinal analgesia with sufentanil and bupivacaine.[13] The main outcome was duration of analgesia. There was no statistical difference between groups, with TENS slightly favored in patients receiving epidural analgesia and sham TENS favored in patients receiving spinal analgesia.

Other analgesic outcomes
Thomas et al.[12] studied TENS patients and sham TENS patients using both groups as their own control. In 40% of TENS patients and in a similar number of sham TENS patients, the pain increased when the machine was turned off. The authors concluded that TENS was similar to placebo for this outcome.

TENS versus active control
Two small studies compared TENS with alternative forms of analgesia. Labrecque et al.[9] compared intradermal sterile water with TENS and a control group in a mixed population of parturients in early labor. They found that intradermal sterile water provided superior analgesia compared with TENS, and TENS was not different from standard care. Chia et al.[6] compared TENS with nitrous oxide in two populations of parturients: mixed parity in spontaneous labor and nulliparous patients undergoing induction of labor. In the latter study, the patients were similar in terms of cervical dilation at the time they requested analgesia, although the patients in the nitrous oxide group had more frequent contractions. Patients in both groups used their assigned treatment modality for approximately 82 min before requesting additional analgesia. They concluded that TENS was as effective as nitrous oxide in providing pain relief in labor.

Table 4.1 Study characteristics and main results.

Study & year	Control group N	Control group Maneuver	Study group N	Study group Maneuver	Quality score	Description	Outcome measures (main outcome if identified)	Results
Tsen 2001[14]	20	Labor epidural + sham TENS Prior to CSE TENS thresholds were determined Pads placed bilaterally T10–L1 and S2–S4	20	Labor epidural + active TENS Prior to CSE TENS thresholds were determined Pads placed bilaterally T10–L1 and S2–S4. 18–20 mA, pulse rate between 66 and 100 Hz, width 310 microseconds	5	Randomized using shuffled envelopes Concealed allocation Blinded (sham TENS vs active TENS) Sample size – to detect a 30-min difference between groups Significantly more multiparous patients received active TENS	Onset of analgesia Duration of analgesia	No significant difference between groups Onset 8.3 vs 7.2 min favoring active TENS Duration 82.3 vs 80.7 min favoring sham TENS
Tsen 2000[13]	20	CSE + sham TENS Prior to CSE TENS thresholds were determined Pads placed bilaterally T10–L1 and S2–S4	20	CSE + active TENS Prior to CSE TENS thresholds were determined. Pads placed bilaterally T10–L1 and S2–S4. 18–20 mA, pulse rate between 66 and 100 Hz, width 310 microseconds	5	Randomized using shuffled envelopes Concealed allocation Blinded (sham TENS vs active TENS) No sample size calculation Significantly more multiparous patients received active TENS	Survival analysis for duration of analgesia from the CSE	No significant difference (91 vs 83 min favoring sham TENS)
Labrecque 1999[9]	12	"Standard care" back massage whirlpool mobilization	12	2 pairs of disposable electrodes on the skin of the lower back "Normal mode" TENS adjusted to tolerance + standard care	3	Randomized in blocks Concealed allocation Balanced demographics No blinding to treatment (after assignment) No sample size calculation	VAS scores for low back pain	Three-group comparison: (i) standard care; (ii) TENS, 0.1 mL intradermal sterile water injected in the lumbosacral area. There was no difference in analgesia scores between standard care and TENS Intradermal sterile water significantly improved pain outcomes compared to both standard care and TENS

Study	n	Control/Sham	n	TENS		Methods	Outcome	Results
van der Ploeg 1996[2]	48	Sham TENS Paired electrodes L1–L3 and L4–S1 Started at level 2 and adjusted at 1–6 IVPCA meperidine and promethazine	46	Paired electrodes L1–L3 and L4–S1 Low frequency (2 bursts of 5 pulses) Started at level 2 and adjusted at 1–6 IVPCA meperidine and promethazine	2	Method of randomization unclear Blinded using sham TENS Patient training (potential for unblinding) No sample size calculation	Meperidine usage	No significant difference (61 ± 22 mg vs 65 ± 16 mg favoring active TENS)
Thomas 1988[12]	148	Sham TENS Pads applied at T10–L1 and S2–S4 Machine rendered inactive	132	Pads applied at T10–L1 and S2–S4	4	Randomization by random number table Blinded using sham TENS Instructed to use TENS during labor. Assessed by blinded assessor. Planned sample size More nulliparous patients in the active TENS group	Differences in pain scores with the machine switched on and off – patient acting as her own control	Patients in both groups experienced an increase in pain when the machine was turned off No difference in absolute scores
Harrison 1986[8]	76	Sham TENS Bilateral paravertebral (5 cm) placement of pads at T10–L1 and S2–S4	74	Bilateral paravertebral (5 cm) placement of pads at T10–L1 and S2–S4 Initial settings – duration 60–80 µs, rate 60–100 Hz Gain = "5" and could be increased	3	Nulliparous and multiparous randomized separately Method unclear Sham TENS, machines rotated to maintain blinding Training at the time of use No sample size calculation	Pain scores and pain relief Use of other pain medications	Similar numbers of patients experienced severe or very severe pain between groups No difference in the amount of pain medications used
Bundsen 1982[5]	9	Control (treatment not described)	15	Electrodes at T10–L1 on the back and over the suprapubic area of the abdomen	2	Randomization unclear Not blinded Cesarean deliveries omitted (n = 1 for each group) No sample size calculation	Analgesic effect	Suprapubic pain was not affected by TENS Back pain was improved with TENS in the first stage of labor (12/15 vs 0/9 in late first stage) 5/9 vs 0/15 patients had good pain relief in second stage of labor with TENS

Continued

Table 4.1 (*continued*)

Study & year	Control group			Study group			Quality		Outcome measures (main outcome if identified)	Results
	N	Maneuver		N	Maneuver		Quality score	Description		
Nesheim 1981[11]	35	Sham TENS Electrodes placed bilaterally T10–L1 and S2–S4, but disconnected "Red light" on to show unit was functioning		35	Electrodes placed bilaterally T10–L1 and S2–S4 "Red light" on to show unit was functioning Current 0–40 mA, at 100 Hz, 250 µs Patient operated for 40–150 Hz		4	Randomization by coin toss Concealed allocation (coin toss after consent) Sample size calculation ? Investigator blinded	Pain relief Additional medication	25/35 (TENS) vs 19/35 (sham) reported at least some pain relief. 2/35 (TENS) vs 0/35 (sham) reported worsening of pain Use of additional medication was similar
Erkkola 1980[7]	100	Usual care		100	Electrodes placed bilaterally T10–L1 and S2–S4. Patient adjusted		Not rated	Quasi-randomization (alphabetical assignment) No concealment of group assignment No blinding No sample size calculation	Pain relief	73% in the TENS group obtained some pain relief No difference in the number of patients who requested medication (23/100 vs 16/100 favoring TENS)
Lee 1990[10]	67	Either sham TENS (n = 33) or "control" (n = 34)		58	Working TENS		3	Randomized No concealment ? Blinding for the sham TENS group No sample size calculation	Outcome of labor Additional pain medication Post-delivery assessment	No difference in labor outcome 77% TENS vs 69% control requested additional pain medication. 32/41 considered TENS helpful in

Study	n	Comparison	n	TENS application	Score	Methods	Outcomes	Results
Chia 1990[6]	53	50% N₂O	48	Electrodes placed bilaterally at T10–T11 and upper sacral. Amplitude adjustment from 0 to 48 mA, burst mode 50–200 Hz	Not rated	Quasi-randomization by order of admission. Not blinded. No sample size calculation	Request for additional medication. Pain intensity	1st stage, 16/26 considered sham TENS helpful in 1st stage. 19/40 considered TENS helpful in 2nd stage, 13/23 considered sham TENS helpful in 2nd stage. 16/41 would ask for TENS in a subsequent labor, 13/26 would ask for sham TENS in a subsequent labor. No difference between groups for any outcomes
Chia 1990[6]	10	50% N₂O	10	Electrodes placed bilaterally at T10–T11 and upper sacral. Amplitude adjustment from 0 to 48 mA, burst mode 50–200 Hz	1	Randomized in concealed envelopes. Not blinded. No sample size calculation	Request for additional medication. Pain intensity	No difference between groups. Nulliparous patients for induction of labor only
Total patients	598		570					

CSE, combined spinal epidural; IVPCA, intravenous patient-controlled analgesia; N₂O, nitrous oxide; TENS, transcutaneous electrical nerve stimulation; VAS, visual analog score.

Maternal satisfaction

None of the studies reported maternal satisfaction directly. Thomas et al.[12] noted that significantly more mothers would choose TENS over sham TENS in a subsequent labor. In contrast, Lee et al.[10] noted that 16/41 (39%) patients would request TENS in a subsequent labor compared with 13/26 (50%) who would request sham TENS ($P = 0.37$).

Fetal and neonatal outcome

An early study noted that interference with fetal heart rate monitoring was a significant practical problem[7]. However, this may depend on the equipment used. Harrison et al.[15] specifically stated that, in their study, interference did not occur. The other studies were silent on this issue.

There was no difference in the 1 and 5 min neonatal Apgar scores in the studies that recorded these outcomes.[2,5,13–15] Further, there was no difference in the neurologic examination of the infant at birth.[5]

Side-effects

Very few side-effects, related to TENS, were reported in the studies. Thomas et al.[12] reported that 41% (vs 35% in the control group) requested removal of the TENS machine because the equipment was annoying or the tingling sensation troublesome. No other study reported side-effects (apart from difficulty in monitoring the fetal heart rate noted above).

Cost

None of the studies addressed economic issues related to the use of TENS.

Discussion

The results of the current studies do not support the theory that TENS provides significantly more analgesia for labor pain than sham (placebo) TENS or "usual care." This finding was consistent in spite of the numerous strategies used by the investigators to measure pain, pain relief and maternal satisfaction. The quality of the studies did not change the result. For example, even when the control group consisted of usual care without patient blinding, no differences could be demonstrated.[5,7,9,10] There is empirical evid-ence that lack of blinding in randomized controlled trials produces significantly biased results in favor of the treatment group.[16] However, both the blinded (sham TENS) and unblinded studies failed to show that TENS was effective. Studies with small sample sizes may not detect significant differences in pain relief. However, four studies had more than 50 patients in each group[7,10,12,15] and three planned the sample size to detect a clinically important difference in the main outcome.[11,12,14]

It is possible that the women that participated in the RCTs were in some way different from the general population. In particular, they may have had different expectations for pain relief or different motivations to avoid medications. One can speculate that this strengthens the argument that TENS has no added benefit compared with sham TENS.

A potentially serious flaw in the design of the studies is that the training of women to use the TENS machines may have been inadequate. It is not possible to tell whether or not a training program could increase the efficacy of TENS during labor. This type of clinical trial would be difficult to design since training would, by definition, result in a study in which the participants were not blinded to group assignment.

In contrast to the RCTs, non-randomized trials reported more positive results. Harrison et al.[15] reported a high satisfaction with TENS, although they noted that only 18% of patients used TENS as a sole modality of pain relief for labor. Bundsen et al.,[17] using multivariate techniques, found that TENS had a significant analgesic effect on back pain. They also found a reduced incidence in the use of alternate methods of analgesia and somewhat better neonatal Apgar scores associated with TENS. However, they noted that half the women could not use TENS optimally because of interference with the fetal heart rate trace. Van der Spank et al.[18] noted a very high satisfaction rate with TENS (96%) accompanied by lower pain scores when the TENS was active compared with when it was turned off. Kaplan et al.[19] noted shorter labors associated with TENS compared with matched controls. They also noted that patients in the TENS group received alternate analgesia later than the controls.

While evidence from non-randomized studies is weaker than that from RCTs, it suggests that TENS may be valuable in some patients, perhaps those with back labor.

Conclusions

Based upon the currently available data, there is no evidence that TENS is more effective than sham TENS as an analgesic for labor. However, it may be appropriate for some patients who have contraindications to other methods of pain relief. None of the available studies have evaluated the use of TENS in trained individuals.

References

1 Stewart P. Transcutaneous nerve stimulation as a method of analgesia in labour. *Anaesthesia* 1979;**34**:361–4.

2 van der Ploeg JM, Vervset HAM, Liem AL, Schagen van Leeuwen JH. Transcutaneous nerve stimulation (TENS) during the first stage of labour: a randomized clinical trial. *Pain* 1996;**68**:75–8.

3 Robertson A. TENS: a marketing triumph. *Practising Midwife* 2003;**6**:20–1.

4 Jadad AR, Moore RA, Carroll D, *et al.* Assessing the quality of reports of randomized clinical trials: is blinding necessary? *Control Clin Trials* 1996;**17**:1–12.

5 Bundsen P, Ericson K, Peterson LE, Thiringer K. Pain relief in labor by transcutaneous electrical nerve stimulation: testing of a modified stimulation technique and evaluation of the neurological and biochemical condition of the newborn infant. *Acta Obstet Gynaecol Scand* 1982;**61**:129–36.

6 Chia YT, Arulkumaran S, Chua S, Ratnam SS. Effectiveness of transcutaneous electric nerve stimulator for pain relief in labour. *Asia-Oceania J Obstet Gynaecol* 1990;**16**:145–51.

7 Erkkola R, Pikkola P, Kanto J. Transcutaneous nerve stimulation for pain relief during labor: a controlled study. *Ann Chir Gynaecol* 1980;**69**:273–7.

8 Harrison RF, Woods T, Shore M, Mathews G, Unwin A. Pain relief in labour using transcutaneous nerve stimulation (TENS): a TENS/TENS placebo controlled study of two parity groups. *Br J Obstet Gynaecol* 1986;**93**:739–46.

9 Labrecque M, Nouwen A, Bergeron M, Rancourt JF. A randomized controlled trial of non-pharmacologic approaches for relief of low back pain during labor. *J Fam Pract* 1999;**48**:259–63.

10 Lee EW, Chung IW, Lee JY, Lam PW, Chin RK. The role of transcutaneous electrical nerve stimulation in management of labour in obstetric patients. *Asia-Oceania J Obstet Gynaecol* 1990;**16**:247–54.

11 Nesheim BI. The use of transcutaneous nerve stimulation for pain relief during labor: a controlled clinical study. *Acta Obstet Gynaecol Scand* 1981;**60**:13–6.

12 Thomas IL, Tyle V, Webster J, Neilson A. An evaluation of transcutaneous electrical nerve stimulation for pain relief in labour. *Aust NZ J Obstet Gynaecol* 1988;**28**:182–9.

13 Tsen LC, Thomas J, Segal S, Datta S, Bader AM. Transcutaneous electrical nerve stimulation does not augment combined spinal epidural labor analgesia. *Can J Anesth* 2000;**47**:38–42.

14 Tsen LC, Thomas J, Segal S, Datta S, Bader AM. Transcutaneous electrical nerve stimulation does not augment epidural labor analgesia. *J Clin Anesth.* 2001;**13**:571–5.

15 Harrison RF, Shore M, Woods T, Mathews G, Gardiner J, Unwin A. A comparative study of transcutaneous electrical nerve stimulation (TENS), Entonox®, pethidine + promazine and lumbar epidural for pain relief in labor. *Acta Obstet Gynaecol Scand* 1987;**66**:9–14.

16 Schulz KF, Chalmers I, Hayes RJ, Altman DG. Empirical evidence of bias: dimensions of methodological quality associated with estimates of treatment effects in controlled trials. *JAMA* 1995;**273**:408–12.

17 Bundsen P, Peterson LE, Selstam U. Pain relief in labor by transcutaneous electrical nerve stimulation: a prospective matched study. *Acta Obstet Gynaecol Scand* 1981;**60**:459–68.

18 van der Spank JT, Cambier DC, De Paepe HM, Danneels LAG, Witvrouw EE, Beerens L. Pain relief in labor by transcutaneous electrical nerve stimulation (TENS). *Arch Gynecol Obstet* 2000;**264**:131–6.

19 Kaplan B, Rabinerson D, Lurie S, Bar J, Krieser UR, Neri A. Transcutaneous electrical nerve stimulation (TENS) for adjuvant pain-relief during labor and delivery. *Int J Gynaecol Obstet* 1998;**60**:251–5.

CHAPTER 5

Is nitrous oxide an effective analgesic for labor?
A qualitative systematic review

Jean E. Kronberg & Dorothy E.A. Thompson

Introduction

The first reported use of nitrous oxide as a labor analgesic was in 1881 from St. Petersburg, Russia. In this report Klikowisch noted that labor pain subsided after two or three deep inhalations, but the patients remained conscious and uterine activity was un-affected.[1,2] In 1934, Minnitt[3] described a demand valve flow apparatus, including a portable model for home births. Nitrous oxide had been in use for some hospital births, but had not been widely available. In 1936, the Central Midwives Board in the UK adopted the use of this apparatus, making available nitrous oxide in air for labor analgesia in the community. Subsequently, the output of these machines was shown to be variable. In some cases the concentration of nitrous oxide was more than 50%.[4] In 1961, Tunstall[5] described pro-duction of a 50 : 50 mixture of liquid nitrous oxide and gaseous oxygen in a single cylinder pressurized to 2000 pounds per square inch. Fifty percent nitrous oxide in oxygen was made commercially available in 1963 by the British Oxygen Company under the trade name Entonox®. A portable apparatus with a demand valve using Entonox® came into use.

Inhaled nitrous oxide is well tolerated, has low blood gas solubility, rapidly equilibrates with blood and brain and is rapidly eliminated after cessation without lasting side-effects. Maximum analgesic effect is achieved within 30 s to 1 min.[1] Data from a rat model suggest that nitrous oxide analgesia is mediated through supraspinal opiate and spinal α_2-adrenoreceptors by way of a descending inhibitory noradrenergic pathway activated by opiate receptors in the periaquaduct of Gray.[6,7]

While regional techniques now represent the "gold standard" for labor analgesia, they are not always indicated, available or desired. Nitrous oxide remains as an alternate analgesic modality. In some practice settings, it is the only labor analgesic available for women.[8] Nitrous oxide has the advantage that it can be used safely without direct medical supervision. The efficacy and safety of nitrous oxide has been reviewed recently by Rosen.[9] His systematic review, limited to publications in the English language, attests to the safety of appropriately administered nitrous oxide for mothers and newborns and also attending healthcare workers. This review examines further the evidence for efficacy of nitrous oxide as an analgesic for labor.

Methods

Randomized controlled trials (RCTs) were sought where nitrous oxide inhalation was used for first and/or second stage labor analgesia. Search strategies for identification of eligible studies included MEDLINE® (1966–August 2003), EMBASE® (1980–August 2003), the Cochrane Central Register of Controlled Trials (issue 2) 2003 and the Cochrane Data Base of Systematic Reviews (issue 2) 2003. The last electronic search was conducted in August 2003. The words [nitrous oxide], [labo(u)r] and [analgesia] were used to find relevant studies, using a combination of free text words without restriction to language. Additional reports were identified from review articles, retrieved reports and specialists textbooks. A hand search of major anesthesia journals for past 5 years was carried out, including *Anesthesiology, Canadian Journal of Anesthesia, British*

Journal of Anaesthesia, Anaesthesia and *Anesthesia and Analgesia.*

Inclusion criteria

Included were all RCTs, reported as full journal publications in laboring parturients in whom nitrous oxide was compared with placebo, other concentrations of nitrous oxide (dose–response) or other inhalational agents. In addition, each included RCT reported the influence of nitrous oxide on labor pain as a main outcome. Excluded were abstracts, letters to the editor and review articles. Studies comparing nitrous oxide with transcutaneous electrical nerve stimulation (TENS) or parenteral narcotics for labor were excluded.[10–12] No RCTs were identified that compared nitrous oxide with narcotics using intravenous patient-controlled analgesia in labor.

Data extraction and analysis

Quality of the data

Each study that possibly could be described as an RCT in which analgesic effects of nitrous oxide in labor were investigated was read independently by each of the authors and given a quality score (0–5) using the three-item Jadad scale[13] (see Appendix for a full description of the scale). The authors then achieved a consensus score that ranged from 0 to 5.

Data extraction

The following data were extracted: date and country of study, parity of and number enrolled, percentage nitrous oxide used, mode of delivery, use of parenteral medication, mode of treatment of a comparison group, stage of labor, duration of use and pain scale used for measurement.

The majority of studies reported measures of global pain relief at the end of labor. Crossover studies also were identified with analgesia measured after each contraction or set of contractions using linear analog scales. Adverse effects were noted also.

Results

Nitrous oxide versus control

Six RCTs studied nitrous oxide inhalation using oxygen or air as the control gas. Five RCTs measured pain relief after inhalation with contractions in the first and second stage of labor.[14–18] Because of overlap of authors and institution, and of similarities in the methods and results, it is possible that a significant number of patients were reported twice.[15,18] However, this could not be confirmed. For this reason, they were treated as independent studies. In total, there were 1944 subjects studied. The study characteristics are shown in Table 5.1. The results of the studies are shown in Table 5.2. Two of the studies[14,16] reported the results using the Mulleetr pain score. This scoring system is the average of the patients' and midwives' pain perception – each on a four-point scale. Using this system, 0 represents excellent analgesia and 3 represents poor analgesia. In these studies, 81%[14] and 97%[16] of women who received nitrous oxide had a score of 1 or less (good to excellent). Only 1% of women in the control group of one study[14] (and 0% in the other)[16] had a score of 1 or less. Two studies[15,17] reported analgesia using a five-category patient rating scale. Of the women who received nitrous oxide, 69.6% and 91.2% rated their labor pain as none or mild compared with 18%[15] and 1.6%[17] in the control group.

An additional study[18] used a verbal analog scale with scores ranging from 0 (no pain) to 5 (extreme pain). Using this score, 81.7% of women who received nitrous oxide and 18% in the control group reported a score of 0 or 1. In contrast, a sixth RCT[19] with crossover design and 29 subjects compared 50% nitrous oxide inhalation in early first stage with compressed air over 10 contractions. A visual analog pain score (0–10), obtained after each contraction, showed no difference between treatment groups and controls. However, 21 of the 29 patients were not truly blinded to the treatment received because they could correctly identify the gas used.

Side-effects reported were nausea and vomiting, dizziness, lethargy, sleepiness, perioral tingling and throat irritation. One large study[14] found no difference in the incidence of nausea and vomiting between women who received nitrous oxide and control groups. In the same study, the most common side-effect was dizziness, reported at 39.4% in the nitrous oxide group and none in the control group. A second large study[17] reported dizziness in 6.4% of women in the nitrous oxide group compared with none in the control group. The second most common side-effect reported in both these studies was sleepiness (3–6%).

Table 5.1 Studies comparing nitrous oxide with oxygen or air.

Author Reference no. Date Country	Primary question	Number enrolled (nulliparous/ multiparous)	% N₂O delivery system Use of parenteral medication	Compared with	Stage of labor	Duration of use	Quality of study
Su[14] 2002 China	Efficacy and safety of N₂O in labor	1300 Nulliparous N_2O N = 658 *Control* N = 642	50%, demand valve, intermittent, on-line gas supply, flow rate 0–20 L/min Both groups: Inhalation 30–40 s before contraction, continued until contraction passed No parenteral medication given Local anesthetic infiltration for episiotomy repair	O_2	Stage 1 & 2 Singleton, term, vertex healthy	*Average time* 4 h 11 min *Range* 46 min–14 h 30 min	*Quality Score 3* Randomization not described Blinding implied not described Withdrawals none
Zhang[15] 2001 China	Efficacy of N₂O in labor and its effects on mother and infant	110 parity not stated N_2O N = 60 *Control* N = 50	30–50%, face mask, no demand valve, administered by nurse Inhalation 3–4 deep breaths 30–50 s before contraction, continued until contraction peak passed	O_2	Stage 1 & 2 Singleton, term, vertex healthy	8.25 ± 3.4 h	*Quality Score 3* Randomization not described Patient blinded 3 withdrawals N₂O group due to nausea
Ou[16] 2001 China	Analgesic effect of 50% N_2O/O_2 inhalation in labor	200 parity not stated N_2O N = 100 *Control* N = 100	50%, demand valve, online gas supply, 0–15 L/min Inhalation 20–30 s before uterine contraction, intermittent inhalation for 2–3 deep breaths during contaction No other analgesia given	O_2	Stage 1 & 2 Singleton, term, vertex, healthy	N_2O 326.27 min *Control* 364.82 min	*Quality Score 2* Randomization not described Blinding not mentioned Withdrawals none in N₂O group Control group 3 patients withdrawn because of cesarean sections

Study	Objective	Participants	Intervention	Control gas	Stage	Results	Comments
Shao[17] 1994 China	Efficacy of N_2O for labor pain relief	250 healthy nulliparous. N_2O N = 115. Control N = 113	50%, (Entonox® cylinders), demand valve, self-administered, identical system for both groups, gas flow rate 4–7 L/min. Mask applied 30–45 s before contraction, intermittent inhalation during contraction for 3–5 breaths. No other analgesia mentioned	Compressed air	Stage 1 & 2	N_2O N = 113. Stage 1: 2.52 ± 1.38 h. Stage 2: 0.71 ± 0.43 h. Control N = 115. Stage 1: 2.99 ± 1.78 h. Stage 2: 2.0 ± 0.53 h	Quality Score 3. Randomization not described. Patient blinded, observer blinded? Withdrawals for cesarean sections 10 with N_2O 12 with control
Wang[18] 1994 China	Efficacy of N_2O for labor pain relief	84. N_2O N = 34. Control N = 50	30–50% N_2O in O_2 anesthesia circuit, flow rate 3–5 L/min demand valve. Mask applied 30–50 s before contraction. Intermittent inhalation during contraction for 3–5 breaths. No other analgesia mentioned	Not stated	Stage 1 & 2	N_2O N = 30. 8 h 49 m ± 3 h 15 m. Control N = 51. 9 h 3 m ± 2 h 51 m	Quality Score 4. Randomization not described. Blinding – unclear who was blinded. Withdrawals described
Carstoniu[19] 1994 Canada	Crossover	29. Nulliparous 14. Multiparous 12. Withdrawn 3	50% (Nitronox®), demand valve, inhalation when contraction first felt. Gas 1 × 5 contractions, then 5 more contractions with Gas 2. Group 1 = N_2O then air. Group 2 = air then N_2O. No washout period	Compressed air	Stage 1. Early labor. All types and presentations	10 contractions	Quality Score 5. Randomization using table. Double blinding (attempted but not effective in 21 of 29 patients). 3 withdrawals. 2 patients unable to give score after each contraction. 1 protocol violation

N_2O, nitrous oxide; O_2, oxygen.

Table 5.2 Analgesia outcomes: studies comparing nitrous oxide with oxygen or air.

Author Reference no. Date Country	Pain measurement	Analgesia outcome			Adverse effects		
Su[14] 2002 China	Combined scale, Patient (Mulleetr pain score) 4-point scale + Midwife 4-point scale Average score computed Categories well defined Score obtained at end of labor?	(a) Labor	N$_2$O (%)	Control (%)		N$_2$O (%)	Control (%)
		Excellent	7.4	0	(a) Nausea, vomiting	4.9	5.6
		Good	73.4	0.9	(b) Dizziness	39.4	0
		Fair	17.3	64.0	(c) Sleepiness	3.3	0
		Poor	8	35	(d) Perioral tingling	1.2	0
		(b) Episiotomy repair	N$_2$O (%)	Control (%)	(e) Throat irritation	1.2	0
					(f) Tachypnea	0.2	0
		Excellent	85.2	69.2	No difference in incidence of nausea and vomiting between groups (4.9% vs 5.6%, not statistically significant)		
		Good	14.8	7.5			
		Fair	17.3	23.4			
		Poor	0	0			
Zhang[15] 2001 China	Patient Verbal rating scale (VRS) 0 = no pain 1 = very little 2 = moderate 3 = severe 4 = extreme Frequency/time of pain scores not stated	VRS scores (%)	N$_2$O (%)	Control (%)	Nausea and vomiting observed in 0.5% of patients in treatment group when inhaling N$_2$O/O$_2$ mixture Resolved when gas discontinued		
		0	26.67	0			
		1	65.00	18.00			
		2	8.33	22.00			
		3	0	56.00			
		4	0	4.00			
Ou[16] 2001 China	Mulleetr pain score Obtained at end of labor		N$_2$O (%)	Control (%)	No side-effects observed in either group		
		Excellent	86	0			
		Good	11	0			
		Fair	3	76			
		Poor	0	24			
Shao[17] 2000 China	5-point categorical scale 0 = no pain 4 = severe, unable to bear Verbal report from patient	Category	N$_2$O (%)	Control (%)		N$_2$O (%)	Control (%)
		0	9.6	0	(a) Dizziness	6.4	0
		1	60	1.6	(b) Lethargic	5.6	0
		2	28	30.4	(c) Sleepiness	1.5	0
		3	2.4	56	All adverse reactions disappeared within 5 min after inhalation discontinued		
		4	0	12			
Wang[18] 1994 China	5-point categorical scale 0 = no pain 4 = severe, unable to bear Verbal report from patient	Category	N$_2$O (%)	Control (%)	1 patient (0.03%) vomited in the group receiving N$_2$O/O$_2$ Resolved after inhalation was discontinued		
		0	26.47	0			
		1	64.71	18			
		2	8.82	22			
		3	0	56			
		4	0	4			
Carstoniu[19] 1994 Canada	VAS 0 = no pain 10 = severe pain Score obtained after each contraction At end, patients asked to identify order of gases	VAS	Group 1	Group 2	None reported		
		Baseline	5.6 ± 2.1	4.9 ± 2.5			
		After 2 contractions	5.2 ± 2.2	5.8 ± 2.7			
		No significant difference in VAS scores between patients receiving N$_2$O or air for any contraction 21 patients could correctly identify the order of gases given					

N$_2$O, nitrous oxide; O$_2$, oxygen.

Table 5.3 Studies comparing different concentrations of nitrous oxide.

Author Reference no. Date Country	Study type	Number enrolled (Nulliparous/ multiparous)	% N$_2$O Mode of delivery Use of parenteral medication	Stage of labor Type of gestation	Duration of use	Quality score
Medical Research Council[20] 1970 UK	Multicentered Efficacy and safety of different concentrations of N$_2$O/O$_2$	506 Mixed parity *N$_2$O 50%* N = 259 *N$_2$O 70%* N = 247	50%, 70% N$_2$O with O$_2$, demand valve Time inhalation begun in relation to contraction onset not specified Use of opioids and tranquilizers permitted and recorded by midwife Both groups showed similar percentage of other drug given	Stage 1 & 2 Singleton, normal labors	Not stated	*Quality score 4* Random allocation to one of two groups – method chosen by site Midwife and patient blinded Exclusions/ withdrawals described (799 enrolled, 506 analyzed)
McAneny[21] 1963 UK	Efficacy and safety of different concentrations of N$_2$O	501 Nulliparous: 342 Multiparous: 159	50%, 60%, 70%, 75%, 80% N$_2$O with O$_2$ demand valve, Lucy Baldwin machine, modified for on-line gases Time inhalation begun in relation to contraction onset not specified Parenteral opioids and tranquilizers were given at the discretion of midwife	End of stage 1 & stage 2	Not stated	*Quality score 3* Randomized by changing concentration every few days by author Midwife, patient and observer blinded Exclusions described. No withdrawals mentioned

N$_2$O, nitrous oxide; O$_2$, oxygen.

Dose–response studies

Two large RCTs measured the analgesic efficacy of different concentrations of nitrous oxide in oxygen. Study characteristics are shown in Table 5.3 and results in Table 5.4. A large Medical Research Council study from the UK[20] compared 50% with 70% nitrous oxide using a four-category pain scale. No difference in scores was found between the two groups; 84% reported satisfaction with pain relief in both groups. A second RCT[21] compared the pain relief from concentrations of 50%, 60%, 70%, 75% and 80% near the end of first stage and in the second stage. Pain relief was assessed using a four-category scale. The dose–response is shown in Fig. 5.1. The number of women who reported considerable or complete pain relief increased from 52% in the 50% nitrous oxide group to 74% with 70%

nitrous oxide. There was no further increase with higher concentrations of nitrous oxide.

Side-effects were reported in both studies and are shown in Table 5.4. In the first study,[20] the incidence of nausea and vomiting reported by midwives was 5% and 9% at both concentrations. The mothers reported higher rates for nausea (22% vs 16%) and vomiting (18% vs 14%) at 50% compared with 70% concentration, but the difference was not statistically significant. Similarly, there was no significant difference in rates of somnolence (21–16%). Discontinuation of nitrous oxide resulting from loss of consciousness or inability to cooperate was small but significantly higher in the 70% group (one patient vs seven patients). Hazy memory of labor was reported by approximately 36% in both groups, while hazy

Table 5.4 Analgesic outcomes of studies comparing different concentrations of nitrous oxide.

Author Reference no. Date Country	Pain measurement	Analgesia outcome	Adverse effects
Medical Research Council[20] 1970 UK	*Patient* Questionnaire with 9 questions Postpartum day 3 *Midwife* 4-point scale soon after delivery	1. No difference in maternal pain scores between 50% & 70% groups 2. Satisfied with pain relief 84%, both groups 3. Helped *considerably or completely* more than 70% both groups. Small differences among groups, statistically significant ($P < 0.02$) but not clinically significant 4. 84% both groups satisfied with amount of pain relief	*Midwives report* (soon after delivery) *% N_2O inhalation* *50% 70%* (a) Nausea 9.1 9.4 (b) Vomiting 5.5 6.1 (c) Co-operation Stg 1 9.4 26.2 Fair or poor Stg 2 21.6 24.6 (d) Unconscious 0.4 3.0 (e) Restless/noisy 15.4 18.7 (f) Inhalation discontinued 5.5 10.5 *Mothers' answers* (obtained on 3rd postpartum day) (%) (g) Fell asleep during contractions 16.6 21.7 (h) Hazy memory of labor 18.4 35.1 (i) Did not remember baby being born 18.4 15.0 (j) Had dreams 12.5 10.0 (k) Dreams unpleasant 45.2 6.9 (l) Felt sick 21.2 16.7 (m) Vomited 18.0 14.0 (l) Other sensations 14.8 11.4
McAneny[21] 1963 UK	*Patient* Questionnaire completed in interview 24–48 h postpartum Analgesia assessed using 4-point categorical scale *Midwife* 3-point scale soon after delivery	1. 40% said pain worse than expected at all concentrations 2. *N_2O concentration 50–75%* > 80% of patients would have same analgesia again *N_2O concentration 80%* 75.5% of patients would have same analgesia again 3. Degree of pain relief obtained: *considerable or complete* |	All labors (%)	Primip (%)	Multip (%)
N_2O 50% group	52	51	55
N_2O 60% group	64	71	52
N_2O 70% group	74	71	82
N_2O 75% group	76	79	71
N_2O 80% group	74	73	74	 *Nulliparous* Pain relief considerable or complete significantly higher in 60% N_2O group as compared with 50% N_2O group $P < 0.02$ *Multiparous* Pain relief considerable or complete significantly higher in 70% N_2O group as compared with 50% N_2O group Ceiling effect reached at 70% N_2O No analgesic advantage demonstrated at higher concentrations	*% Inhaled N_2O* 50 60 70 75 80 % Hazy or no memory of labor 43 53 57 53 49 % Hazy or no memory of birth 15 25 26 31 26 % Falling asleep 16 31 33 31 31 % Dreaming 8 12 18 21 26 % Nausea and vomiting 16 15 22 22 18.5 1. Significantly more amnesia for labor and birth in patients that received 70% N_2O or more 2. Significantly less somnolence with 50% N_2O ($P < 0.02$) 3. Increased dreams (including bad dreams with 80% N_2O compared with 50%) 4. Approximately 20% incidence of nausea and vomiting – less with 50% N_2O compared with other concentrations ($P < 0.02$)

N_2O, nitrous oxide.

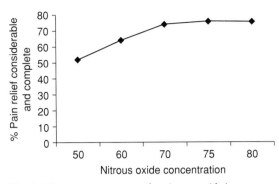

Fig. 5.1 Dose–response curve for nitrous oxide in oxygen. The concentration of nitrous oxide is on the x axis, and the number of patients (in percent) who experienced considerable or complete analgesia is on the y axis.[21]

memory of delivery in both groups was reported in approximately 17%.

The second study[21] reported an approximate 20% incidence of nausea and vomiting with no significant difference between concentration groups. The incidence of somnolence was significantly less at 50% (16%) compared with higher concentrations (31–33%). The incidence of "hazy or no memory" of labor showed a dose–response relationship. Nitrous oxide 50%, 60% and 70% produced a 43%, 53% and 57% incidence of impaired memory, respectively.

Nitrous oxide versus other inhalational agents

Eleven RCTs compared nitrous oxide with another inhalational agent. The study characteristics are shown in Table 5.5 and the results in Table 5.6. Five were crossover studies in the first stage of labor; four[22,23,26,31] compared nitrous oxide with another agent (isoflurane + Entonox®, isoflurane, enflurane, methoxyflurane, desflurane) and were limited to 3–5 contractions per agent. Three studies determined that the other agent provided better analgesia (Arora et al.[22] N = 41, McLeod et al.[23] N = 32, McGuiness & Rosen[26] N = 20) and in one there was no difference (Bergsjø[31] N = 63). All reported some analgesia with nitrous oxide alone. One study, Wee et al.[24] (N = 18), compared Entonox® with Entonox® with 0.2% isoflurane. In this study, patients were randomly assigned to one of the two groups and then crossed over at 1 and 3 h. There was no wash-out period. Baseline pain scores were similar

for both groups and subsequent measurement showed lower pain scores in both groups. Entonox® with isoflurane inhalation produced significantly lower pain scores than Entonox® alone.

Two RCTs compared nitrous oxide with a second agent in the second stage: nitrous oxide 30–50% compared with desflurane 1–4.5% by continuous administration (Abboud et al.[25] N = 80) and nitrous oxide 30–60% compared with enflurane 0.25–1.25% by continuous administration (Abboud et al.[27] N = 105). The duration of both studies was 10–20 min. Good to excellent analgesia was reported by more than 75% of patients in the desflurane study for both agents and in the enflurane study by 63% with higher ratings for enflurane (P < 0.02). A third RCT compared nitrous oxide with 3–5% cyclopropane given in continuous administration during the second and third stage of labor.[32] Patients reported good to excellent analgesia in 61% of both treatment groups.

Two RCTs (Jones et al.[28,29] N = 48, N = 50) compared nitrous oxide with methoxyflurane; one study by continuous administration and the other by self-administration using a demand valve, for first and second stage. Pain ratings of complete or considerable pain relief were obtained in 76% of patients given nitrous oxide and in 79% given methoxyflurane by continuous administration. Similar rating of 80% and 84%, respectively, were obtained in the second study with self-administration and intermittent inhalation.

One large multicentered clinical trial, which assigned the groups using a quasi-randomization scheme, compared the effectiveness of methoxyflurane with either trichloroethylene or nitrous oxide by intermittent inhalation. Ratings of considerable or complete pain relief measured 15 min after delivery were reported by 70% of patients receiving all three agents.

Side-effects mentioned in this group of studies varied as did the sample size and study design. However, nausea, dizziness and drowsiness were the most frequently reported. In general, the addition of a potent inhalational agent such as enflurane or desflurane increased the incidence of dizziness and drowsiness. The incidence of nausea and vomiting was variable but the addition of an inhalation agent to nitrous oxide did not change incidence. Amnesia for delivery was reported in three small studies.[25,27,29] In one study, the incidence was 25% with desflurane with none reported for nitrous oxide alone.

Table 5.5 Studies comparing nitrous oxide with other inhalational agents.

Author Reference no. Date Country	Study type	Number enrolled (parity)	% N$_2$O Delivery system Use of parenteral medication	Compared with	Stage of labor Type of gestation Presentation	Duration of use	Quality score
Arora[22] 1992 UK	Crossover Study	41 Nulliparous 23 Multiparous 16	50% N$_2$O (Entonox®) Demand valve, draw over vaporizer with switch in circuit for delivery of isoflurane Calibration with Datex Agent Analyzer Mixture 1 × 5 contractions Room air × 1 contraction Mixture 2 × 5 contractions	Isoflurane 0.25% in Entonox®	Stage 1	11 contractions	*Quality score 4* Randomized using table Double blind? patient and investigator except for smell of isoflurane Withdrawals described (2)
McLeod[23] 1985 UK	Crossover study Comparison of N$_2$O with isoflurane	32 Mixed parity	50% N$_2$O (Entonox®), demand valve Continuous inhalation during contractions × 5 contractions Washout period × 2 contractions, then inhalation during contractions with other gas Inhalation start related to onset of contraction not mentioned No other sedatives or analgesics	Isoflurane 0.75%	Stage 1	12 contractions	*Quality score 2* Randomization not described Single blind Withdrawal/exclusions described (1)
Wee[24] 1993 UK	Crossover study Comparison of analgesic efficacy of N$_2$O with a mixture of N$_2$O/ isoflurane	18 Nulliparous 6 Multiparous 11	50% N$_2$O (Entonox®), demand valve *Group 1* Entonox® × 1 h, Entonox® + Isoflurane 2% × 1 h, Entonox® × 1 h (EIE) *Group 2* Entonox® + Isoflurane 2% × 1 h Entonox® × 1 h, Entonox® + Isoflurane 2% × 1 h (IEI) No other analgesics given Calibration with Datex Agent Analyzer	Entonox® + Isoflurane 0.2%	Stage 1	3 h	*Quality score 2* Randomization not described Blinding not mentioned Withdrawal described (1)

Study	Aim/design	N/parity	Intervention	Comparison	Stage	Duration/result	Quality
Abboud[25] 1995 USA	No crossover Analgesic effect of subanesthetic doses of desflurane	80 N₂O = 40 Nulliparous 13 Multiparous 27 Desflurane 40 Nulliparous 12 Multiparous 28	N₂O 30–50% in O₂ (usual 46%) Continuous administration by anesthesiologist; circle absorber system Concentration adjusted to provide "optimal analgesia" ?% Concentrations obtained from flowmeters and vaporizer Use of analgesics or sedatives not stated	Desflurane/O₂ 1–4.5% (usual 2%)	Stage 2	N₂O 10.1 ± 7.0 min Desflurane 11.8 ± 7.0 min	Quality score 3 Randomization using table Patient and obstetrician blinded No withdrawals
McGuiness[26] 1984 UK	Crossover Effectiveness of enflurane as an analgesic compared with N₂O	20 Mixed parity	N₂O 50% (Entonox®), demand valve Gases delivered by same tubing and mouthpiece Operator blinded to agent One agent inhaled for 3 consecutive contractions followed by the second agent for 3 contractions No washout period	Enflurane 1% in air	Stage 1	6 contractions	Quality score 3 Method of randomization not described Double blind No withdrawals
Abboud[27] 1981 US	Investigation of subanalgesic concentrations of enflurane as an analgesic	105 N₂O = 50 Nulliparous 19 Multiparous 31 Enflurane = 55 Nulliparous 28 Multiparous 27	N₂O 30–60% in O₂ (usual 52%) Continuous administration until delivery; circle absorber system Concentration adjusted by anesthesiologist to provide "optimal analgesia while keeping the patient awake" % Concentrations obtained from flowmeters and vaporizer 40% in each group received narcotics 50% received local for perineal analgesia for delivery	Enflurane/O₂ 0.25–1.25% usual dose 0.50%	Stage 2	11–20 min no significant difference in mean duration for each group	Quality score 2 Method of randomization not described Patient and obstetrician blinded No withdrawals

Continued

Table 5.5 (*continued*)

Author Reference no. Date Country	Study type	Number enrolled (parity)	% N$_2$O Delivery system Use of parenteral medication	Compared with	Stage of labor Type of gestation Presentation	Duration of use	Quality score
Jones[28] 1969 UK	Comparison of MOF with N$_2$O by *continuous administration*	48 *N$_2$O = 24* Nulliparous 11 Multiparous 13 *MOF = 24* Nulliparous 11 Multiparous 13	N$_2$O/O$_2$ Continuous administration Magill circuit at 40 L/min Concentration adjusted by anesthesiologist to maintain response to contraction % N$_2$O titrated in 5% increments: mean concentration 41.2% Meperidine less than 4 h before N$_2$O = 11, MOF = 14	MOF Venturi system run on 40% O$_2$ at 30 L/min MOF titrated 0.05% steps median concentration 0.22%	Stage 1 & 2 Normal deliveries	*Total* N$_2$O 83 ± 66.3 min MOF 82.5 ± 72.8 min *Stage 2* N$_2$O 32.0 ± 23.4 min MOF 36.7 ± 25.3 min Times comparable in each group	*Quality score 2* Randomization not described Midwife and patient blinded (? odor of MOF) No withdrawals
Jones[29] 1969 UK	Comparison of MOF and N$_2$O by self-administered *intermittent inhalation*	50 *N$_2$O = 25* Nulliparous 11 Multiparous 14 *MOF = 25* Nulliparous 9 Multiparous 16	N$_2$O 50% (Entonox®) Intermittent demand valve Instructed to breath during contraction *Meperidine* N$_2$O N = 16 MOF N = 17	MOF 0.35% Mask and handset same as N$_2$O	Stage 1 & 2 Normal deliveries	*Total* N$_2$O 66.1 ± 39.2 min *MOF* 90.1 ± 67.5 min	*Quality score 3* Randomization not described Midwife and patient blinded Anesthetists not blinded No withdrawals

Study	Design/objective	N/Parity	Intervention	Comparator	Stage	Duration	Quality
Rosen[30] 1969 UK	8 centers. Randomized by day of the week to either MOF or midwives choice of N_2O or TCE. On Sundays midwives agent of choice. Effectiveness of MOF compared with TCE or N_2O	1257 Nulliparous 554 Multiparous 703 *MOF* N = 598 *TCE* N = 394 *N_2O* N = 265 Number multiparous in N_2O group less $P < 0.02$	N_2O 50% (Entonox®) demand valve TCE 0.35% & 0.50% in air, drawover vaporizer Administration during contractions Meperidine and other drugs permitted %/group who received parenteral meds *MOF group* 60% *TCE group* 62% *N_2O group* 37%	MOF 0.35% in air, drawover vaporizer	Stage 1 & 2 All deliveries	Mean duration of use (min) MOF 91.19 N_2O 103.14 TCE 97.15 Range 0–4 h	*Quality score 0* Randomized by day of week Not double blind Exclusions/withdrawals not described
Bergsjo[31] 1971 Norway	Crossover sequential analysis Comparison of analgesia between MOF and N_2O	63 Nulliparous 39 Multiparous 24	N_2O 50%: Entonox® or preset regulator system, demand valve, face mask Inhalation started "as soon as contraction felt but before pain developed" Agent 1 × 3 contractions then 1 contraction on room air followed by 3 contractions with agent 2 4 patients omitted washout contraction 9 patients took agent for 2 or 4 contractions Diazepam and meperidine used before trial "as necessary"	MOF (0.5–0.8%) delivered by mouthpiece Drawover vaporizer	Stage 1 All patients	7 contractions	*Quality score 3* Random number table used to determine order of drug for each patient Physician and patient blinded(?) (smell of MOF mentioned, apparatus different) Exclusions described
Shnider[32] 1963 USA	To compare cyclopropane with N_2O analgesia for labor and delivery	718 Mixed parity Cyclopropane = 319 N_2O = 382	40% N_2O semi-closed circle absorbed system by continuous administration Approximately 80% of mothers both groups received premedication 75% of mothers received either pudendal block or local infiltration with 1% lidocaine	Cyclopropane in O_2 3–5% by continuous administration Concentration titrated to maintain patient oriented and conversant	Stage 2 & 3 All vaginal deliveries	Stage 2 89% < 15 min	*Quality score 3* Randomized – method not described Blinded? Withdrawals described N_2O – 4 (1%) Cyclopropane – 13 (4%)

MOF, methoxyflurane; N_2O, nitrous oxide; O_2, oxygen; TCE, trichloroethylene.

Table 5.6 Analgesia outcomes for studies comparing nitrous oxide with other inhalational agents.

Author Reference no. Date Country	Comparison agent	Pain measurement	Analgesia outcome	Adverse effects
Arora[22] 1992 UK	Isoflurane	Linear analog scale (10 cm) 0 = severe pain, 10 = no pain. Measured after each set of 5 contractions	*Mean/median pain score* Entonox® alone 5.8 ± 1.5/5.0. Isoflurane 0.25% + Entonox® 7.0 + 1.5/7.0. Order of agent did not affect pain scores. Isoflurane/Entonox® mixture provided significantly more pain relief than Entonox® alone ($P = 0.001$). Wilcoxon Ranked Sum Test for paired samples	*Dizziness* Both both agents 5/41. Entonox® + Isoflurane 4/41. Entonox® 1/41. *Sedation* 5 subjects increased sedation by 1 level (4-point scale) after completing both inhalations. No patient became unresponsive
McLeod[23] 1985 UK	Isoflurane	Linear analog score 0–100. 0 = no pain. Baseline and after each contraction	1. Baseline scores range 44–99, most common 60–80, mean 75.4. 2. N_2O scores range 24–92, most common 60–80, mean 63.0. 3. Isoflurane 0.75% scores, range 19–86 most common 20–40, mean 46. Pain scores recorded for Isoflurane were significantly lower that those recorded for Entonox® ($P < 0.001$)	*Drowsiness* 58% had higher scores for drowsiness with isoflurane, 32% has equal drowsiness with both agents. 10% had more drowsiness with Entonox®. No patient became unresponsive. *Other* Nausea 3%, dizziness 2%
Wee[24] 1993 UK	Isoflurane	Visual analog pain score 0–200 mm. Baseline and at 20-min intervals, measurement just after a contraction	Group 1/group 2 no significant difference in baseline pain scores. Subsequent lower pain scores in both groups. Significantly lower pain scores with Isoflurane/Entonox® mixture in both groups ($P < 0.001$)	*Drowsiness* No significant difference between two groups end of 1st hour. Significant increases in drowsiness between hour 1 & 2 and between hour 2 & 3 ($P = 0.004$). Higher score for Isoflurane/Entonox® mixture. All subjects remained alert. *Amnesia* None reported
Abboud[25] 1995 USA	Desflurane	*Patient* 5-point categorical scale 0 = no pain relief. *Anesthesiologist & obstetrician* 5-point categorical scale	1. Mothers: analgesia scores: (3+,4+) 63% in each group. 2. Obstetricians: 55% N_2O/50% Desflurane. 3. Anesthesiologists: 63% N_2O/58% Desflurane no difference in analgesia outcomes at $P < 0.05$	*Breathholding* 2/40 in Desflurane group. *Amnesia for delivery* 9/40 in Desflurane group. None in N_2O group

Study	Agent	Measurement	Results	Side effects
McGuiness[26] 1984 UK	Enflurane	Linear analog scores 0–100 0 = No pain Scores obtained before and after use of each agent Analgesic given after score > 40 reported	1. N₂O (Entonox®) scores: Range 29–79, most common scores 40–60, median 52 2. Enflurane scores: Range: 13–79, most common scores 20–40, median 50 3. Scores no analgesic used: Range 47–87, median 61 Comparative effect: Enflurane > N₂O > none $P < 0.02$	*Drowsiness* Significantly higher drowsiness scores for Enflurane ($P < 0.02$) No mother became unresponsive *Nausea* Enflurane 3/20 Entonox® 1/20
Abboud[27] 1981 USA	Enflurane	*Patient* 5-point categorical scale 0 = no pain relief 4 = no pain *Anesthesiologist & obstetrician* Same 5-point categorical scale	Analgesia scores (3 or 4) 　　　　　　　Enflurane (%)　N₂O (%) Mother　　　　　89　　　　76 Anesthesiologist　80　　　　70 Obstetrician　　　84　　　　68 Obstetrician score significantly lower $P = 0.05$ Would patient have same agent again? Yes Enflurane/N₂O (98%/86%) $P < 0.02$	*Amnesia for delivery* Enflurane group　7% N₂O group　　10% 1 patient became agitated and vomited
Jones[28] 1969 UK	Methoxyflurane	*Patient* Interview at 15 min & 36–48 h after delivery 4-point categorical scale *Midwife* 4-point categorical scale *Anesthesiologist* Satisfactory/unsatisfactory	*Mother immediate*　　　　　　N₂O (%)　MOF (%) Pain relief complete　　　　　18　　　29 Pain relief considerable　　　68　　　50 Not different ($P > 0.2$) *Midwife* Pain relief complete　　　　　9　　　38 Pain relief considerable　　　65　　　83 MOF better ($P = >0.2$) *Anesthesiologist* mean % time satisfactory: N₂O/MOF: 77.2 ± 14.7/81.4 ± 22.3% not significant ($P = > 0.2$) *Mother at 48 h* Pain relief complete or considerable. N₂O/MOF = 83%/92%	*Nausea during labor* 8% of each group reported nausea during labor *Nausea in first 24 h* 54% of N₂O group 21% of MOF group significant ($P < 0.05$) *Vomiting* 25% of N₂O group 17% of MOF group *Sleepiness during labor* 33% in N₂O group, 22% dreamed, 2 reported nightmares. 41% in MOF group 17% dreamed

Continued

Table 5.6 (continued)

Author Reference no. Date Country	Comparison agent	Pain measurement	Analgesia outcome	Adverse effects
Jones[29] 1969 UK	Methoxyflurane	*Patient* Interview 15 min & 36– 48 h after delivery 4-point categorical scale *Midwife* 4-point categorical scale *Anesthesiologist* Satisfactory/unsatisfactory	*Mother immediate* N_2O (%) MOF (%) Pain relief complete 16 28 Pain relief considerable 64 56 *Midwife* Pain relief complete 8 16 Pain relief considerable 72 84 $P > 0.03$ *Anesthesiologist* Satisfactory: N_2O/MOF $62.3 \pm 29.9/79.3 \pm 20\%$ Mothers at 48 h 18% changed opinion. Slightly more in favor of MOF	*Nausea and vomiting* *Immediate interview:* N_2O group: 32% nauseated and 8% vomited MOF group 0 Significant $(P < 0.01)$ *Later interview:* N_2O group: 32% reported nausea and vomiting MOF group 16% reported nausea and vomiting Statistically significant *Memory of labor & delivery* Remembered clearly 68% both groups. 68% in MOF group remembered delivery clearly, compared with 40% in N_2O group Statistically significant *Dreams* N_2O group, 24%. MOF group 16%
Rosen[30] 1969 UK	Methoxyflurane with TCE or N_2O	*Patient* Interview 15 min & 36– 48 h after delivery 4-point categorical scale *Midwife* 4-point categorical scale *Anesthesiologist* Satisfactory/unsatisfactory	Mothers at 15 min MOF (%) TCE (%) N_2O (%) Complete 11.5 12 11 Considerable 59 60 61 Slight 26 25 25 None 3.5 3 3 Overall conclusion MOF, a better obstetric analgesic than TCE	*Nausea and vomiting* No significant difference between groups: Incidence of nausea 20%, vomiting 7% *Restlessness* "Slightly more" restlessness in patients receiving MOF if meperidine had also been given. Inhalation abandoned in significantly fewer cases using N_2O
Bergsjo[31] 1971 Norway	Methoxyflurane	*Patient* After 7th contraction patient asked which drug was better. If no answer, asked to say which one she would choose *Physician* 4-point scale: excellent/ good/moderate/poor	Both drugs gave excellent or good analgesia in 92% Significant preference for N_2O $(0.1 < P < 0.05)$. 33 out of 40 patients continued to use N_2O 18 out of 20 patients continued to use MOF *Physician* Degree of analgesia good or excellent in 92% or all cases. Distribution not related to preference of patient	N_2O group MOF group (%) (%) Nausea 6.5 3.1 Dizziness 17 17 Dry mouth 9.5 0 Bad taste/Smell 0 14 Numbness 1.6 0 No side-effects 67 70
Shnider[32] 1963 USA	Cyclopropane	*5-category score* (observer) 4 = excellent 3 = good 2 = fair 1 = poor 0 = no pain relief	Category Cyclopropane (%) N_2O (%) 4 29.5 16.5 3 31.7 45.3 2 28.5 28.0 0 & 1 6.3 9.2 Good to excellent analgesia in 61% of both groups	Nausea and vomiting rare No other statements on adverse effects made

MOF, methoxyflurane; N_2O, nitrous oxide; TCE, trichloroethylene.

In a second study, the incidence was reported as 7% with enflurane and 10% with nitrous oxide alone. A third study using methoxyflurane reported a higher incidence of amnesia for delivery in the group receiving nitrous oxide alone (Table 5.6).

Discussion

Nitrous oxide clearly has an analgesic effect for relief of labor pain when compared with inhalation of oxygen or air. The effect was measured, in all but one study,[19] with nitrous oxide used from the first stage of labor until delivery. While complete analgesia was not reported, a marked improvement in pain assessments was obtained from the majority receiving nitrous oxide. Recent studies, which would not be feasible in settings where alternative modalities of analgesia are available, were carried out in China in large regional hospitals where previously there was no expectation of analgesia for labor.

The only RCT that did not report any analgesic effect of nitrous oxide compared with compressed air was a short study in early first stage.[19] While this study received the highest quality score and represents the strongest study design, problems include a small sample size (N = 29), measurements obtained over 10 contractions in early first stage with relatively low baseline pain scores, and timing of inhalation at the onset of the contraction (a peak analgesic effect may not have been attained). Further, there was no washout period in the crossover between gases. These features of the study design may have precluded the measurement of important differences. Alternately, the Chinese studies[14–18] may have overestimated analgesic effect, although there is no reason to expect this type of bias from the study design. Two of these studies (N = 1500)[14,16] reported high scores used a combined scoring system (Mulleetr's score) with midwife and patient scores averaged; all studies measured analgesia at a single point only, after delivery.

Two RCTs with large enrollments differed in their estimation of analgesic effect although this was not the primary purpose of either study. The first study,[21] measuring analgesia outcomes at 24–48 h after delivery, compared five concentrations of nitrous oxide (50%, 60%, 70%, 75% and 80%). There was a dose–response effect with a ceiling effect at 70% (Fig. 5.1). In contrast, a multicenter study conducted by the

Medical Research Council in the UK[20] comparing 50% with 70% nitrous oxide, found a majority (75%) rated their pain relief as considerable or complete with no significant difference in efficacy between groups. In both studies, pain measurements were obtained using a questionnaire. In the study by McAneny & Doughty[21] responses were obtained within 24–48 h after delivery, while in the Medical Research Council study[20] responses were obtained on the third postpartum day, which may have resulted in attenuation of memory of pain. Both studies report an analgesia effect for inhaled nitrous oxide. McAneny & Doughty[21] studied more concentration points and separated data by parity. The demonstration of increasing efficacy with increasing concentration of inhaled nitrous oxide is evidence that nitrous oxide provided pain relief.

Most RCTs that compare nitrous oxide alone with another inhalational agent or nitrous oxide with a mixture of nitrous oxide and second agent measured an analgesic effect in addition to nitrous oxide. Of four reports of short exposure with crossover in the first stage of labor,[22,23,26,31] three measured improved analgesia with an inhalational agent combined with nitrous oxide compared with nitrous oxide alone. In the two RCTs that studied the second stage of labor,[24,32] nitrous oxide compared favorably with desflurane and cyclopropane. Neither agent was found to provide better analgesia than nitrous oxide. A third study, in the second stage of labor, reported that enflurane[27] provided better analgesia than 50% nitrous oxide. Methoxyflurane was found to provide slightly better analgesia than nitrous oxide throughout first and second stage of labor in two RCTs. A third large trial[30] in which analgesia was not the primary outcome reported good analgesia in a majority of subjects with methoxyflurane, trichloroethylene or nitrous oxide. All studies in this group reported some analgesic effect for nitrous oxide.

In reviewing the reported side-effects from all three groupings of RCTs, the most frequently reported are nausea and vomiting, somnolence, dizziness and amnesia. Of these, somnolence, dizziness and amnesia appear to be related to nitrous oxide or inhalational agent use and may be concentration-dependent. Reports of study withdrawals because of intolerance to a side-effect were very few, with somnolence the most common reason. In a large placebo-controlled study,[14] the incidence of nausea and vomiting with nitrous oxide compared with control groups was found to be similar (5%). Rates of up to 20% were reported in the two large dose–response studies[20,21] but no dose-related effect was found. Nitrous oxide likely does not further contribute to the nausea and vomiting associated with labor.

Rosen,[9] in his recent review, has summarized the adverse effects of nitrous oxide. Nitrous oxide use in labor does not appear to alter the force of uterine contractions or the progress of labor. While nitrous oxide is rapidly equilibrated across the placenta, it also is rapidly eliminated once the newborn starts breathing. Adverse neonatal outcomes associated with the use of nitrous oxide have not been demonstrated. Minimum maternal oxygen saturation with nitrous oxide use does not differ significantly from controls. Nitrous oxide has minimal cardiovascular or respiratory depressant effects. The greatest maternal risk is loss of consciousness and loss of protective airway reflexes. A MAC awake for nitrous oxide in pregnant women has been estimated at 50%. Although loss of consciousness at this concentration is rare, self-administration of 50% nitrous oxide with the use of a demand valve appears to be safe. Nitrous oxide should be used with scavenging in well-ventilated rooms to minimize occupational exposure to healthcare workers.

Conclusions

Self-administered nitrous oxide inhalation is a simple, safe and inexpensive form of pain relief in labor which does not require physician supervision and is acceptable to patients. The findings of most of the RCTs in this review showed that inhaled nitrous oxide has analgesic efficacy for relief of labor pain. The addition of other inhalational agents to inhaled nitrous oxide and the use of more than 50% nitrous oxide may improve efficacy but increases somnolence and theoretical risk of aspiration. The variety of measures and study designs used presents difficulty in arriving at a precise evaluation of the efficacy of nitrous oxide as a labor analgesic. However, efficacy reported ranged from 55% to more than 90% of patients. Further, an RCT[21] measuring efficacy over a range of concentrations obtained data that demonstrated a dose–response with a maximum effect at a concentration of approximately 70%.

Is nitrous oxide an effective analgesic for labor? The evidence obtained from this systematic review would suggest that inhaled nitrous oxide relieves labor pain to a significant degree in most patients but does not provide complete analgesia for many. It is especially useful in practice settings where other modalities of labor analgesia are unavailable.

Acknowledgments

We are grateful to Dr Margaret Lin, Xiaodong Li and Leiming Xu for their expert translation of the articles in Chinese.

References

1 Klikowitsch S. Über das Stickstoffoxydul als Anaesthetikum bei Geburten. *Arch Gynaekol* 1881;**18**:81–108.

2 Marx GF, Katsnelson T. The introduction of nitrous oxide analgesia into obstetrics. *Obstet Gynecol* 1992;**80**:715–8.

3 Minnitt RJ. Self-administered analgesia for the midwifery of general practice. *Proc R Soc* 1934;**27**:1313–8.

4 Cole PV, Nainby-Luxmore RC. The hazards of gas and air in obstetrics. *Anaesthesia* 1962;**17**:505–18.

5 Tunstall ME. Use of fixed nitrous oxide and oxygen from one cylinder. *Lancet* 1961;**2**:964.

6 Guo TZ, Poree L, Golden W, Stein, J, Fujinaga M, Maze M. Antinociceptive response to nitrous oxide is mediated by supraspinal opiate and spinal α_2-adrenergic receptors in the rat. *Anesthesiology* 1996;**85**:846–52.

7 Chousheng Z, Davies MF, Guo TZ, Maze M. The analgesic action of nitrous oxide dependent on the release of norepinephrine in the dorsal horn of the spinal cord. *Anesthesiology* 1999;**91**:1401–7.

8 Soyannwo OA. Self-administered Entonox® (50% nitrous oxide in oxygen) in labour: report of the experience in Ibadan. *African J Med Med Sci* 1985;**14**:95–8.

9 Rosen MA. Nitrous oxide for relief of labor pain: a systematic review. *Am J Obstet Gynecol* 2002;**186**:S110–30.

10 Holdcroft A, Morgan M. An assessment of the analgesic effect in labour of pethidine and 50% nitrous oxide in oxygen (Entonox®). *J Obstet Gynaecol Br Comm* 1974;**81**:603–7.

11 Harrison RF, Shore M, Woods T, Mathews G, Gardiner J, Unwin A. A comparative study of transcutaneous electrical nerve stimulation (TENS), Entonox®, pethidine + promazine and lumbar epidural for pain relief in labor. *Acta Obstet Gynaecol Scand* 1987;**66**:9–14.

12 Chia YT, Arulkumaran S, Chua S, Ratnam SS. Effectiveness of transcutaneous electric nerve stimulator for pain relief in labour. *Asia-Oceania J Obstet Gynaecol* 1990;**16**:145–51.

13 Jadad AR, Moore RA, Carroll D, *et al.* Assessing the quality of reports of randomized clinical trials: is blinding necessary? *Control Clin Trials* 1996;**17**:1–12.

14 Su F, Wei X, Chen X, Hu Z, Xu H. Clinical study on efficacy and safety of labor analgesia with inhalation of nitrous oxide in oxygen. *Chin J Obstet Gynecol* 2002;**37**:584–7.

15 Zhang X. Inhalation of nitrous oxide for labor analgesia and its effects on mothers and infants. *J Henan Med Univ* 2001;**36**:7–9.

16 Ou X, Li B, Du H. Clinical study: the effects of inhaling nitrous oxide for analgesia labor on pregnant women and fetus. *Chin J Obstet Gynecol* 2001;**36**:399–401.

17 Shao HJ, Lu X, Cheng W. Clinical study on analgesic labor with inhaling laughing gas. *Chin J Pract Gynecol Obstet* 2000;**16**:83–5.

18 Wang B, Zhang X, Wei L. Application of nitrous oxide in labor analgesia. *Chin J Obstet Gynecol* 1994;**29**:330–1.

19 Carstoniu J, Levytam S, Norman P, Daley D, Katz J, Sandler AN. Nitrous oxide in early labor: safety and analgesic efficacy assessed by a double-blind, placebo-controlled study. *Anesthesiology* 1994;**80**:30–5.

20 Council of the Committee on Nitrous Oxide and Oxygen Analgesia in Midwifery. Clinical trials of different concentrations of oxygen and nitrous oxide for obstetric analgesia. *BMJ* 1970;**1**:709–13.

21 McAneny TM, Doughty AG. Self-administered nitrous oxide/oxygen analgesia in obstetrics. *Anaesthesia* 1963;**18**:488–97.

22 Arora S, Tunstall M, Ross J. Self-administered mixture of Entonox® and isoflurane in labor. *Int J Obstet Anesth* 1992;**1**:119–202.

23 McLeod DD, Ramayya GP, Tunstall ME. Self-administered isoflurane in labour. *Anaesthesia* 1985;**40**:424–6.

24 Wee MYK, Hasan MA, Thomas TA. Isoflurane in labour. *Anaesthesia* 1993;**48**:369–72.

25 Abboud TK, Swart F, Zhu J, Donovan MM, Peres DS, Yakal K. Desflurane analgesia for vaginal delivery. *Acta Anaesthesiol Scand* 1995;**39**:259–61.

26 McGuinness C, Rosen M. Enflurane as an analgesic in labour. *Anaesthesia* 1984;**39**:24–6.

27 Abboud TK, Shnider SM, Wright RG, *et al.* The use of enflurane in obstetrics. *Anesth Analg* 1981;**80**:133–7.

28 Jones PL, Rosen M, Mushin WW, Jones EV. Methoxyflurane and nitrous oxide as obstetric analgesics. I. A comparison by continuous administration. *BMJ* 1969;**3**:255–9.

29 Jones PL, Rosen M, Mushin WW, Jones EV. Methoxyflurane and nitrous oxide as obstetric analgesics II. A comparison by self-administered inhalation. *BMJ* 1969;**3**:259–62.

30 Rosen M, Mushin WW, Jones PL, Jones EV. Field trial of methoxyflurane, nitrous oxide and trichloroethylene as obstetric analgesics. *BMJ* 1969;**3**:263–7.

31 Bergsjø P. Comparison between nitrous oxide and methoxyflurane for obstetrical analgesia. *Acta Obstet Gynaecol Scand* 1971;**50**:285–90.

32 Shnider SM, Moya F, Thorndike V, Bossers A, Morishima H, James LS. Clinical and biochemical studies of cyclopropane analgesia in obstetrics. *Anesthesiology* 1963;**24**:11–7.

CHAPTER 6

Choice of local anesthetic for labor and delivery – bupivacaine, ropivacaine and levobupivacaine

Stephen H. Halpern

Introduction

Epidural bupivacaine has been used for many years for labor analgesia. While this agent provided excellent sensory analgesia, some patients experienced unacceptable motor block when high concentrations were used. Further, excessive cardiac toxicity with death has resulted from accidental intravenous injection of high concentrations of bupivacaine in parturients.

Ropivacaine was developed originally to reduce the incidence of cardiac toxicity in the unlikely event of accidental intravenous injection. Early studies indicated that epidural ropivacaine was associated with a reduced incidence of instrumental vaginal delivery and better neonatal outcomes as measured by the neuroadaptive capacity score. In addition, there appeared to be less motor block associated with ropivacaine compared with bupivacaine.[1] Another local anesthetic – levobupivacaine – purports to have similar advantages to ropivacaine compared with bupivacaine.

Since 1995 numerous studies compared epidural ropivacaine with bupivacaine for labor analgesia and recently data comparing bupivacaine with levobupivacaine have become available. Most investigators compared the drugs with respect to mode of delivery, incidence of motor block of the lower extremities, maternal satisfaction and neonatal outcome. Disagreement as to whether ropivacaine and bupivacaine are equipotent has resulted in a large number of studies comparing these drugs. Further, the pattern of anesthetic practice changed following the introduction of ropivacaine, with lower concentrations of local anesthetics being used for epidural labor analgesia over the

course of time. Therefore the results of some of the older studies may not be directly applicable to current practice.

This chapter examines the studies that were designed primarily to compare potencies among bupivacaine, ropivacaine and levobupivacaine. In addition, it discusses whether or not there are important differences in the effects of these drugs when used for labor analgesia. The data comes from randomized controlled trials, retrieved from MEDLINE® and EMBASE® using a broad text-word based search strategy. First, studies with the terms [bupivacaine], [ropivacaine], and/or [levobupivacaine] combined with [labour] or [labor] in the title were retrieved. The Science Citation Index® was used to obtain additional studies that had cited those found in the first search. Finally, the bibliographies of review articles were scanned for appropriate studies. The last systematic search was carried out in January 2004. The articles retrieved were given a numeric score for quality according to a validated scoring system. This system gives a maximum of 5 points, depending on how the randomization, blinding and patient flow through the study is described[2] (see Appendix for a full description of the scale). Other important aspects of study design such as concealment of randomization, statistical analysis and the presentation of results are not included as items in this scale and are described separately where appropriate.

Currently, the issue of cardiac toxicity is not an important aspect of labor epidural analgesia because low doses of local anesthetic are commonly employed. This issue will not be considered further.

Potency of bupivacaine, ropivacaine and levobupivacaine

There are primarily two methods of determining the relative potencies of the local anesthetics used for labor epidural analgesia and there are advantages and disadvantages to each. These are described in detail below.

Minimum local anesthetic concentration

These studies determine the minimum local anesthetic concentration (MLAC, analogous to the "minimum alveolar concentration") that provides comfort for 50% of laboring patients. Typically, patients in early labor are randomized to receive a bolus dose of one of the local anesthetics of interest. After carrying out pilot investigations to determine the approximate amount of local anesthetic required, a concentration is chosen by the investigator for the first patient. Subsequent concentrations are determined by the outcome of the preceding patient. If the patient was comfortable at a given concentration, the next patient received a reduced concentration of local anesthetic. If she was not, the concentration was increased.

The MLAC (with its 95% confidence intervals) can be determined after studying a sufficient number of patients. Statistically, MLAC is established using the method of Dixon and Massey and/or Wilcoxon and Lichfield probit regression (when both of these were performed on the same population, the results were similar).[3] Once the value of MLAC is calculated, differences between the drugs studied can be calculated.

The use of MLAC to compare drugs has several advantages. The analysis is well known and relatively few patients are required to determine its value. When the method is standardized (e.g. investigators use similar volumes, the patients are of similar parity and cervical dilation) the results are applicable to much of the normal laboring population.

In all the studies cited, the patients were in early labor (less than 5 cm dilation) and 20 mL of solution was used to initiate labor analgesia. The primary drawback is that the rest of the dose–response curve is not measured. Clinicians need to be at least 95% confident (not 50%) that the concentration of local anesthetic will relieve labor pain. It cannot be assumed from MLAC studies alone that the clinical effectiveness of the drugs at higher, clinically relevant concentrations will reflect the MLAC of the local anesthetic.

The studies that determined potency of local anesthetics using MLAC are shown in Table 6.1. All are high quality, randomized trials that allocated patients to receive either two different drugs or a single drug with different concentrations of additives. All were double blinded and had between 25 and 40 patients per group.

There were seven studies that contained an estimate of the MLAC of bupivacaine,[3–9] five for ropivacaine[3,4,10–12] and three for levobupivacaine.[7,10,11] As can be seen in Fig. 6.1, the estimated MLAC for bupivacaine is approximately 0.081%, ropivacaine 0.11% and levobupivacaine 0.083%. When bupivacaine and ropivacaine were compared in the same study, ropivacaine was significantly less potent than bupivacaine.[3,4] However, when bupivacaine was compared with levobupivacaine, there was no difference.[7] Of interest, when ropivacaine was compared with levobupivacaine, there was also no significant difference.[10,11]

Lacassie et al.[13] used the MLAC technique to compare the motor blocking potency of bupivacaine with that of ropivacaine and bupivacaine compared with levobupivacaine.[14] Both of these studies used much higher concentrations of local anesthetic compared with the analgesic studies. Of note, the MLAC for motor block of bupivacaine was approximately 0.37% compared with 0.5% for ropivacaine, a difference of approximately 25%.[13] When bupivacaine was compared with levobupivacaine by the same investigators, the MLAC of bupivacaine was approximately 10% lower than levobupivacaine (0.27% vs 0.31%, $P = 0.02$). Assuming that the sensory and motor blocking capabilities of each of these drugs are similar, these observations would lend weight to the finding that bupivacaine is slightly more potent than levobupivacaine and significantly more potent than ropivacaine.

Analgesic requirements in clinical trials

While the MLAC technique allowed comparisons of epidural local anesthetics at very low concentrations for initiation of labor analgesia, a number of investigators compared bupivacaine with ropivacaine as these drugs are used commonly in clinical practice. In some cases, local anesthetics were combined with opioids such as fentanyl or sufentanil. The investigators determined the relative potency of the drugs by comparing the hourly requirements of parturients. There were eight studies that maintained labor analgesia using a

Table 6.1 Minimum local anesthetic concentration (MLAC) studies.

Study	Quality score	Drugs	Parity	Number of patients included	Mean or median cervical dilation (cm)	Comments
Primary outcome – maternal comfort						
Polley 2002[8]	5	Bupivacaine vs bupivacaine + epinephrine	Mixed	35/35	4	Initial bolus
Polley 2003[11]	5	Levobupivacaine vs ropivacaine	Mixed	35/35	4–5	Initial bolus 29 exclusions from the levobupivacaine group, 6 exclusions from the ropivacaine group
Benhamou 2003[10]	3	Levobupivacaine vs ropivacaine	Mixed	40/40	3–4	Replacement patients (for those rejected) were allocated with the same randomization number. It is unclear whether or not the allocation was completely blinded in these patients
Capogna 1999[4]	3	Bupivacaine vs ropivacaine	Nulliparous	40/40	4	
Columb 1995[5]	3	Bupivacaine vs lidocaine	Mixed	30/30	4.5	
Lyons 1998[7]	3	Bupivacaine vs levobupivacaine	Mixed	30/30	3	
Polley 1998[9]	4	Bupivacaine vs 3 different concentrations of sufentanil + bupivacaine	Mixed	30/30/30/30	4.2–4.3	Only one of the study groups had bupivacaine without added opioid
Lyons 1997[6]	2	Bupivacaine vs 3 different concentrations of fentanyl + bupivacaine	Mixed	40/40/40/40	3–4	Only one of the study groups received bupivacaine without added opioid
Aveline 2002[12]	3	Ropivacaine with different concentrations of sufentanil or clonidine	Mixed	30/28/19	3.6	Only one of the study groups (n = 30) received ropivacaine without added clonidine
Polley 1999[3]	4	Ropivacaine vs bupivacaine	Mixed	25/25	4.4–4.6	
Primary outcome – maternal motor block						
Lacassie 2002[13]	3	Bupivacaine vs ropivacaine	Mixed	30/30	3.0–3.5	Cervical dilation in the ropivacaine group was statistically greater than the bupivacaine group
Lacassie 2003[14]	3	Bupivacaine vs levobupivacaine	Mixed	30/30	2.7–2.9	

patient-controlled device and a continuous infusion rate of less than 10 mL/h.[15–22] In six of these studies,[15,17,18,20–22] the concentration of bupivacaine and ropivacaine were the same, in two[16,19] the concentration of bupivacaine was reduced by approximately 40% based on the results of the MLAC studies. One study maintained analgesia using clinician top-up doses, according to patient demand.[23] In all cases, the

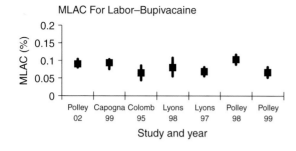

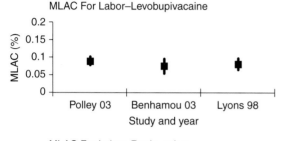

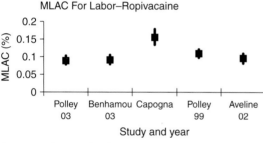

Fig. 6.1 Minimum local anesthetic concentration (MLAC) (mean and 95% confidence intervals) for bupivacaine, levobupivacaine and ropivacaine. The MLAC in percent is shown on the *y*-axis, the source of the data is shown on the *x*-axis.

studies were randomized and appropriately blinded but the potency of the drugs was not the primary outcome. There were no studies of this type that compared levobupivacaine with either bupivacaine or ropivacaine.

A summary of these studies is shown in Table 6.2. In the studies that compared equal concentrations of bupivacaine and ropivacaine, the amount of drug used was similar between groups. However, both studies that used a higher concentration of ropivacaine reported a highly statistically significant increase in the amount of ropivacaine used between the groups. This may reflect the fact that the volume of local anesthetic used in patient-controlled epidural analgesia (PCEA)

is more important in maintaining analgesia than the concentration of the drugs used.

Summary

MLAC studies indicate that ropivacaine is significantly less potent than bupivacaine but levobupivacaine is similar in potency to bupivacaine. Clinical studies did not confirm that there was a difference in potency at commonly used concentrations. This may be because the measurement of potency was too crude or the difference between drugs is not important clinically. All three drugs provide excellent analgesia at clinically relevant concentrations.

Obstetric, neonatal and anesthetic outcomes

Twenty-nine studies compared the epidural use of bupivacaine, ropivacaine and/or levobupivacaine for labor analgesia.[15,16,18–45] Two of these included two separate comparisons,[16,38] and one investigator reported different outcomes in two manuscripts.[36,37] As can be seen in Table 6.3, most of the patients were enrolled in high-quality studies as defined by a Jadad score of 3 or more. All investigators reported that their study was randomized and blinded. There are many small clinical trials, but some larger trials have been published recently.[16–18,40] The conduct of these trials is sufficiently similar to justify combining the main results in a meta-analysis (Table 6.3). The risk differences for dichotomous data and the weighted mean differences for continuous variables are presented. Significant statistical heterogeneity is present for a number of outcomes. These are identified and discussed below.

Obstetric outcomes

In contrast to earlier data,[1] there is no difference in the mode of delivery when bupivacaine and ropivacaine are compared. Specifically, the incidence of instrumental vaginal delivery is very similar (Table 6.4). There is significant heterogeneity in two of the outcomes (instrumental vaginal delivery and the length of second stage). This likely relates to clinical factors. For example, none of the studies controlled for the indication for instrumental vaginal delivery and therefore the indication for this intervention may have differed among institutions and over time.

Table 6.2 Studies using patient-controlled doses to determine analgesic potencies of local anesthetics. See Table 6.3 for a description of the quality of the studies.

Study	Parity	Ropivacaine concentration, additives and maintenance infusion	Bupivacaine concentration, additives and maintenance infusion	Ropivacaine (mg/h ± SD where available)	Bupivacaine (mg/h ± SD where available)	Comments
Ropivacaine concentrations = Bupivacaine concentrations						
Owen 2002[21]	Mixed	0.075% with 2 µg/mL fentanyl. PCEA + 6 mL/h infusion	0.075% with 2 µg/mL fentanyl. PCEA + 6 mL/h infusion	15.3 (3.1)	14.5 (4.1)	
Owen 1998[22]	Mixed	0.125%. PCEA + 6 mL/h infusion	0.125%. PCEA + 6 mL/h infusion	19.8 (6.2)	18.3 (5.5)	
Meister 2000[20]	Mixed	0.125% with 2 µg/mL fentanyl. PCEA + 6 mL/h infusion	0.125% with 2 µg/mL fentanyl. PCEA + 6 mL/h infusion	13.7 (5.2)	13.7 (6.9)	
Halpern 2003[18]	Nulliparous	0.1% with 2 µg/mL fentanyl PCEA + 5 mL/h infusion	0.1% with 2 µg/mL fentanyl PCEA + 5 mL/h infusion	11.7	10.2	Derived from the total amount of local anesthetic used divided by the number of hours of epidural analgesia
Fischer 2000[17]	Mixed	0.1% with 0.5 µg/mL sufentanil. PCEA with no infusion	0.1% with 0.5 µg/mL sufentanil. PCEA with no infusion	12.9	12.3	Derived from the total amount of local anesthetic used divided by the number of hours of epidural analgesia
Chua 2001[15]	Nulliparous	0.125%. PCEA with no infusion	0.125%. PCEA with no infusion	12.5 (6.25–15.7)	10.8 (6.7–20)	Data presented as median and range
Asik 2002[23]	Nulliparous	0.2% with fentanyl 2 µg/mL. Clinician top-up on patient demand	0.2% with fentanyl 2 µg/mL. Clinician top-up on patient demand	10.1 (2.6)	11.2 (3.1)	
Ropivacaine concentrations > Bupivacaine concentrations						
Hofmann-Kiefer 2002[19]	Mixed	0.2% with 0.75 µg/mL sufentanil. PCEA with no infusion	0.125% with 0.75 µg/mL sufentanil. PCEA with no infusion	14.8 (4.4)	12.1 (5.1)	Ropivacaine > bupivacaine, $P < 0.01$
Evron 2004[16]	Nulliparous multiparous	0.2%. PCEA with 5 mL/h	0.125%. PCEA with 5 mL/h	22.1(12) 24.8 (13)	15.7 (9.5) 18.6 (14)	Nulliparous and multiparous parturients were reported separately. Ropivacaine > bupivacaine, $P < 0.0001$

PCEA, Patient-controlled epidural analgesia; SD, standard deviation.

Table 6.3 Description of studies.

Reference & year	Quality score	Population	Bupivacaine			Ropivacaine			Levobupivacaine	Remarks
			N	Concentration	Maintenance	N	Concentration	Maintenance		
McCrae 1995[36,37]	4*	Mixed	20	0.25–0.5%	Clinician top-up	20	0.25–0.5%	Clinician top-up	No	Study ended at delivery or 2nd top-up
Stienstra 1995[43]	4*	Mixed	37	0.25%	Continuous infusion	39	0.25%	Continuous infusion	No	
Gatt 1996[31]	Abstract	Mixed	38	0.25%	Clinician top-up	38	0.25%	Clinician top-up	No	
Eddleston 1996[26]	4*	Mixed	51	0.25%	Clinician top-up	52	0.25%	Clinician top-up	No	
Gaiser 1997[30]	3	Mixed	38	0.25%	Continuous infusion	37	0.25%	Continuous infusion	No	
Muir 1997[39]	2	Mixed	26	0.25%	Clinician top-up	34	0.25%	Clinician top-up	No	
Irestedt 1998[34]	3	Nulliparous	12	0.25%	Continuous infusion	12	0.25%	Continuous infusion	No	Lidocaine test dose
Owen 1998[22]	4	Mixed	25	0.125%	Patient-controlled	26	0.125%	Patient-controlled	No	
Gautier 1999[32]	4	Mixed	45	0.125% + 0.75 µg/mL sufentanil	Single bolus	45	0.125% + 0.75 µg/mL sufentanil	Single bolus	No	
Campbell 2000[24]	5	Nulliparous	20	0.08% + 2 µg/mL fentanyl	Patient-controlled	20	0.08% + 2 µg/mL fentanyl	Patient controlled	No	
Finegold 2000[29]	4	Nulliparous	50	Initiation 0.25% Maintenance 0.125%, 2 µg/mL fentanyl	Continuous infusion	50	Initiation 0.2% Maintenance 0.1% 2 µg/mL fentanyl	Continuous infusion	No	
Fischer 2000[17]	4*	Mixed	94	0.1% + 0.5 µg/mL sufentanil	Patient-controlled	95	0.1% + 0.5 µg/mL sufentanil	Patient-controlled	No	

Continued

61

Table 6.3 (*continued*)

Reference & year	Quality score	Population	Bupivacaine			Ropivacaine			Levobupivacaine	Remarks
			N	Concentration	Maintenance	N	Concentration	Maintenance		
Hughes 2000[33]	Abstract	?	28	0.1% + 2 µg/mL fentanyl	Continuous infusion	32	0.1% + 2 µg/mL fentanyl	Continuous infusion	No	
Kessler 2000[35]	Abstract	Mixed	30	Initiation 0.25% Maintenance 0.125% + 0.5 µg/mL sufentanil	Patient-controlled	30	Initiation 0.2% Maintenance 0.1% + 0.5 µg/mL sufentanil	Patient-controlled	No	More nulliparous in ropivacaine group
Meister 2000[20]	5	Mixed	25	0.125% + 2 µg/mL fentanyl	Patient-controlled	25	0.125% + 2 µg/mL fentanyl	Patient-controlled	No	20 excluded after randomization
Parpaglioni 2000[40]	3	Nulliparous	97	0.0625% + 10 µg sufentanil	Initiation bolus only	93	0.1% + 10 µg sufentanil	Initiation bolus only	No	Study of initial bolus only
Smiley 2000[42]	Abstract	Nulliparous	21	0.0625% + 2 µg/mL fentanyl	Patient-controlled	23	0.0625% + 2 µg/mL fentanyl	Patient-controlled	No	
Chua 2001[15]	3	Nulliparous	16	0.125%	Patient-controlled	16	0.125%	Patient-controlled	No	
Fernandez-Guisasola 2001[28]	4	Mixed	51	0.0625% + 2 µg/mL fentanyl	Continuous infusion	47	0.1% + 2 µg/mL fentanyl	Continuous infusion	No	Initiation with lidocaine
Merson (low dose) 2001[38]	5*	Nulliparous	16	0.125% loading 0.1% + 0.6 µg/mL sufentanil	Continuous infusion	16	0.125% loading 0.1% + 0.6 µg/mL sufentanil	Continuous infusion	No	2 comparisons in 1 manuscript (see below)
Merson (high dose) 2001[38]	5*	Nulliparous	17	0.25% loading 0.1% + 0.6 µg/mL sufentanil	Continuous infusion	19	0.25% loading 0.1% + 0.6 µg/mL sufentanil	Continuous infusion	No	
Hofmann-Kiefer 2002[19]	3	Mixed	50	0.125% with 0.75 µg/mL sufentanil	PCEA	50	0.2% with 0.75 µg/mL sufentanil	PCEA	No	Lidocaine test dose

Study		Parturient	N	Regimen	Mode	N	Regimen	Mode	Concealment	Comments
Owen 2002[21]	3	Nulliparous	25	0.075% + 2 µg/mL fentanyl	Patient-controlled	25	0.075% + 2 µg/mL fentanyl	Patient-controlled	No	9 patients eliminated from analysis
Asik 2002[23]	5	Nulliparous	28	0.2% + 2 µg/mL fentanyl	Intermittent clinician bolus	25	0.2% + 2 µg/mL fentanyl	Intermittent clinician bolus	No	Maintained with low volume, frequent clinician boluses
Pirbudak 2002[41]	2	Nulliparous	20	Initiation 0.125% + 50 µg fentanyl Maintenance 0.05% + 1.5 µg/mL fentanyl	Patient-controlled	20	Initiation 0.125% + 50 µg fentanyl Maintenance 0.05% + 1.5 µg/mL fentanyl	Patient-controlled	No	
Halpern 2003[18]	5*	Nulliparous	276	Initiation 0.1% + 5 µg/mL fentanyl Maintenance 0.08% + 2 µg/mL fentanyl	Patient-controlled	279	Initiation 0.1% + 5 µg/mL fentanyl Maintenance 0.08% + 2 µg/mL fentanyl	Patient-controlled	No	
Camorcia 2003[45]	4	Nulliparous	35	0.0625% + 10 µg sufentanil 20 mL	Initiation bolus only	37	0.1% + 10 µg sufentanil 20 mL	Initiation bolus only	No	3-group comparison levobupivacaine N = 34, concentrations were the same as the bupivacaine group
El Moutaz 2003[27]	2	Mixed	30	10 mL 0.25%	Initial bolus only	–	–	–	No	10 mL 0.25% initial bolus only
Evron (nulliparous) 2004[16]	4	Nulliparous	165	Test dose of 3 mL 2% lidocaine followed by 0.125% bupivacaine	Patient-controlled	113	Test dose of 3 mL 2% lidocaine followed by 0.2% ropivacaine	Patient-controlled	No	Nulliparous and multiparous parturients studied separately
Evron (multiparous) 2004[16]	4	Multiparous	148	Test dose of 3 mL 2% lidocaine followed by 0.125% bupivacaine	Patient-controlled	139	Test dose of 3 mL 2% lidocaine followed by 0.2% ropivacaine	Patient-controlled	No	

* Concealment of allocation explicitly stated.
PCEA, patient-controlled epidural analgesia.

Table 6.4 Obstetric, anesthetic and neonatal outcomes (bupivacaine versus ropivacaine).

Outcome	No. studies included	Bupivacaine n/N or N	Ropivacaine n/N or N	Percentage risk difference or weighted mean difference (± 95% CI)	P value
Obstetric outcomes					
Spontaneous vaginal delivery	25[15–23,25,26,28–32,34,36–39,41,43,45,47]	886/1393	875/1340	3 (–1 to 6)	0.16
Instrumental delivery	24[15–23,25,26,28–30,32,34,36–39,41,43,45,47]	299/1320	304/1270	1 (–5 to 6)	0.81*
Cesarean section	25[15–23,25,26,28–30,32,34,36–39,41–43,45,47]	198/1332	166/1297	1 (–3 to 1)	0.49
Length of second stage of labor (min)	11[15–19,21,26,28,29,41,47]	957	895	1.2 (–8.0 to 5.6)	0.73*
Neonatal outcomes					
Apgar score at 1 min <7	15[15,17,18,20–22,26,28–31,36,37,41,43]	86/762	99/772	–1 (–3 to 1)	0.36
Apgar score at 5 min <7	18[15,17–22,26,28–31,34,36,37,39,41,43,47]	25/876	19/867	1 (–1 to 2)	0.43
Umbilical artery pH	9[16–19,26,28,30,34]	809	871	0 (0–0.01)	0.25
Anesthetic outcomes					
Time to block onset (min)	12[23,25,26,29,30,32,33,36,37,40,43,45,47]	506	513	0.42 (0.7–1.53)	0.45*
Good or excellent analgesia	14[18,20–22,26,28,32–34,36,37,39,43,47]	564/628	565/639	–1 (–4 to 1)	0.34
Ambulation	5[18,19,40,45,47]	338/466	359/471	4 (–1 to 9)	0.14
Detectable motor block (reported by the investigators or at 2 h postinjection	30[15–23,25,26,28–36,38–43,45,47]	873/1424	739/1472	9 (2–15)	0.007*
Maternal satisfaction (VAS score in mm)	2[25,46]	346	343	–0.29 (–2.96 to 2.38)	0.83

* Statistically significant heterogeneity.

CI, clearance interval; VAS, visual analog score.

Similarly, in some institutions the second stage of labor is shortened by operative obstetric interventions. Finally, the indications for oxytocin were different. While these factors may cause heterogeneity in the magnitude of change, it is unlikely that bias would result as complete blinding to treatment group was reported in the studies.

Only one study with 30 patients in each group compared levobupivacaine with racemic bupivacaine. There was no difference between groups for any obstetric outcomes.[27] This finding should be interpreted with caution because of the small sample size.

Neonatal outcomes

In all studies, the neonatal outcomes were good for both bupivacaine and ropivacaine. The incidence of an Apgar score ≤ 7 at 1 or 5 min was extremely low (Table 6.4). In addition, the umbilical artery cord blood gases were similar. An earlier meta-analysis found that the neuroadaptive capacity scores were better in neonates of ropivacaine-treated mothers.[1] However, this test is no longer considered reliable.[46]

Anesthesic outcomes

After epidural injection, both ropivacaine and bupivacaine provide good to excellent analgesia in a relatively short period of time. The onset time varies between 10 and 20 min among studies, but pooled mean difference between treatment groups is less than 30 s (Table 6.4). The statistical heterogeneity among studies can be explained on the basis of differences among concentrations of the drugs used, the use of a lidocaine test dose and the addition of additives, such as opioids. In addition, heterogeneity is seen in the two studies that reported the onset of action of levobupivacaine.[27,45] The onset time was approximately 20 min when 20 mL of 0.0625% levobupivacaine with sufentanil was used to initiate epidural labor analgesia, which was similar to the onset time for the same concentration of bupivacaine.[45] However, when 10 mL of 0.25% levobupivacaine was used, the onset time was approximately 13 min (compared with 14 min for bupivacaine).[27]

Of the other parameters measured, the only difference between bupivacaine and ropivacaine was the incidence of detectable motor block of the lower extremities. This was statistically significant and favored ropivacaine. The statistical heterogeneity came from two main sources. First, the investigators used varying concentrations of local anesthetics and additives. While many studies used equal concentrations of local anesthetics between groups,[15,17,18,20–23,26,30–34,36–39,42,43,47] some used higher concentrations of ropivacaine[16,19,28,35,40,45] and one used a higher concentration of bupivacaine[29] (Table 6.3). Second, motor block was assessed in different ways by different investigators. Some reported an overall incidence of motor block over the entire course of labor while others reported the incidence at specific times after initial injection. It should be noted that very few patients had total motor block of the lower extremities with either drug.

Three studies reported motor block after 2 h of use.[18,25,32] These studies found progressive differences in the incidence of motor block over time. When compared with bupivacaine, ropivacaine appears to produce a lower incidence of motor block after approximately 6 h of labor.[18] This observation has little clinical significance to most patients because there was no difference in the incidence of ambulation, maternal satisfaction or any of the obstetric outcomes (Table 6.4). The incidence of motor block associated with levobupivacaine appears similar to bupivacaine and ropivacaine.[27,45]

Summary

There has been an enormous amount of research comparing epidural ropivacaine with bupivacaine for epidural labor analgesia. MLAC studies have consistently shown that ropivacaine is less potent than bupivacaine at concentrations that provide analgesia for 50% of parturients. The clinical significance of this finding is uncertain, because randomized trials comparing higher, more relevant concentrations did not find a difference in total drug use. While data for levobupivacaine are sparse, MLAC studies indicate its potency is similar to bupivacaine.

Current data do not support the contention that ropivacaine is superior to bupivacaine for any obstetric or neonatal outcome. It is possible that ropivacaine may produce less motor block than bupivacaine after prolonged use. There are insufficient data available to determine the role of epidural levobupivacaine for labor analgesia.

References

1 Writer WD, Stienstra R, Eddleston JM, *et al*. Neonatal outcome and mode of delivery after epidural analgesia for labour with ropivacaine and bupivacaine: a prospective meta-analysis. *Br J Anaesth* 1998;**81**:713–7.

2 Jadad AR, Moore RA, Carroll D, *et al*. Assessing the quality of reports of randomized clinical trials: is blinding necessary? *Control Clin Trials* 1996;**17**:1–12.

3 Polley LS, Columb MO, Naughton NN, Wagner DS, van de Ven CJ. Relative analgesic potencies of ropivacaine and bupivacaine for epidural analgesia in labor: implications for therapeutic indexes. *Anesthesiology* 1999;**90**:944–50.

4 Capogna G, Celleno D, Fusco P, Lyons G, Columb M. Relative potencies of bupivacaine and ropivacaine for analgesia in labour. *Br J Anaesth* 1999;**82**:371–3.

5 Columb MOF, Lyons GF. Determination of the minimum local analgesic concentrations of epidural bupivacaine and lidocaine in labor. *Anesth Analg* 1995;**81**:833–7.

6 Lyons G, Columb M, Hawthorne L, Dresner M. Extradural pain relief in labour: bupivacaine sparing by extradural fentanyl is dose dependent. *Br J Anaesth* 1997;**78**:493–7.

7 Lyons G, Columb M, Wilson RC, Johnson RV. Epidural pain relief in labour: potencies of levobupivacaine and racemic bupivacaine. *Br J Anaesth* 1998;**81**:899–901.

8 Polley LSM, Columb MOF, Naughton NNM, *et al*. Effect of epidural epinephrine on the minimum local analgesic concentration of epidural bupivacaine in labor. *Anesthesiology* 2002;**96**:1123–8.

9 Polley LSM, Columb MOF, Wagner DSP, Naughton NNM. Dose-dependent reduction of the minimum local analgesic concentration of bupivacaine by sufentanil for epidural analgesia in labor. *Anesthesiology* 1998;**89**:626–32.

10 Benhamou DMD, Ghosh CMD, Mercier FJM. A randomized sequential allocation study to determine the minimum effective analgesic concentration of levobupivacaine and ropivacaine in patients receiving epidural analgesia for labor. *Anesthesiology* 2003;**99**:1383–6.

11 Polley LSM, Columb MOF, Naughton NNM, *et al*. Relative analgesic potencies of levobupivacaine and ropivacaine for epidural analgesia in labor. *Anesthesiology* 2003;**99**:1354–8.

12 Aveline C, El Metaoua S, Masmoudi A, Boelle PY, Bonnet F. The effect of clonidine on the minimum local analgesic concentration of epidural ropivacaine during labor. *Anesth Analg* 2002;**95**:735–40.

13 Lacassie HJ, Columb MO, Lacassie HP, Lantadilla RA. The relative motor blocking potencies of epidural bupivacaine and ropivacaine in labor. *Anesth Analg* 2002;**95**:204–8.

14 Lacassie HJ, Columb MO. The relative motor blocking potencies of bupivacaine and levobupivacaine in labor. *Anesth Analg* 2003;**97**:1509–13.

15 Chua NP, Sia AT, Ocampo CE. Parturient-controlled epidural analgesia during labour: bupivacaine vs ropivacaine. *Anaesthesia* 2001;**56**:1169–73.

16 Evron S, Glezerman M, Sadan O, Boaz M, Ezri T. Patient-controlled epidural analgesia for labor pain: effect on labor, delivery and neonatal outcome of 0.125% bupivacaine vs 0.2% ropivacaine. *Int J Obstet Anesth* 2004;**13**:5–10.

17 Fischer C, Blanie P, Jaouen E, *et al*. Ropivacaine, 0.1%, plus sufentanil, 0.5 µg/mL, versus bupivacaine, 0.1%, plus sufentanil, 0.5 µg/mL, using patient-controlled epidural analgesia for labor: a double-blind comparison. *Anesthesiology* 2000;**92**:1588–93.

18 Halpern SH, Breen TW, Campbell DC, *et al*. A multicentered randomized controlled trial comparing bupivacaine to ropivacaine for labor analgesia. *Anesthesiology* 2003;**98**:1431–5.

19 Hofmann-Kiefer K, Saran K, Brederode A, *et al*. Ropivacaine 2 mg/mL vs bupivacaine 1.25 mg/mL with sufentanil using patient-controlled epidural analgesia in labour. *Acta Anaesthesiol Scand* 2002;**46**:316–21.

20 Meister GC, D'Angelo R, Owen M, Nelson KE, Gaver R. A comparison of epidural analgesia with 0.125% ropivacaine with fentanyl versus 0.125% bupivacaine with fentanyl during labor. *Anesth Analg* 2000;**90**:632–7.

21 Owen MD, Thomas JA, Smith T, Harris LC, D'Angelo R. Ropivacaine 0.075% and bupivacaine 0.075% with fentanyl 2 µg/mL are equivalent for labor epidural analgesia. *Anesth Analg* 2002;**94**:179–83.

22 Owen MD, D'Angelo R, Gerancher JC, *et al*. 0.125% ropivacaine is similar to 0.125% bupivacaine for labor analgesia using patient-controlled epidural infusion. *Anesth Analg* 1998;**86**:527–31.

23 Asik I, Goktug A, Gulay I, Alkis N, Uysalel A. Comparison of bupivacaine 0.2% and ropivacaine 0.2% combined with fentanyl for epidural analgesia during labour. *Eur J Anaesthesiol* 2002;**19**:263–70.

24 Campbell DC, Breen TW, Kronberg J, Nunn RT, Fick G. Comparison of the effects of ropivacaine vs bupivacaine on maternal ambulation and spontaneous micturition. *Anesthesiology* 2000;A1044.

25 Clement HJ, Caruso L, Lopez F, *et al*. Epidural analgesia with 0.15% ropivacaine plus sufentanil 0.5 µg/mL versus 0.10% bupivacaine plus sufentanil 0.5 µg/mL: a double-blind comparison during labour. *Br J Anaesth* 2002;**88**:809–13.

26 Eddleston JM, Holland JJ, Griffin RP, *et al*. A double-blind comparison of 0.25% ropivacaine and 0.25% bupivacaine for extradural analgesia in labour. *Br J Anaesth* 1996;**76**:66–71.

27 El Moutaz H, El Said A, Fouad M. Comparative study between 0.25% levobupivacaine and 0.25% racemic bupivacaine for epidural analgesia in labour. *Egypt J Anaesth* 2003;**19**:417–23.

28 Fernandez-Guisasola J, Serrano ML, Cobo B, *et al*. A comparison of 0.0625% bupivacaine with fentanyl and 0.1% ropivacaine with fentanyl for continuous epidural labor analgesia. *Anesth Analg* 2001;**92**:1261–5.

29 Finegold H, Mandell G, Ramanathan S. Comparison of ropivacaine 0.1% fentanyl and bupivacaine 0.125%: fentanyl infusions for epidural labor analgesia. *Can J Anaesth* 2000;**47**:740–5.

30 Gaiser RR, Venkateswaren P, Cheek TG, *et al*. Comparison of 0.25% ropivacaine and bupivacaine for epidural analgesia for labor and vaginal delivery. *J Clin Anesth* 1997;**9**:564–8.

31 Gatt S, Crooke D, Lockley S, Anderson A, Armstrong P, Aveline C. A double-blind, randomized parallel investigation into the neurobehavioral status and outcome of infants born to mothers receiving epidural ropivacaine 0.25% and bupivacaine 0.25% for analgesia in labor. *Anaesth Intensive Care* 1996;**24**:108–9.

32 Gautier P, De Kock M, Van Steenberge A, *et al.* A double-blind comparison of 0.125% ropivacaine with sufentanil and 0.125% bupivacaine with sufentanil for epidural labor analgesia. *Anesthesiology* 1999;**90**:772–8.

33 Hughes D, Hill D, Fee H. A comparison of bupivacaine–fentanyl with ropivacaine–fentanyl by epidural infusion for labor analgesia. *Anesthesiology* 2000;**93**:A1051.

34 Irestedt L, Ekblom A, Olofsson C, Dahlstrom AC, Emanuelsson BM. Pharmacokinetics and clinical effect during continuous epidural infusion with ropivacaine 2.5 mg/mL or bupivacaine 2.5 mg/mL for labour pain relief. *Acta Anaesthesiol Scand* 1998;**42**:890–6.

35 Kessler BV, Thomas H, Gressler S, Probst S, Vettermann J. PCEA during labor: no difference in pain relief between ropivacaine 0.1% and bupivacaine 0.125% when sufentanil 0.5 µg/mL is added. *Anesthesiology* 2000;**93**:A1068.

36 McCrae AF, Jozwiak H, McClure JH. Comparison of ropivacaine and bupivacaine in extradural analgesia for the relief of pain in labour. *Br J Anaesth* 1995;**74**:261–5.

37 McCrae AF, Westerling P, McClure JH. Pharmacokinetic and clinical study of ropivacaine and bupivacaine in women receiving extradural analgesia in labour. *Br J Anaesth* 1997;**79**:558–62.

38 Merson N. A comparison of motor block between ropivacaine and bupivacaine for continuous labor epidural analgesia. *AANA J* 2001;**69**:54–8.

39 Muir HA, Writer D, Douglas J, *et al.* Double-blind comparison of epidural ropivacaine 0.25% and bupivacaine 0.25%, for the relief of childbirth pain. *Can J Anaesth* 1997;**44**:599–604.

40 Parpaglioni R, Capogna G, Celleno D. A comparison between low-dose ropivacaine and bupivacaine at equianalgesic concentrations for epidural analgesia during the first stage of labor. *Int J Obstet Anesth* 2000;**9**:83–6.

41 Pirbudak L, Tuncer S, Kocoglu H, Goksu S, Celik C. Fentanyl added to bupivacaine 0.05% or ropivacaine 0.05% in patient-controlled epidural analgesia in labour. *Eur J Anaesthesiol* 2002;**19**:271–5.

42 Smiley RM, Kim-Lo SH, Goodman SR, Jackson MA, Landau R. Patient-controlled epidural analgesia with 0.625% ropivacaine versus bupivacaine with fentanyl during labor. *Anesthesiology* 2000;**93**:A1065.

43 Stienstra R, Jonker TA, Bourdrez P, *et al.* Ropivacaine 0.25% versus bupivacaine 0.25% for continuous epidural analgesia in labor: a double-blind comparison. *Anesth Analg* 1995;**80**:285–9.

44 Vercauteren MP, Hans G, De Decker K, Adriaensen HA. Levobupivacaine combined with sufentanil and epinephrine for intrathecal labor analgesia: a comparison with racemic bupivacaine. *Anesth Analg* 2001;**93**:996–1000.

45 Camorcia M, Capogna G. Epidural levobupivacaine, ropivacaine and bupivacaine in combination with sufentanil in early labour: a randomized trial. *Eur J Anaesthesiol* 2003;**20**:636–9.

46 Halpern SH, Littleford JA, Brockhurst NJ, Youngs PJ, Malik N, Owen HC. The neurologic and adaptive capacity score is not a reliable method of newborn evaluation. *Anesthesiology* 2001;**94**:958–62.

47 Campbell DC, Zwack RM, Crone LA, Yip RW. Ambulatory labor epidural analgesia: bupivacaine versus ropivacaine. *Anesth Analg* 2000;**90**:1384–9.

CHAPTER 7

Intrathecal opioids in labor – do they increase the risk of fetal bradycardia?

Chahé Mardirosoff & Martin R. Tramèr

Introduction

Intrathecal opioid administration is a way, among others, to initiate pain relief during labor. Its advantages are supposed to be a lack of motor blockade, a faster onset of analgesia and the reliability of the intrathecal injection.[1] However, reliability of the intrathecal injection has been challenged by some authors who documented a 11% failure rate to identify the cerebrospinal fluid with the intrathecal needle.[2] A recent meta-analysis compared intrathecal opioids with epidural local anesthetics in labor; analgesia at 15–20 min after injection was shown to be similar.[3]

Soon after the advent of this innovative analgesic technique, obstetric anesthesiologists were alerted by reports of fetal heart rate abnormalities, particularly bradycardia, following intrathecal injection of opioids during labor.[4] These abnormalities did not seem to be related to cardiovascular changes in the mother. Because these accusations came from uncontrolled observations, two questions arise. First, is there a causal link between the intrathecal injection of an opioid during labor and the occurrence of fetal bradycardia? As this question is about causation, it can be answered by applying the "rules of causation":[5]

1 the association should be consistently present in different types of studies;

2 the temporal relationship should be correct;

3 there should be a dose–response association; and

4 there should be a biologic reason that makes sense.

The second question concentrates on the importance of this event (assuming that a true association exists). This question is about the clinical relevance of the adverse event. How often does it happen? How severe is it? What are the consequences in terms of morbidity and mortality? It has to be kept in mind that we are discussing the additional risk of this potential adverse event. This means that fetal bradycardia may happen spontaneously, i.e. without any intervention. For rational decision-making it is important to know about this underlying risk.

We address these issues in this chapter. In a previously published systematic review we reported on the evidence base of a link between maternal intrathecal opioids and fetal bradycardia; in that analysis we concentrated on data from randomized controlled trials.[6] However, not all questions can be addressed in randomized trials.[7] Thus, in this chapter we include data from relevant reports independent of their study architecture, i.e. observational studies, such as uncontrolled case series, non-randomized comparative trials and randomized studies.

Methods

We performed a comprehensive search in the MEDLINE® (PubMed) and Cochrane Central Register of Controlled Trials databases for relevant reports that were published before September 2003. We used the free text terms [fetal *or* foetal], [bradycardia], [intrathecal], [intrathecal *or* subarachnoid], [opioid], [labor *or* labour] and [anesthesia *or* anaesthesia]. We hand-searched all issues of the *International Journal of Obstetric Anesthesia* which is peer reviewed but, at the time of writing, not indexed in MEDLINE®. This search retrieved approximately 350 citations. We also screened bibliographies of relevant papers. Finally, anesthesia journals were scanned for randomized controlled trials until April 1, 2004. Studies were selected that reported on the number of parturients in whom fetal bradycardia was diagnosed after an intrathecal injection of any opioid regimen during labor. Definition of fetal bradycardia was taken as reported in the original reports. However, we only analyzed events of fetal bradycardia if they happened within 1 h of the intrathecal injection of the opioid and if there was no associated maternal hypotension. Data from abstracts were not included. We divided the relevant reports into three groups: case series, non-randomized controlled trials (e.g. studies with historical controls) and randomized controlled trials.

Results

Intrathecal opioids and fetal bradycardia in case series

Fifteen relevant uncontrolled case series were identified (Table 7.1).[2,8–21] In those, 1121 parturients received a variety of intrathecal opioid regimens, and in 48, fetal bradycardia was diagnosed. In some studies, no event occurred, and in others there was a 30% incidence of fetal bradycardia. The average incidence of fetal bradycardia was approximately 4%. In these studies there was no standard way of monitoring the fetus, nor was there a standard definition of fetal bradycardia. Therefore, the incidence might be expected to vary widely. For the same reason, a dose–response could not be

Table 7.1 Intrathecal opioids and risk of fetal bradycardia. Evidence from uncontrolled case series.

Reference	Opioid regimen	Event	Number of events/ total number of parturients
Arkoosh et al.[8]	IT sufentanil 1–10 µg	Fetal bradycardia	0/50 (0.0%)
Camann et al.[9]	IT sufentanil 10 µg ± epinephrine	Fetal bradycardia	0/40 (0.0%)
Cheng et al.[10]	IT bupivacaine + fentanyl or sufentanil	Fetal distress	0/40 (0.0%)
Clarke et al.[11]	IT fentanyl 50 µg	Fetal bradycardia	9/30 (30%)
Cohen et al.[12]	IT sufentanil 10 µg	Fetal bradycardia	1/73 (1.4%)
Collis et al.[2]	IT fentanyl 25 µg + bupivacaine 2.5 mg	Fetal bradycardia	0/300 (0.0%)
Goodman et al.[13]	IT fentanyl 35 µg ± bupivacaine 2.5 mg ± epinephrine 100 µg	Fetal bradycardia	7/67 (9.2%)
Herman et al.[14]	IT fentanyl 2–25 µg	Fetal bradycardia	2/90 (2.2%)
Honet et al.[15]	IT fentanyl 10 µg or sufentanil 5 µg or meperidine 10 mg	Fetal bradycardia	0/65 (0.0%)
Hughes et al.[16]	IT fentanyl 25 µg + bupivacaine or ropivacaine 2.5 mg	Fetal bradycardia	0/40 (0.0%)
Nelson et al.[17]	IT fentanyl 36 µg or sufentanil 8 µg	Fetal bradycardia	3/55 (5.5%)
Palmer et al.[18]	IT fentanyl 5–45 µg	Fetal bradycardia	0/84 (0.0%)
Vaughan et al.[19]	IT bupivacaine 2.5 mg + fentanyl 25 µg or diamorphine 250 µg	Fetal bradycardia	8/59 (13.6%)
Vercauteren et al.[21]	IT sufentanil 1.5 µg + bupivacaine 2.5 mg ± epinephrine 2.25 µg	Fetal bradycardia	6/44 (13.6%)
Vercauteren et al.[20]	IT sufentanil 1.5 µg + epinephrine 2.5 µg ± levobupivacaine or racemic bupivacaine 2.5 mg	Fetal bradycardia	12/75 (16.0%)

IT, intrathecal.

Table 7.2 Intrathecal opioids and the risk of fetal bradycardia. Evidence from controlled trials.

Reference	IT opioid regimen	Control	Event	No. events/total no. parturients		Odds ratio (95% CI)
				IT opioid	Control	
Palmer et al.[4]	IT fentanyl 25 μg or IT fentanyl 25 μg + bupivacaine 2.5 mg	Epi lidocaine 90 mg + fentanyl 50 μg + epinephrine 33 μg	Fetal bradycardia	5/100 (5.0%)	1/99 (1.0%)	3.89 (0.77–19.7)
Nielsen et al.[23]	IT sufentanil 10 μg	Epi bupivacaine 0.25% titration until (T8–10) sensory level	Fetal bradycardia	11/65 (16.9%)	11/64 (17.2%)	0.98 (0.39–2.45)
Van de Velde et al.[24]	IT sufentanil 7.5 μg or IT sufentanil 1.5 μg + bupivacaine 2.5 mg	Epi bupivacaine 12.5 mg + sufentanil 7.5 μg	Fetal bradycardia + prolonged decelerations	47/838 (5.6%)	13/346 (3.8%)	1.47 (0.83–2.60)
Eberle et al.[22]	IT sufentanil 10 μg	Epi bupivacaine 32.5 mg	Prolonged and severe decelerations	6/153 (3.9%)	5/128 (3.9%)	1.00 (0.30–3.36)

CI, confidence interval; Epi, epidural; IT, intrathecal.

demonstrated. In one of the studies, fentanyl 50 μg was injected intrathecally, and the authors reported a very high incidence of uterine hyperactivity in those patients with fetal bradycardia (five out of nine patients), suggesting a potential mechanism for its occurrence.[11]

Intrathecal opioids and fetal bradycardia in controlled trials

Four relevant reports were identified (Table 7.2).[4,22–24] In all four studies, an intrathecal opioid regimen was compared with an analgesia technique that did not include an intrathecal injection. Two were retrospective analyses using historical controls,[4,24] and two were prospective comparative controlled trials without randomization.[22,23] With intrathecal opioids, fetal bradycardia was diagnosed in 69 of 1156 parturients, corresponding to an average rate of 6%. Among the 637 parturients who did not receive intrathecal opioids, fetal bradycardia was diagnosed in 30 (4.7%). There was less variability in the rates of events with intrathecal opioids compared with case series; in three of the four trials, the absolute risk of fetal bradycardia with intrathecal opioids was between 3.9% and 5.6%.[4,22,24] However, in the smallest trial (n = 129), the incidence of bradycardia with or without intrathecal

opioids was approximately three times higher than in the other studies (16.9%).[23] In two trials, the risk with intrathecal opioids was higher compared with controls. In the others, there was equivalence. No trial reported a decreased risk of bradycardia with intrathecal opioids.

Intrathecal opioids and fetal bradycardia in randomized controlled trials

Sixteen potentially relevant randomized controlled trials were identified.[25–40] Of these, four trials were comprised of one group that did not receive intrathecal opioid (control group) and more than one treatment group.[26,31,36,38] For the purposes of this review, the incidence of fetal bradycardia was pooled among the treatment groups within each study.

Some of the studies reported cesarean section[40] or fetal heart rate abnormalities[39] but not fetal bradycardia. Three studies that did report fetal bradycardia were subsequently excluded by us.[28,29,32] The study by Gambling et al.[29] analyzed the rates of operative deliveries with a combined spinal epidural technique compared with intravenous meperidine. Profound fetal bradycardia was reported in nine of 616 (1.5%) parturients who had received an intrathecal opioid injection compared with none of 607 who had received intravenous meperidine. This difference was statistically significant; the odds ratio was 7.38 (95% confidence interval, 1.99–27.4). In all women in whom profound fetal bradycardia was diagnosed, an emergency cesarean section was performed. We regarded this trial as invalid for the purpose of our analysis because the method of fetal monitoring was not strictly controlled between the two groups: parturients who received an intrathecal opioid injection had continuous fetal heart rate monitoring recorded during the first 30 min after the injection, whereas those who received intravenous meperidine had intermittent Doppler auscultation only. Finally, two large randomized controlled trials[28,32] were not included in our analysis because the authors did not report on the number of parturients in whom fetal bradycardia was diagnosed.

Thus, two new studies[36,37] could be added to our previously published systematic review of randomized trials (Table 7.3).[6] One of the additional trials reported on fetal heart rate abnormalities only but did not specify the number of episodes of fetal bradycardia within 1 h after the intrathecal injection.[36] We therefore contacted the main author who was kind enough to provide the necessary data; there were 6% fetal bradycardia in controls receiving epidural bupivacaine, 10% with intrathecal sufentanil 1.5 μg and bupivacaine, and 16% with intrathecal sufentanil 7.5 μg alone (S. Halpern and M. Van de Velde, personal communication). A total of 1340 parturients were randomized in 11 trials; the average size of the control groups was 50 parturients (range 20–100). The methodologic quality of the trials was limited. Two trials described the method of randomization, and one described a method of concealment of allocation. In two trials, no method of blinding was used; in the others, there were different degrees of blinding, sometimes involving the parturient, sometimes the anesthesiologist, the midwife or the obstetrician. The fetal heart rate was assessed by a blinded observer in four of the trials.[31,35,36,38] Data for all but six of the patients who were recruited into the trials were available (see Table 7.3).[31,36,37]

Of 789 parturients who had received an intrathecal opioid, 66 (8.3%) had fetal bradycardia. Of 551 controls who had not received any intrathecal opioid, 26 (4.7%) had an episode of fetal bradycardia (Table 7.3).

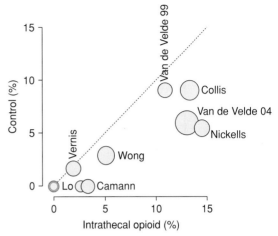

Fig. 7.1 Incidence of fetal bradycardia in randomized controlled trials. The size of the symbol represents the size of the trial. Three trials did not report on any events: Caldwell *et al.*,[25] Hepner *et al.*[30] and Pham *et al.*[34]

The event rate scatter suggested relative homogeneity of the data (Fig. 7.1). When data from all 11 trials were pooled, the combined odds ratio (fixed effect model) was 1.87 (95% confidence interval, 1.20–2.92), and the number-needed-to-harm (NNH) was 27. In three trials, no events were reported in both intrathecal opioid and control groups.[25,30,34]

In four trials, the absolute risk of having an episode of fetal bradycardia with intrathecal opioids was between 1.9% and 5.1%.[26,31,37,38] Finally, in four trials, the rate of fetal bradycardia with intrathecal opioids was between 10.9% and 14.5%.[27,33,35,36] Among the four trials that reported on the highest rates of fetal bradycardia with intrathecal opioids, the opioid regimens included fentanyl 25 μg,[27,33] sufentanil 1.5 μg[35] or sufentanil 7.5 μg.[36]

All eight trials that reported episodes of fetal bradycardia (omitting the trials with no events) found an increased risk with intrathecal opioids, and the difference reached statistical significance in one (Table 7.3).[36] Absolute risk differences ranged from 0.16%[37] to 9%[33]; corresponding NNH were 625 and 11. None of the randomized trials reported a decreased risk of fetal bradycardia with intrathecal opioids compared with control.

Table 7.3 Intrathecal opioids and the risk of fetal bradycardia. Evidence from randomized controlled trials. Where there was a statistically significant difference, the number-needed-to-harm (NNH) is reported with its 95% confidence interval.

Reference	IT opioid regimen	Control	Event	Randomization and concealment of allocation	Blinding Parturient	Caregiver	Fetal heart rate assessor	Exclusions (n)	No. of events/total number of parturients IT opioids	Control	Absolute difference (95% confidence interval)	NNH/NNB
Caldwell et al.[25]	IT fentanyl 25 µg + morphine 0.25 mg	Epi bupivacaine 0.25% + sufentanil 10 µg	Bradycardia	Not described	No	No	No	None	0/26 (0%)	0/33 (0%)	0.0%	∞
Camann et al.[26]	IT sufentanil 2, 5 or 10 µg or IT sufentanil 1 µg + Epi bupivacaine 2.5 mg or IT sufentanil 2.5 µg + Epi bupivacaine 6.25 mg or IT sufentanil 5 µg + Epi bupivacaine 12.5 mg	Epi bupivacaine 5, 12.5 or 25 mg	Transient fetal bradycardia	Not described	Yes	Yes	No	None	2/66 (3.0%)	0/34 (0%)	3% (−1.1 to 7.2%)	NNH = 33
Collis et al.[27]	IT fentanyl 25 µg + bupivacaine 2.5 mg	Epi bupivacaine 25 mg	Fetal bradycardia	Not described	No	No	No	None	13/98 (13.3%)	9/99 (9.1%)	4.2% (−4.6 to 13%)	NNH = 24
Hepner et al.[30]	IT fentanyl 25 µg + bupivacaine 2.5 mg	Epi bupivacaine 10 mg + fentanyl 32 µg + epinephrine 1/200,000	Fetal bradycardia	Not described	No	Yes	No	None	0/26 (0%)	0/24 (0%)	0.0%	∞
Lo et al.[31]	IT sufentanil 10 µg or IT fentanyl 10 µg + bupivacaine 2.5 mg	IT bupivacaine 2.5 mg + saline	Fetal bradycardia	Not described	Yes	Yes	Yes	One	1/39 (2.6%)	0/20 (0%)	2.6% (−2.4 to 7.5%)	NNH = 39

Study	Intervention	Comparator	Outcome	Randomization				Complications/exclusions				
Nickells et al.[33]	IT fentanyl 25 µg + bupivacaine 2.5 mg	Epi bupivacaine 12.5 mg + fentanyl 50 µg	Fetal bradycardia	Not described	Yes	Yes	No	None	10/69 (14.5%)	4/73 (5.5%)	9% (−0.8 to 18%)	NNH = 11
Pham et al.[34]	IT sufentanil 10 µg + Epi saline	Epi bupivacaine 30 mg + IT saline	Fetal bradycardia	Not described	Yes	Yes	No	None	0/20 (0%)	0/20 (0%)	0.0%	∞
Van de Velde et al.[35]	IT sufentanil 1.5 µg + epinephrine 2.5 µg + bupivacaine 2.5 mg	Epi bupivacaine 12.5 mg + sufentanil 7.5 µg + epinephrine 12.5 µg	Fetal bradycardia	Not described	Yes	Yes	Yes	None	6/55 (10.9%)	5/55 (9.1%)	1.8% (−9.4 to 13%)	NNH = 55
Wong et al.[38]	IT sufentanil 2.5 µg + bupivacaine 2.5 mg or IT sufentanil 5 µg + epinephrine 2.5 mg or IT sufentanil 10 µg + bupivacaine 2.5 mg	Epi bupivacaine 2.5 mg	Late decelerations	Computer-generated table	Yes	Yes	Yes	None	7/136 (5.1%)	1/34 (2.9%)	2.2% (−4.6 to 9%)	NNH = 45
Van de Velde et al.[36]	IT sufentanil 7.5 µg or IT sufentanil 1.5 µg + epinephrine 2.5 µg + bupivacaine 2.5 mg	Epi bupivacaine 12.5 mg + epinephrine 12.5 µg + sufentanil 7.5 µg	Fetal bradycardia	Computer-generated, stratified for parity, double-blind design	Yes	Yes	Yes	4 patients (3 in the CSE, 1 in the epidural group)	26/200 (13%)	6/100 (6%)	7% (0.6 to 14%)	NNH = 14 (7 to 166)
Vernis et al.[37]	IT sufentanil 5 µg + bupivacaine 2.5 mg	Epi bupivacaine 0.125% + epinephrine 2.5 µg/mL + sufentanil 7.5 µg	Fetal bradycardia	Randomization not described. "Blinded allocation"	Yes	Yes	No	1 patient in the epidural group was given a CSE and excluded	1/54 (1.9%)	1/59 (1.7%)	0.16% (−4.7% to 5%)	NNH = 637

CI, confidence interval; CSE, combined spinal epidural; Epi, epidural; IT, intrathecal; NNB, number needed to benefit; NNH, number needed to harm.

Comment

Do intrathecal opioids cause (as defined by the "rules of causation") fetal bradycardia within the first hour of administration?

1 The data appear to be relatively consistent. In all the comparative trials, there was an increase or no change in the incidence of fetal bradycardia in parturients who received intrathecal opioid.

2 The temporal relationship appears to be appropriate because many of the studies monitored the fetal heart rate before and after the intervention.

3 There is some weak evidence of dose–responsiveness. Recent data suggest an increased incidence of a non-reassuring fetal heart rate trace and fetal bradycardia in patients who receive a higher dose of intrathecal sufentanil compared with a lower dose.[36]

4 There is a potential biologic basis for the observation. Rapid relief of pain quickly reduces circulating catecholamine levels. Because catecholamines, particularly β-sympathomimetics, are known to reduce uterine tone, one could postulate that rapid withdrawal could increase uterine activity and tone. When this occurs, oxygen delivery to the fetus is reduced, leading to fetal bradycardia. The situation can rapidly be reversed by relaxing the uterus.[41]

It is therefore plausible that intrathecal opioids may cause an increased incidence of fetal bradycardia.

This analysis included data from 30 reports with different study architecture: 3066 parturients received different regimens of intrathecal opioids during labor and, of those, 143 had at least one episode of fetal bradycardia. Several issues need to be addressed.

First, there was a relationship between study architecture and the magnitude of the reported rates of fetal bradycardia in parturients who had received an intrathecal opioid injection. In uncontrolled case series, an episode of fetal bradycardia was reported in approximately 4% of parturients who had received an intrathecal opioid. In non-randomized controlled trials, this number was 6%. In adequately randomized controlled trials, the rate was above 8%. The question then is whether uncontrolled observations underestimated the risk or whether randomized trials overestimated the risk of fetal bradycardia with intrathecal opioids. Clinicians tend to blame clinical factors for differences in event rates. However, it is possible that factors related to study architecture contributed to this discrepancy. Uncontrolled observations are prone to multiple biases and confounding factors. In addition, the quality and validity of patient follow-up and data recording may not be as thorough in a retrospective chart review compared to a prospective randomized trial. Conversely, a properly conducted prospective cohort study with appropriately blinded assessors may yield more accurate results than a randomized trial in which fetal bradycardia was a secondary outcome.

Secondly, and partially related to the first issue, blinding has to be taken into account. Proper blinding controls for observer bias. There is empirical evidence that unblinded (open) studies tend to overestimate the efficacy of a treatment.[42] However, we do not know how this translates into the assessment of the risk of an intervention. We cannot exclude that the studies that lacked adequate blinding overestimated the risk with intrathecal opioids.

Thirdly, some randomized trials did not report any episodes of fetal bradycardia independent of the analgesic treatment. Zero-event trials occur when the event is very rare or when the trials are of limited size. Indeed, fetal bradycardia is a relatively rare event, and these trials were small; group sizes rarely exceeded 40 patients. Two randomized trials were large enough to identify an increased risk with intrathecal opioids that reached statistical significance.[29,36] One of those was disregarded by us because the method of fetal heart rate monitoring was not well controlled between groups.[29] There is no general agreement on how to report a zero event rate. It is possible that the event occurred but, because it was not an outcome of interest to the investigator, it was not reported. Alternatively, the trial may have been too small to detect a rare event. There is then an argument to regard small trials as inappropriate to assess this outcome.

Fourthly, these data need to be put into a clinical context. The risk of fetal bradycardia with intrathecal opioids has to be balanced against the potential benefit of this analgesic method; for instance, the gain of some minutes in the onset of adequate pain relief. We may quantify the additional risk that is related to the intrathecal opioid injection, and we may search for further opioid-related morbidity. The magnitude of the absolute risk difference (or its reciprocal, the NNH) indicated that between 20 and 30 women have to receive an intrathecal opioid during labor for one fetus to have an episode of bradycardia within 1 h of the injection. This risk may be reduced by reducing the dose of opioid.[36] However, the minimal effective opioid dose that still improves analgesia to a clinically relevant degree but does not increase the risk of fetal bradycardia remains unknown. Obstetricians, anesthesiologists and mothers may consider this additional risk to have clinical relevance. This begs the question as to whether these episodes of fetal bradycardia lead to additional morbidity. In the randomized trials, there were no more cesarean sections, instrumental deliveries, oxytocin usage or babies with a low Apgar score associated with intrathecal opioids.[6] This is reassuring, although in some practice settings an episode of fetal bradycardia is likely to be interpreted as a sign of fetal distress. As a consequence, additional treatments such as supplemental oxygen, left lateral position, vasopressors or uterine relaxation may be initiated. Also, parturients who receive intrathecal opioids may be discouraged from ambulation during labor because of the concern that fetal bradycardia may occur. Indeed, some may argue that parturients who receive intrathecal opioids should have continuous fetal heart rate monitoring for up to 1 h after the injection. Continuous monitoring itself may increase the incidence of cesarean section and operative vaginal delivery.[43]

Finally, the majority of women who receive an intrathecal opioid will have pruritus.[6] Itching is a well-known adverse effect of intrathecal opioid administration, and it may not be considered as a true medical problem; it never becomes chronic and it does not kill. However, some parturients may be extremely bothered by it. In addition to pruritus, any intrathecal injection carries a small but finite risk of neurologic damage to and infection of the central nervous system.[37]

In conclusion, multiple published reports of different study architecture suggest that there may be an additional risk of fetal bradycardia in women who receive intrathecal opioids during labor. While it appears that intrathecal opioids cause an increase in the incidence of fetal bradycardia, the magnitude of the increase is difficult to determine and may be small. In many settings where intrathecal opioids are used commonly, there appears to be no additional maternal or fetal morbidity. Because there is some evidence that the risk of fetal bradycardia may be related to the dose of the intrathecally administered opioid, clinicians have started to use very small doses of opioids on an empirical basis. In addition, it is unclear whether or not a difference exists between the different opioids that are currently used in clinical practice (e.g. fentanyl and sufentanil). Ideally, valid randomized and double-blind trials of appropriate size should be designed to address these issues. These trials, which will most likely be multicenter studies, should report on clinically relevant endpoints such as fetal and maternal morbidity associated with fetal bradycardia. In the meantime, clinicians should be aware of these findings when weighing the risks and benefits of administering intrathecal opioids in parturients.

References

1 Eisenach JC. Combined spinal–epidural analgesia in obstetrics. *Anesthesiology* 1999;**91**:299–302.

2 Collis RE, Baxandall ML, Srikantharajah ID, Edge G, Kadim MY, Morgan BM. Combined spinal epidural (CSE) analgesia: technique, management, and outcome of 300 mothers. *Int J Obstet Anesth* 1994;**3**:75–81.

3 Bucklin BA, Chestnut DH, Hawkins JL. Intrathecal opioids versus epidural local anesthetics for labor analgesia: a meta-analysis. *Reg Anesth Pain Med* 2002;**27**:23–30.

4 Palmer CM, Maciulla JE, Cork RC, Nogami WM, Gossler K, Alves D. The incidence of fetal heart rate changes after intrathecal fentanyl labor analgesia. *Anesth Analg* 1999;**88**:577–81.

5 Sackett DL, Hayes RB, Guyatt GH, Tugwell P. *Clinical Epidemiology: A Basic Science for Clinical Medicine.* Boston, Toronto, London: Little Brown and Co, 1991.

6 Mardirosoff C, Dumont L, Boulvain M, Tramèr MR. Fetal bradycardia due to intrathecal opioids for labour analgesia: a systematic review. *Br J Obstet Gynaecol* 2002;**109**:274–81.

7 Black N. Why we need observational studies to evaluate the effectiveness of health care. *BMJ* 1996;**312**:1215–8.

8 Arkoosh VA, Cooper M, Norris MC, *et al.* Intrathecal sufentanil dose response in nulliparous patients. *Anesthesiology* 1998;**89**:364–70.

9 Camann WR, Minzter BH, Denney RA, Datta S. Intrathecal sufentanil for labor analgesia: effects of added epinephrine. *Anesthesiology* 1993;**78**:870–4.

10 Cheng CJ, Sia AT, Lim EH, Loke GP, Tan HM. Either sufentanil or fentanyl, in addition to intrathecal bupivacaine, provide satisfactory early labour analgesia. *Can J Anesth* 2001;**48**:570–4.

11 Clarke VT, Smiley RM, Finster M. Uterine hyperactivity after intrathecal injection of fentanyl for analgesia during labor: a cause of fetal bradycardia? *Anesthesiology* 1994;**81**:1083.

12 Cohen SE, Cherry CM, Holbrook Jr RH, El Sayed YY, Gibson RN, Jaffe RA. Intrathecal sufentanil for labor analgesia: sensory changes, side-effects, and fetal heart rate changes. *Anesth Analg* 1993;**77**:1155–60.

13 Goodman SR, Kim-Lo SH, Ciliberto CF, Ridley DM, Smiley RM. Epinephrine is not a useful addition to intrathecal

fentanyl or fentanyl–bupivacaine for labor analgesia. *Reg Anesth Pain Med* 2002;**27**:374–9.

14 Herman NL, Choi KC, Affleck PJ, *et al.* Analgesia, pruritus, and ventilation exhibit a dose–response relationship in parturients receiving intrathecal fentanyl during labor. *Anesth Analg* 1999;**89**:378–83.

15 Honet JE, Arkoosh VA, Norris MC, Huffnagle HJ, Silverman NS, Leighton BL. Comparison among intrathecal fentanyl, meperidine, and sufentanil for labor analgesia. *Anesth Analg* 1992;**75**:734–9.

16 Hughes D, Hill D, Fee JP. Intrathecal ropivacaine or bupivacaine with fentanyl for labour. *Br J Anaesth* 2001;**87**:733–7.

17 Nelson KE, Rauch T, Terebuh V, D'Angelo R. A comparison of intrathecal fentanyl and sufentanil for labor analgesia. *Anesthesiology* 2002;**96**:1070–3.

18 Palmer CM, Cork RC, Hays R, Van Maren G, Alves D. The dose–response relation of intrathecal fentanyl for labor analgesia. *Anesthesiology* 1998;**88**:355–61.

19 Vaughan DJ, Ahmad N, Lillywhite NK, Lewis N, Thomas D, Robinson PN. Choice of opioid for initiation of combined spinal epidural analgesia in labour: fentanyl or diamorphine. *Br J Anaesth* 2001;**86**:567–9.

20 Vercauteren MP, Jacobs S, Jacquemyn Y, Adriaensen HA. Intrathecal labor analgesia with bupivacaine and sufentanil: the effect of adding 2.25 μg epinephrine. *Reg Anesth Pain Med* 2001;**26**:473–7.

21 Vercauteren MP, Hans G, De Decker K, Adriaensen HA. Levobupivacaine combined with sufentanil and epinephrine for intrathecal labor analgesia: a comparison with racemic bupivacaine. *Anesth Analg* 2001;**93**:996–1000.

22 Eberle RL, Norris MC, Eberle AM, Naulty JS, Arkoosh VA. The effect of maternal position on fetal heart rate during epidural or intrathecal labor analgesia. *Am J Obstet Gynecol* 1998;**179**:150–5.

23 Nielsen PE, Erickson JR, Abouleish EI, Perriatt S, Sheppard C. Fetal heart rate changes after intrathecal sufentanil or epidural bupivacaine for labor analgesia: incidence and clinical significance. *Anesth Analg* 1996;**83**:742–6.

24 Van de Velde M, Vercauteren M, Vandermeersch E. Fetal heart rate abnormalities after regional analgesia for labor pain: the effect of intrathecal opioids. *Reg Anesth Pain Med* 2001;**26**:257–62.

25 Caldwell LE, Rosen MA, Shnider SM. Subarachnoid morphine and fentanyl for labor analgesia: efficacy and adverse effects. *Reg Anesth* 1994;**19**:2–8.

26 Camann W, Abouleish A, Eisenach J, Hood D, Datta S. Intrathecal sufentanil and epidural bupivacaine for labor analgesia: dose–response of individual agents and in combination. *Reg Anesth Pain Med* 1998;**23**:457–62.

27 Collis RE, Davies DW, Aveling W. Randomised comparison of combined spinal–epidural and standard epidural analgesia in labour. *Lancet* 1995;**345**:1413–6.

28 Dresner M, Bamber J, Calow C, Freeman J, Charlton P. Comparison of low-dose epidural with combined spinal–epidural analgesia for labour. *Br J Anaesth* 1999;**83**:756–60.

29 Gambling DR, Sharma SK, Ramin SM, *et al.* A randomized study of combined spinal–epidural analgesia versus intravenous meperidine during labor: impact on cesarean delivery rate. *Anesthesiology* 1998;**89**:1336–44.

30 Hepner DL, Gaiser RR, Cheek TG, Gutsche BB. Comparison of combined spinal–epidural and low dose epidural for labour analgesia. *Can J Anesth* 2000;**47**:232–6.

31 Lo WK, Chong JL, Chen LH. Combined spinal epidural for labour analgesia: duration, efficacy and side-effects of adding sufentanil or fentanyl to bupivacaine intrathecally vs plain bupivacaine. *Sing Med J* 1999;**40**:639–43.

32 Nageotte MP, Larson D, Rumney PJ, Sidhu M, Hollenbach K. Epidural analgesia compared with combined spinal–epidural analgesia during labor in nulliparous women. *N Engl J Med* 1997;**337**:1715–9.

33 Nickells JS, Vaughan DJ, Lillywhite NK, Loughnan B, Hasan M, Robinson PN. Speed of onset of regional analgesia in labour: a comparison of the epidural and spinal routes. *Anaesthesia* 2000;**55**:17–20.

34 Pham LH, Camann WR, Smith MP, Datta S, Bader AM. Hemodynamic effects of intrathecal sufentanil compared with epidural bupivacaine in laboring parturients. *J Clin Anesth* 1996;**8**:497–501.

35 Van de Velde M, Mignolet K, Vandermeersch E, Van Assche A. Prospective, randomized comparison of epidural and combined spinal epidural analgesia during labor. *Acta Anaesthesiol Belg* 1999;**50**:129–36.

36 Van de Velde M, Teunkens A, Hanssens M, Vandermeersch E, Verhaeghe J. Intrathecal sufentanil and fetal heart rate abnormalities: a double-blind, double placebo-controlled trial comparing two forms of combined spinal epidural analgesia with epidural analgesia in labor. *Anesth Analg* 2004; **98**:1153–9.

37 Vernis L, Duale C, Storme B, Mission JP, Rol B, Schoeffler P. Perispinal analgesia for labour followed by patient-controlled infusion with bupivacaine and sufentanil: combined spinal–epidural vs epidural analgesia alone. *Eur J Anaesthesiol* 2004;**21**:186–92.

38 Wong CA, Scavone BM, Loffredi M, Wang WY, Peaceman AM, Ganchiff JN. The dose–response of intrathecal sufentanil added to bupivacaine for labor analgesia. *Anesthesiology* 2000;**92**:1553–8.

39 Campbell DC, Camann WR, Datta S. The addition of bupivacaine to intrathecal sufentanil for labor analgesia. *Anesth Analg* 1995;**81**:305–9.

40 Harsten A, Gillberg L, Hakansson L, Olsson M. Intrathecal sufentanil compared with epidural bupivacaine analgesia in labour. *Eur J Anaesthesiol* 1997;**14**:642–5.

41 Mercier FJ, Dounas M, Bouaziz H, Lhuissier C, Benhamou D. Intravenous nitroglycerin to relieve intrapartum fetal distress related to uterine hyperactivity: a prospective observational study. *Anesth Analg* 1997;**84**:1117–20.

42 Schulz KF, Chalmers I, Hayes RJ, Altman DG. Empirical evidence of bias: dimensions of methodological quality associated with estimates of treatment effects in controlled trials. *JAMA* 1995;**273**:408–12.

43 Thacker SB, Stroup D, Chang M. Continuous electronic heart rate monitoring for fetal assessment during labor. *Cochrane Database of Systematic Reviews* 2001;CD000063.

CHAPTER 8

Epidural catheter design and the incidence of complications

Margaret Srebrnjak & Stephen H. Halpern

Introduction

Continuous epidural analgesia is an excellent modality for pain relief in labor. However, success rates are hampered by a measurable incidence of complications. The presumed causes of these complications are varied. While controlling for patient-related factors, investigators have studied epidural needle insertion techniques, the direction and depth of catheter placement, the physical properties of the catheters and the way solutions are injected.

Early epidural catheters were simply crude rubber ureteral catheters.[1,2] They were round-nosed with two orifices approximately 1 cm from the end. Over time, manufacturers developed specialized epidural catheters that were manufactured with various grades of plastic or incorporated a soft, flexible, stainless steel wire. Some of these required a stylet for proper insertion.[3] Other manufacturers modified the distal end, incorporating more than one orifice proximal to a blunt end. It was during this evolution that anesthesiologists recognized that catheter design had significant effects on the incidence of complications.[4,5] The purpose of this systematic review is to determine whether the design of epidural catheters, both in the number of distal holes and the material from which they are manufactured, influences the incidence of successful labor analgesia and complications.

Methods

Search strategy

The data for this chapter comes from a comprehensive, systematic computerized search from January 1985 to December 2003 of MEDLINE®, EMBASE® and the Cochrane Register of Controlled Trials, in English, that compared epidural catheters of different designs in women in labor or having cesarean section. We used the following medical subject headings (MeSH) [regional anesthesia], [obstetrical anesthesia], [neuraxial anesthesia] and [epidural catheters]. Other text terms used were [epidural catheter], [uniport catheter], [multiport catheter], [endhole catheter], [terminal hole catheter] and [single-endhole catheter].

We hand searched the major anesthesia journals and abstract supplements for the same time interval, including *Anesthesiology, Anesthesia and Analgesia, Canadian Journal of Anesthesia, Anaesthesia and Intensive Care, British Journal of Anaesthesia, Anaesthesia, International Journal of Obstetric Anesthesia* and *Regional Anesthesia and Pain Medicine*. Finally, we hand searched the reference lists of review articles and all articles considered for eligibility, as well as relevant articles in our own personal files. We did not seek unpublished data.

Inclusion criteria

We included all English language, published controlled trials (both randomized controlled trials and cohort studies) and abstracts of scientific meetings that compared catheters of different designs in obstetric patients. These differences included the number and/or position of the distal holes and the material from which the catheters were made. The two authors independently searched and assessed all titles and abstracts identified from the literature search for relevance.

Validity assessment

Following selection of the eligible articles, each reviewer extracted data and performed the quality score independently. We rated all full manuscripts of randomized studies for quality using a previously validated 5-point scale (see Appendix for a full description of the scale).[6] Studies with a score of 3 or more were considered to be of good quality. The abstracts and cohort studies were not rated.

Outcome measurements

The main outcomes were:

1 incidence of paresthesias;
2 incidence of intravascular cannulation; and
3 incidence of inadequate labor analgesia.

We included pain on catheter insertion in the definition of paresthesia. We defined intravascular cannulation as either documented "blood in the catheter" or "signs of systemic toxicity," only if the two outcomes were reported to be mutually exclusive. In cases of doubt, we reported the incidence of "blood in the catheter." Patients with inadequate labor analgesia were uncomfortable and/or had objective evidence of unilateral or missed segment analgesia. This outcome did not include patients in whom there was no analgesia or in whom the epidural catheter could not be passed.

Results

We found 10 randomized controlled trials in English that met the inclusion criteria and separated them into two categories. The first category was made up of five studies that compared uniport with multiport catheters made from the same material and by the same manufacturer (Table 8.1).[7–11] The second category was made up of five studies (three were available only as abstracts) that compared catheters made from different materials and different manufacturers.[12–16] We also identified four cohort studies that compared catheters made from different materials (Table 8.1).[3,17–19]

All studies were carried out on laboring patients[8–16] but one also included emergency and elective cesarean section patients.[7] D'Angelo et al.[8] and Michael et al.[10] limited their participants to those who were ASA 1 and ASA 2, while the remaining eight studies included all patients regardless of ASA status.[7–16] Only one randomized controlled trial had a quality score of 3 or higher (Table 8.2).[8]

Nylon uniport and nylon multiport catheters and the incidence of complications

Each of the five studies[7–11] compared catheters from the same manufacturer. D'Angelo et al.[8] used Braun® catheters, the remaining four studies used Portex® catheters.[7,9–11] Before the study began, one center supplied multiport catheters,[7] one supplied uniport catheters,[8] one supplied either type at the discretion of the anesthesiologist.[9] In two, the type of catheter was unknown.[10,11]

The incidence of paresthesia and intravenous cannulation are shown in Table 8.3. All five studies reported the incidence of paresthesias.[7–11] The incidence ranged from 8.5% to 42% with little difference between catheters within each study. Four investigators reported data for intravascular cannulation.[7–10]. Blood vessel trauma occurred in 4–12% of patients with a consistently higher incidence with multiport catheters. The difference was statistically significant in two studies.[9,10] One study reported the incidence of "blood in the catheter" as well as "blood on aspiration at catheter insertion."[11] While it was not possible to tell whether these categories were mutually exclusive, there was a higher incidence of both in the multiport group. This was statistically significant for the outcome "blood in the catheter" (3.3% vs 11.4%, $P < 0.0001$) as described by the authors.

All five studies reported the incidence of inadequate analgesia[7–11] (Table 8.4). Collier and Gatt[7], D'Angelo et al.[8] and Michael et al.[10] found a statistically significant increase of inadequate analgesia in uniport catheters with values ranging from 31–32.7% for the uniport catheters to 11–21.2% for the multiport catheters.[7,8,10] Dickson et al.[9] and Morrison et al.[11] found a slight trend to poorer analgesia with uniport catheters with values of 14.1% and 16.7% compared with 13.7% and 14.8% with multiport catheters, respectively. The diagnosis of "inadequate analgesia" varied among studies and was assessed by the patient, nurse and/or the physician. One study reported objective sensory testing as the sole measure of inadequate analgesia.[8] The management of inadequate analgesia also varied among studies. Some studies described withdrawal of the catheter and top-ups[7–9] and others described only top-ups.[10] Morrison et al.[11] did not discuss the management of inadequate analgesia.

The best indication of the success of the maneuvers was reflected in the incidence of "resiting a catheter due to inadequate analgesia." Three studies reported

Table 8.1 Characteristics of studies comparing epidural catheters.

Study	Quality score	Patient sample size for specific catheter types	Comments
RCT Category 1. Catheters made from the same material			
Collier & Gatt (1994)[7]	2	50 nylon uniport Portex® 52 nylon multiport Portex®	Included cesarean section and labor epidurals "Inadequate analgesia" outcome included only labor epidurals (35 uniport, 36 multiport). Study stopped early because obstetricians and midwives complained of inadequate analgesia in patients who received uniport catheters. All epidurals performed by the authors
D'Angelo et al. (1997)[8]	3	242 nylon uniport Braun® 245 nylon multiport Braun®	Not blinded. Catheters passed 6 cm into the epidural space
Dickson et al. (1997)[9]	2	Total N = 364 188 nylon uniport Portex® 176 nylon multiport Portex®	Different number of patients (denominator) included in each outcome. Denominator estimated, leading to some rounding imprecision
Michael et al. (1989)[10]	1	401 nylon uniport Portex® 401 nylon multiport Portex®	Number of patients randomized is not known. Uniport catheter passed 1.5 cm into the epidural space, multiport 2.5 cm Anesthesiologist not blinded
Morrison & Buchan (1990)[11]	2	245 nylon uniport Portex® 229 nylon multiport Portex®	Sample size based on the number of questionnaires returned, not the number of patients randomized Study did not include 14 patients in each group who had catheters resited because of inadequate analgesia These were added for the outcome "inadequate analgesia"
RCT Category 2. Catheters made from different materials			
Banwell et al. (1998)[12]	2	103 spring-wound uniport Arrow® 97 nylon multiport Portex®	Outcomes recorded attempts rather than patients Patients who had failed blocks and venous cannulation were counted twice for the repeated attempt "Inadequate analgesia" not recorded
Herbstman & Newman (1997)[13]*	Not rated	103 variety of uniport (BD®, Arrow®, Abbott®, Braun®) 82 variety of multiport (BD®, Abbott®, Braun®)	All labor epidurals part of CSE 7 varieties of catheters studied
Juneja et al. (1995)[15]*	Not rated	735 nylon uniport Braun® 742 spring-wound uniport Arrow® 739 copolymer bullet-tip Kendall®	Paresthesias recorded only Unclear if Kendall® bullet-tip a multiport catheter
Juneja et al. (1996)[14]*	Not rated	1110 nylon uniport Braun® 1122 spring-wound uniport Arrow® 1122 copolymer Kendall®	Vascular cannulation recorded only Unclear if Kendall® bullet-tip a multiport catheter
Rolbin et al. (1987)[16]	2	75 nylon multiport Portex® 75 polyurethane multiport Vas-Cath®	"Inadequate analgesia" outcome not recorded
Non-RCT studies			
Hayashi et al. (2001)[17]*	Not rated	1060 spring-wound uniport Arrow® 961 polyamide multiport Braun®	Included small number of elective cesarean section patients.
Jaime et al. (2000)[18]	Not rated	1352 spring-wound uniport Arrow® 1260 nylon multiport Portex®	Prospective quality assurance study
Spriggs et al. (1995)[19]*	Not rated	50 spring-wound uniport Arrow® 51 polyamide uniport Braun®	
Segal et al. (1997)[3]	Not rated	433 stylet uniport Baxter® 439 multiport Burron®	Cohort "catastrophic " study

CSE, combined spinal epidural; RCT, randomized controlled trial.

* Studies are published abstracts from scientific meeting.

Table 8.2 Validity score for randomized controlled trials (see Appendix for rating scale).

	Randomization		Blinding		Description of withdrawals and drop-outs
Study	Stated	Appropriate	Double-blinded	Blinding appropriate	
RCT Category 1. Catheters made from the same material					
Collier & Gatt[7]	1	0	0	0	1
D'Angelo et al.[8]	1	1	0	0	1
Dickson et al.[9]	1	1	0	0	0
Michael et al.[10]	1	0	0	0	0
Morrison & Buchan[11]	1	1	0	0	0
RCT Category 2. Catheters made from different materials					
Banwell et al.[12]	1	1	0	0	0
Herbstman & Newman[13]*	Not rated				
Juneja et al. (1995)[15]*	Not rated				
Juneja et al. (1996)[14]*	Not rated				
Rolbin et al.[16]	1	0	0	0	1

RCT, randomized controlled trial.
* Studies are published abstracts from scientific meeting.

this outcome.[7,10,11] The incidence ranged from 5.4–11.4% with uniport catheters to 0–5.8% with multiport catheters. The incidence consistently favored multiport catheters and was statistically significant in two studies[7,10] (Table 8.3). Dickson et al.[9] managed inadequate analgesia in a number of ways, including local anesthetic and opioid top-ups, catheter withdrawal and postural changes. Out of his 364 patients, only two required resiting because of inadequate analgesia, although the group(s) to which these patients belonged was not reported.[9] Finally, although D'Angelo et al.[8] did not report the incidence of resiting because of inadequate analgesia, they provided an overall resiting incidence of 10.7% for the uniport catheters and 10.2% for the multiport catheters. This group reported a significantly higher incidence of inadequate analgesia in the uniport group before the maneuvers.[8]

Catheter material and the incidence of complications

Four studies compared a flexible spring-wound uniport catheter (Arrow®) with a traditional nylon catheter.[12–15] The remaining study by Rolbin et al.[16] compared a soft polyurethane multiport catheter with a firm nylon multiport catheter.

The studies comparing the Arrow® catheter found a significant decrease in paresthesias in these catheters with values ranging from 0% to 2.7% as compared with 15.2–35.5% for the firm catheters.[12,13,15] The study by Rolbin et al.[16] also found a significant decrease in paresthesia with the soft polyurethane catheter (24%) compared to the firm nylon catheter (44%)[16] (Table 8.3).

Banwell et al.,[12] Herbstman & Newman[13] and Juneja et al.[14,15] found less intravascular cannulation with soft catheters, with values ranging from 0% to 1% as compared with 4.9% to 11.3% for the firmer catheters.[12–14] Rolbin et al.[16] also found a trend to less intravascular cannulation in the soft polyurethane catheters as compared with the firm catheters, 6.7% versus 12%[16] (Table 8.3).

Only Herbstman & Newman[13] looked at the incidence of inadequate analgesia in two types of catheters (uniport and multiport) made from different materials. Their uniport group of four types of catheters had an inadequate analgesia rate of 10.7% as compared with 2.4% of the multiport group of three catheters ($P = 0.02$) (Table 8.4). They did not carry out a subgroup analysis to see if one catheter material was better than another.[13]

Table 8.3 Summary of the incidence of paresthesias and intravascular cannulation.

Study	Paresthesias	Intravascular cannulation	Comments
RCT Category 1. Catheters made from the same material			
Collier & Gatt[7]	28.0% uniport Portex® 17.3% multiport Portex®	4.0% uniport Portex® 7.7% multiport Portex®	Management of intravascular catheters not noted
D'Angelo *et al.*[8]	41% uniport Braun® 42% multiport Braun®	7.0% uniport Braun® 6.5% multiport Braun®	"Bloody catheters" incrementally withdrawn but did not report degree of success
Dickson *et al.*[9]	23.0% uniport Portex® 19.4% multiport Portex®	4.3% uniport Portex® 12.1% multiport Portex® $P < 0.05$ In addition, 3 patients in each group experienced "toxic symptoms on test dose." Of these, two required catheter replacement (uniport group), one needed manipulation (multiport group)	Management of intravascular catheters unclear
Michael *et al.*[10]	12.2% uniport Portex® 8.5% multiport Portex®	5.7% uniport Portex® 10.5% multiport Portex® $P = 0.01$	In all cases of intravascular cannulation the problem was recognized and the catheter adjusted
Morrison & Buchan[11]	31.3% uniport Portex® 29.2% multiport Portex® These data represent the total of "right leg paresthesia + left leg paresthesia"	"Blood in catheter" 3.3% uniport 11.4% multiport $P < 0.0001$ Blood on aspiration after catheter insertion 4.1% uniport 7.4% multiport $P = NS$	The difference between the two ways of detecting intravascular placement were not explained in the text
RCT Category 2. Catheters made from different materials			
Banwell *et al.*[12]	2.7% uniport Arrow® 35.5% multiport Portex® $P < 0.05$	0% uniport Arrow® 11.3% multiport Portex® $P < 0.05$	"Bloody catheters" were withdrawn automatically and resited
Herbstman & Newman[13]*	28.0% uniport – all 4 catheters 31.7% multiport – all 3 catheters	1.0% uniport – all 4 catheters 15.9% multiport – all 3 catheters $P < 0.05$	"Bloody catheters" repositioned with good effect in 77%
Juneja *et al.* (1995)[15]*	2.1% uniport Arrow® 32.0% uniport Braun® 15.2% bullet tip Kendall® $P < 0.05$	Not reported	
Juneja *et al.* (1996)[14]*	Not reported	0.53% uniport Arrow®* 4.68% uniport Braun® 5.61% bullet tip Kendall® *$P < 0.05$ compared with the other two types of catheter	
Rolbin *et al.*[16]	44% multiport Portex® 24% multiport Vas-Cath® $P < 0.05$	12 .0% multiport Portex® 6.7% multiport Vas-Cath® $P < 0.05$	

NS, not significant; RCT, randomized controlled trial.
* Studies are published abstracts from scientific meeting.

Table 8.4 Summary of the incidence of inadequate analgesia and management.

Study	Distance in epidural space	Test dose	Initial bolus solution after test dose	Incidence of inadequate analgesia	Management of inadequate analgesia		Resiting due to inadequate analgesia effect	Overall resiting effect	Comments
					Catheter manipulated	Top-up solution			
Collier & Gatt[7]	3–4 cm uniport 3–4 cm multiport	3 mL via needle 4 mL via catheter 0.375% bupivacaine	6–10 mL 0.375% bupivacaine	31% uniport 11% multiport $P < 0.05$	Catheter withdrawal, after failure of 1st top-up	4–8 mL 0.375% bupivacaine	11.4% uniport 0% multiport $P < 0.05$	?	
D'Angelo et al.[8]	6 ± 4.6 cm uniport 6 ± 4.6 cm multiport	2 + 5 mL 2% lidocaine	3 mL 2% lidocaine	31.8% uniport 21.2% multiport $P < 0.05$	Catheter withdrawn 3 cm	10 mL 2% lidocaine	?	10.7% uniport 10.2% multiport	Inadequate analgesia defined as inadequate sensory level
Dickson et al.[9]	2–4 cm uniport 3–5 cm multiport	4 mL 2% lidocaine	8 mL 0.25% or 0.5% bupivacaine	Initial 14.1% uniport 13.7% multiport (NS) Developing after infusion: 16.4% uniport 8.4% multiport $P = 0.02$	Inconsistently used	8 mL 0.25% bupivacaine Inconsistent use of opioids	Two catheters resited but unclear which group(s)	?	Concentration of bupivacaine determined by clinical judgment of the anesthesiologist
Michael et al.[10]	1.5 cm uniport 2.5 cm multiport	2 mL 0.5% bupivacaine + 5 µg/cc epinephrine	8 mL 0.25% bupivacaine	32.7% uniport 13.7% multiport $P < 0.05$	No	16 mL 0.125% bupivacaine	5.7% uniport 1.0% multiport $P < 0.05$	?	
Morrison & Buchan[11]	< 3 cm uniport < 3 cm multiport	4 mL 2% lidocaine	?	16.7% uniport 14.8% multiport	?	?	5.4% uniport 5.8% multiport	?	
Banwell et al.[12]	5 cm uniport 5 cm multiport	Outcome not documented							
Herbstman & Newman[13]*	5 cm uniport 5 cm multiport	Outcome not documented		10.7% uniport 2.4% multiport $P < 0.05$					
Juneja et al. (1995)[15]*		Outcome not documented							
Juneja et al. (1996)[14]*		Outcome not documented							
Rolbin et al.[16]*		Outcome not documented							

NS, not significant.

* Studies are published abstracts from scientific meeting.

Discussion

In order to put these results into a context that one can use clinically, one needs to be aware of how methodologic differences within the studies could affect their outcomes. The following sections briefly review the literature about spinal anatomy, the path of epidural catheters and the spread of fluids that have been introduced into the epidural space. Using this information, one can draw some conclusions about the outcomes we discovered in the two categories of studies.

The anatomy and physiology of the epidural space

The epidural space is a fat- and vessel-filled space surrounding the dural sac. It is bordered by bony vertebral structures superficially. At the intervertebral foramina, the epidural space is continuous with para-vertebral fascial planes, resembling a long cylinder with regular holes along its length. Each of these holes represents the area where spinal nerves pass through to the periphery from the spinal cord. The epidural space is not symmetrical, rather it is divided by the dural sac and its nerve roots into a small anterior area and larger posterior space. Computed tomographic (CT) studies of the lumbar spine at the level of the vertebral disc show the surface of the anterior dura is in immediate contact with the posterior longitudinal ligament. This results in two anterior epidural areas that do not communicate with each other directly. Anatomic studies of the larger posterior epidural space are more controversial, with some investigators reporting the presence of inconsistent bands of tissue that may act as a barrier to the flow of solutions in the area.[20–23]

While it would be preferable to have catheter tips in the middle of the posterior epidural space, less than half of catheter tips end up there.[21] Radiologic studies show that epidural catheters frequently loop and coil. Some may pass out intervertebral foramina or lodge in the epidural space.[21] Stiffer catheters tend to resist curling but often coil within 5 cm.[2,24–26] The soft Arrow® catheter coils within 2.8 cm and only 14% remain straight at 4 cm.[27] This suggests that softer catheters are easily deflected by blood vessels and nerve roots, likely causing less trauma. Attempts to reliably direct catheters into ideal positions have been unsuccessful.[28]

Spread of local anesthetics to the appropriate nerve roots is important when providing analgesia. Using radiologic contrast, Collier showed that solutions preferentially spread cephalad from the injection site over a number of vertebral levels.[29] He also showed contrast extending out a variable distance through the intervertebral foramina producing a "Christmas tree" pattern.[29] However, detailed CT scan studies by Hogan[21] showed a great variability in the distribution of solution particularly with small volumes. Magides *et al.*[30] demonstrated that the distribution was not dependent on whether the catheter was uniport or multiport. When greater volumes of solution were injected the uniformity of spread improved. Clinically it has been observed that additional local anesthetic volumes improve epidural analgesia.[31] Hogan's most striking conclusion was that a variety of catheter tip positions and patterns of solution spread often resulted in normal epidural analgesia.[21]

The distance catheters are fed into the epidural space has significant implications on the functioning of those catheters. The distance can also change unpredictably because catheters are not static below the skin. With non-specific patient movements, catheters can move up to several centimeters both in and out of the back. In fact, they move with changing from a sitting to a lying position and with body habitus.[32,33] Although the initial catheter "movement" may be related to the readjustment of back tissues, over the long-term, migrating catheters have been associated with poorer analgesia overall.[33–35] In the study by Beilin *et al.*[36] patients were randomized to receive multiport catheters, inserted to a depth of 3, 5 and 7 cm. They found that the incidence of intravascular cannulation increased as the depth of insertion increased. There was no difference in the incidence of paresthesia among the groups. Finally, catheters passed 3 and 7 cm had an increased incidence of inadequate labor analgesia (approximately 33%) compared with 5 cm (6%). They postulate that all three ports of the 3-cm multiport catheters were not completely in the epidural space for the duration of the testing period and the 7-cm catheters were too deep.[36] D'Angelo *et al.*[37] randomized patients who had received uniport catheters inserted to a depth of 2, 4, 6 and 8 cm. They found a low rate of inadequate labor analgesia in the 2-cm group but 8% of the catheters dislodged over the course of labor. There was a high incidence (9–13%) of unilateral analgesia in patients of the 4, 6 and 8 cm groups but only 1.5% of these dislodged.[37]

Nylon uniport and multiport catheters

The number of holes in a catheter or their location had no impact on the paresthesia rates, indicating that the manufacturing differences between open-tip nylon catheters and closed blunt tipped catheters were insignificant for this outcome.[7–11] Blood vessel trauma occurred more frequently in multiport catheters.[7–11] Michael et al.[10] and Dickson et al.[9] fed their multiport catheters 1 cm deeper than uniport catheters. This may have caused the increased incidence of intravascular cannulation in these studies.[36,37] The clinical significance of an intravascular catheter depends on how that complication is managed. The options may include resiting the epidural catheter or partial withdrawal of the catheter. Finally, some authors have suggested that rather than causing more trauma, multiport catheters are simply more likely to detect intravascular cannulation and injury, but this has yet to be confirmed.[7,9–11]

The incidence of adequate analgesia was consistently higher with nylon multiport catheters compared with nylon uniport catheters; in three studies[8–10] the difference was statistically significant.[7,8,10] In these studies, the catheters were inserted a variable distance into the epidural space: less than 5 cm in four studies[7,9–11] and 6 cm in the fifth.[8] The initial local anesthetic volumes were 10–12 mL in three studies and 13–17 mL in one. The fifth study did not report the dose.[11] There was no relationship between the volume of local anesthetic and the incidence of inadequate analgesia. However, the majority of patients in each study responded to local anesthetic top-ups. Collier & Gatt[7] hypothesized that the proximal holes of a multiport catheter may allow for delivery of solution closer to the midline, resulting in more uniform spread at smaller volumes. In uniport catheters, a top-up (a larger volume) may compensate for the limitations of the end-hole. None of our selected studies looked specifically at how opioid solutions would affect analgesia with the two catheters. Other studies have shown that epidural opioids not only reduce the amount of local anesthetic required for analgesia but they may improve the quality as well.[38–40]

The need to replace the epidural catheter can be the result of blood in the catheter or inadequate analgesia, and this outcome may be an important measure of possible patient dissatisfaction and inconvenience. Unfortunately, not all of the investigators reported this outcome. D'Angelo et al.[8] noted the incidence of resiting catheters overall and found no difference. Whether or not the increased incidence of intravascular cannulation associated with multiport catheters in the other studies resulted in an increased number of epidural catheters that needed to be replaced is unknown.

Catheter material

There is little doubt that catheter material has significant effects on the incidence of complications. All the studies looking at the spring-wound catheter found much lower paresthesia and intravascular cannulation rates.[12–15] These findings are supported by the cohort studies of Hayashi et al.[17] and Jaime et al.[18] The soft catheters used by Rolbin et al.[16] also produced a lower incidence of paresthesias and vascular cannulation, although only the former outcome was statistically significant. These results are not surprising because soft spring-wound catheters deflect off epidural structures relatively early and easily from needle exit.[27]

Only one randomized controlled trial, reported as an abstract, compared the incidence of effective labor analgesia between spring-wound catheters and nylon catheters.[13] However, the study was relatively small and there were seven different types of catheters. They found no difference in the incidence of poor analgesia when they compared uniport with multiport catheters (all manufacturers). The results from two larger cohort studies confirmed that there was no difference among the catheter types.[17,18] The advantage possessed by multiple apertures in a multiport catheter may be less important in soft catheters, because they tend to curl up relatively easily at the site of insertion rather than traveling into peripheral compartments.

Conclusions

Epidural catheter design influences the incidence of paresthesia, intravascular cannulation and poor analgesia when used for labor. Compared with uniport catheters of the same material, nylon multiport catheters are associated with a higher incidence of satifactory analgesia. This comes with an increased risk of intravascular cannulation. Soft catheters are associated with a reduced incidence of paresthesia and blood vessel damage compared with stiffer catheters. Unfortunately, there are few data from randomized controlled trials concerning the incidence of adequate analgesia. The clinical significance of these findings depends on the subsequent clinical management of the complications.

References

1 Curbelo MM. Continuous peridural segmental anesthesia by means of a ureteral catheter. *Anesth Analg* 1949;**28**:13–23.

2 Frumin MJ, Schwartz H. Continuous segmental peridural anesthesia. *Anesthesiology* 1952;**13**:488–95.

3 Segal S, Eappen S, Datta S. Superiority of multi-orifice over single-orifice epidural catheters for labor analgesia and cesarean delivery. *J Clin Anesth* 1997;**9**:109–12.

4 Ward CF, Osborne R, Benumof JL, Saidman LJ. A hazard of double-orifice epidural catheters. *Anesthesiology* 1978;**48**:362–4.

5 Beck H, Brassow F, Doehn M, *et al*. Epidural catheters of the multi-orifice type: dangers and complications. *Acta Anaesthesiol Scand* 1986;**30**:549–55.

6 Jadad A, Moore R, Carroll D. Assessing the quality of reports of randomized clinical trials: is blinding necessary? *Control Clin Trials* 1996;**17**:1–12.

7 Collier CB, Gatt SP. Epidural catheters for obstetrics; terminal hole or lateral eyes? *Reg Anesth* 1994;**19**:378–85.

8 D'Angelo R, Foss ML, Livesay CH. A comparison of multiport and uniport epidural catheters in laboring patients. *Anesth Analg* 1997;**84**:1276–9.

9 Dickson MAS, Moores C, McClure JH. Comparison of single, end-holed and multi-orifice extradural catheters when used for continuous infusion of local anaesthetic during labour. *Br J Anaesth* 1997;**79**:279–300.

10 Michael S, Richmond MN, Birks RJS. A comparison between open-end (single hole) and closed-end (three lateral holes) epidural catheters. *Anaesthesia* 1989;**44**:578–80.

11 Morrison LMM, Buchan AS. Comparison of complications associated with single-holed and multi-holed extradural catheters. *Br J Anaesth* 1990;**64**:183–5.

12 Banwell BR, Morley-Forster P, Krause R. Decreased incidence of complications in parturients with the Arrow® (FlexTip Plus) epidural catheter. *Can J Anaesth* 1998;**45**:370–2.

13 Herbstman CH, Newman LM. Evaluation of single versus multiple orifice epidural catheters in laboring women. *Anesthesiology* 1997;**87**:A908.

14 Juneja M, Kargas G, Miller D, Perry E, Botic Z, Rigor B. Incidence of epidural vein cannulation in parturients with three different epidural catheters. *Reg Anesth* 1996;**21**:A4.

15 Juneja M, Kargas GA, Miller DL, *et al*. Comparison of epidural catheters induced paresthesia in parturients. *Reg Anesth* 1995;**20**:A152.

16 Rolbin SH, Hew E, Ogilvie G. A comparison of two types of epidural catheters. *Can J Anaesth* 1987;**34**:459–61.

17 Hayashi RD, Cross JS, Jones BR. Efficacy and complications of two types of epidural catheters for obstetric anesthesia. *Anesthesiology* 2001;**94**:A26.

18 Jaime F, Mandell GFL, Vallejo MC, Ramanathan S. Uniport soft-tip, open-ended catheters versus multiport firm-tipped close-ended catheters for epidural labor analgesia: a quality assurance study. *J Clin Anesth* 2000;**12**:89–93.

19 Spriggs LE, Vasdev GM, Leicht CH. Clinical evaluation of wire impregnated epidural catheter with standard epidural catheter for labor analgesia. *Reg Anesth* 1995;**20**:A154.

20 Usubiaga JE, Dos Reis A, Usubiaga LE. Epidural misplacement of catheters and mechanisms of unilateral blockade. *Anesthesiology* 1970;**32**:158–61.

21 Hogan Q. Epidural catheter tip position and distribution of injectate evaluated by computed tomography. *Anesthesiology* 1999;**90**:964–70.

22 Fukushige T, Kano T, Sano T. Radiographic investigation of unilateral epidural block after single injection. *Anesthesiology* 1997;**87**:1574–5.

23 Blomberg R. The dorsomedian connective tissue band in the lumbar epidural space of humans. *Anesth Analg* 1986;**65**:747–52.

24 Bridenbaugh LD, Moore DC, Bagdi P, Bridenbaugh PO. The position of plastic tubing in continuous-block techniques: an X-ray study of 552 patients. *Anesthesiology* 1968;**29**:1047–9.

25 Sanchez R, Acuna L, Rocha F. An analysis of the radiological visualization of the catheters placed in the epidural space. *Br J Anaesth* 1967;**39**:485–9.

26 Muneyuki M, Shirai K, Inamoto A. Roentgenographic analysis of the positions of catheters in the epidural space. *Anesthesiology* 1970;**33**:19–24.

27 Lim YJ, Bahk JH, Ahn WS, Lee SC. Coiling of lumbar epidural catheters. *Acta Anaesthesiol Scand* 2002;**46**:603–6.

28 Tiso R, Thomas P, Macadaeg K. Epidural catheter direction and local anesthetic dose. *Reg Anesth* 1993;**18**:308–11.

29 Collier CB. Why obstetric epidurals fail: a study of epidurograms. *Int J Obstet Anesth* 1996;**5**:19–31.

30 Magides AD, Sprigg A, Richmond MN. Lumbar epidurography with multi-orifice and single orifice epidural catheters. *Anaesthesia* 1996; **51**: 757–63.

31 Beilin Y, Zahn J, Bernstein HH, Zucker-Pinchoff B, Zenzen W, Andres LA. Treatment of incomplete analgesia after placement of an epidural catheter and administration of local anesthetic for women in labor. *Anesthesiology* 1998;**88**:1502–6.

32 Hamilton CL, Riley ET, Cohen SE. Changes in the position of epidural catheters associated with patient movement. *Anesthesiology* 1997;**86**:778–84.

33 Bishton IM, Martin PH, Vernon JM, Liu WHD. Factors influencing epidural catheter migration. *Anaesthesia* 1992; **47**:610–2.

34 Crosby ET. Epidural catheter migration during labour: an hypothesis for inadequate analgesia. *Can J Anaesth* 1990;**37**:789–93.

35 Phillips DC, MacDonald R. Epidural catheter migration during labour. *Anaesthesia* 1987;**42**:661–3.

36 Beilin Y, Bernstein HH, Zucker-Pinchoff B. The optimal distance that a multiorifice epidural catheter should be threaded into the epidural space. *Anesth Analg* 1995;**81**:301–4.

37 D'Angelo R, Berkebile BL, Gerancher JC. Prospective examination of epidural catheter insertion. *Anesthesiology* 1996;**84**:88–93.

38 Lyons G, Columb M, Hawthorne L, Dresner M. Extradural pain relief in labour: bupivacaine sparing by extradural fentanyl is dose dependent. *Br J Anaesth* 1997;**78**:493–7.

39 Russell R, Reynolds F. Epidural infusion of low-dose bupivacaine and opioid in labour. *Anaesthesia* 1996;**51**:266–73.

40 Debon R, Allaouchiche B, Duflo F, Boselli E, Chassard D. The analgesic effect of sufentanil combined with ropivacaine 0.2% for labor analgesia: a comparison of three sufentanil doses. *Anesth Analg* 2001;**92**:180–3.

PART 2

Anesthesia for cesarean section

CHAPTER 9

The effect of increasing central blood volume to decrease the incidence of hypotension following spinal anesthesia for cesarean section

Pamela J. Morgan

Introduction

Hypotension following spinal anesthesia is a well-recognized physiologic response. In the parturient, the concerns about the effects of hypotension on both mother and fetus have led to a number of studies in the literature addressing potential preventative measures. The incidence of hypotension in women receiving spinal anesthesia for cesarean section is reported to be as high as 81%.[1] The pathophysiological mechanism of the hypotension relates to the sympathetic block resulting in arterial and venous dilatation. The subsequent decrease in venous return to the right side of the heart leads to a fall in mean arterial blood pressure. This phenomenon may be further exacerbated by pressure of the gravid uterus on the aorta and inferior vena cava. One of the earliest approaches in the prevention of hypotension was the rapid administration of a crystalloid bolus. Marx *et al.*[2] demonstrated a zero incidence of hypotension when fluid preload was administered before spinal anesthesia, a result that no other investigator has been able to reproduce. Nonetheless, historically, this reference represents one of the reasons many anesthesiologists were taught to preload patients prior to spinal anesthesia.

In addition to the physiologic effects on the peripheral vasculature, the sympathetic blockade induced by spinal anesthesia can affect the cardioaccelerator output if the block reaches the upper thoracic dermatomes, a level often achieved during cesarean section anesthesia. It has been demonstrated that the sympathetic blockade is often two to three dermatomal levels higher than the associated sensory block.[3,4] The height of the block therefore may impair the tachycardic response to a decrease in venous return that would otherwise improve cardiac output. The incidence of severe maternal bradycardia with spinal anesthesia for cesarean section has been reported at 6.7%.[5]

The effect of maternal hypotension on uteroplacental perfusion has been the subject of many investigations. A decrease in uteroplacental perfusion can have significant effects on fetal well being as reflected by acid–base status and Apgar scores. Some of the earliest studies demonstrated a higher incidence of base deficits in neonates whose mothers had become hypotensive following regional anesthesia[2,6] but Datta *et al.*[7] reported no significant differences in neonatal outcome if maternal hypotension following spinal anesthesia was promptly treated.

The literature is replete with suggested methods of both preventing and treating spinal-induced hypotension in the obstetric population. The common triad of prehydration, left uterine displacement and vasopressors remain the standard of practice for many anesthesiologists. Whether or not a prophylactic fluid bolus reliably prevents hypotension is controversial.

Factors leading to difficulty in interpretation of published studies include the differences in the definition of hypotension. Some investigators have defined hypotension as a systolic blood pressure (SBP) less than 90–100 mmHg or SBP less than 70–80% of baseline recording, while others define hypotension as a fall in mean arterial pressure (MAP) of more than 20% or 30% of resting MAP. Another confounding factor is the definition of resting MAP. Some investigators have used the blood pressure of the parturient immediately before the induction of spinal anesthesia as the "resting" blood pressure. Others have used a mean of three blood pressures taken outside the operating theater as the resting blood pressure. In one survey, approximately 40% of clinicians used the most recent antenatal blood pressure, or that recorded in the clinic at the time of booking of the cesarean section as most appropriate.[8] It is difficult therefore to determine the exact incidence of hypotension and to judge the success of treatment because the endpoint differs from study to study.

Increasing central blood volume would seem to be the appropriate physiologic intervention to prevent spinal-induced hypotension. This volume increase could be achieved by:

1 intravenous infusion of crystalloid or colloid; or
2 a mechanical increase in preload by leg elevation, leg wrapping or adoption of the head down position.

A survey, conducted in 1999, of 558 UK anesthesiologists indicates that approximately 77% administer a preload of at least 500 mL of solution before spinal anesthesia for cesarean section. Of those who administer fluids intravenously, less than 10% use colloid alone or in combination of crystalloid. The survey did not enquire about other methods of increasing central blood volume.[8] The purpose of this chapter is to review the evidence concerning the efficacy of increasing central blood volume before spinal anesthesia for cesarean section.

Search strategy

Randomized controlled trials (RCTs) investigating any method of increasing central blood volume prior to initiation of obstetric spinal anesthesia were sought using MEDLINE® (1966–2003), EMBASE® (January 1988–April 2003) and the Cochrane Library (Issue 3, 2003) using text terms [cesarean or caesarean], [spinal anesthesia or spinal anaesthesia], [complication] and [hypotension]. Additional terms, such as [leg wrapping] and [Trendelenberg], were used to capture other methods of increasing preload. Additional reports from retrieved and review articles, hand searching of non-MEDLINE® journals and abstracts of major anesthesia meetings (1997–2003) were located. The last search was conducted in August 2003.

Quality of trials

The studies were assessed for the quality of the randomization, blinding and flow of patients through the study (see Appendix for a complete description of the Jadad scoring system). In addition, a description of concealment of randomization until the time of recruitment and an *a priori* sample size calculation were sought.[9]

Outcome measurements

The primary outcome was the incidence of hypotension as defined by the authors of the original papers. Secondary outcomes included: ephedrine use, maternal nausea and vomiting, increase in central venous pressure and neonatal outcomes.

Increasing central blood volume using crystalloid solutions

Eleven studies in 10 manuscripts fulfilled the criteria and are summarized in Table 9.1[2,10–19] One manuscript contained two studies.[10] One study used a quasi-randomization schedule of alternate assignment.[2] An additional study randomized the first 40 patients but then used a "play the winner" strategy for the remaining recruitment. This design was chosen to ensure that, if there was harm in the omission of a crystalloid preload, the harm would be minimized by reducing the number of patients in that group assignment.[18]

There were a total of 587 patients enrolled in the studies comparing crystalloid preload, 339 in the larger volume preload group and 248 in the low volume or no preload group (control). Sample sizes ranged from 16 to 140 subjects. Of the eight studies, only two reported allocation concealment[11,19] and only one study performed a sample size calculation.[14] In all of the retrieved studies that compare differing volumes of crystalloid, a balanced salt solution was used and in two studies[2,10] the solution contained dextrose. Clark *et al.*[10] divided the patients into those having a cesarean section following labor and the second group who had an elective cesarean section. This study may be less applicable to current clinical practice because left uterine displacement was not consistently part of the anesthetic technique.

Table 9.1 Crystalloid preload and the incidence of hypotension.

Reference	Quality score	Fluid protocol		Definition of hypotension	Incidence of hypotension n/N (%)		Comments
		Fluid group (mL)	Control group (mL)		Fluid group	Control group*	
Marx et al. 1969[2]	0	1000 D5RL	0	Any decrease in blood pressure	0/18 (0%)	18/18 (100%)	Quasi-randomized / Alternating assignment / Significant difference
Clark et al. 1976[10]	1	1000 D5RL	0	Systolic blood pressure less than 100 mmHg	43/76 (57%)	25/27 (92%)	Elective cesarean / No prophylactic left uterine displacement / Significant difference noted favoring preload
Clark et al. 1976[10]	1	1000 D5RL	0	Systolic blood pressure less than 100 mmHg	18/39 (46%)	9/18 (50%)	Cesarean following labor / No prophylactic left uterine displacement / No significant difference
Kangas-Saarela et al. 1990[13]	2	20 mL/kg RL	15 mL/kg RL	More than 10% decrease in systolic blood pressure	4/8 (50%)	4/8 (50%)	Control group received therapeutic ephedrine boluses / No significant difference
Rout et al. 1992[17]	2	20 mL/kg RL over 10 min	20 mL/kg over 20 min	Systolic blood pressure less than 100 mmHg and systolic blood pressure to less than 80% of baseline	7/10 (70%)	6/10 (60%)	No significant difference
Rout et al. 1993[18]	Not rated	1413 PL	0	Systolic blood pressure less than 100 mmHg and systolic blood pressure to less than 80% of baseline	43/78 (55%)	44/62 (71%)	Play the winner after the first 40 randomized patients / Not blinded / Prophylactic ephedrine in the no preload group / Significant difference favoring preload
Olsen et al. 1994[15]	2	2700 Saline	1800 Saline	Decrease of 10 mmHg in mean arterial blood pressure	4/13 (30%)	5/13 (37%)	Prophylactic ephedrine in both groups / No significant difference
Jackson et al. 1995[12]	4	997 Hartmann's solution	204 Hartmann's solution	More than 3% decrease in systolic blood pressure from baseline or a systolic blood pressure of less than 90 mmHg	10/30 (33%)	9/30 (30%)	No significant difference

Continued

Table 9.1 (*continued*)

Reference	Quality score	Fluid protocol		Definition of hypotension	Incidence of hypotension n/N (%)		Comments
		Fluid group (mL)	Control group (mL)		Fluid group	Control group*	
Park et al. 1996[16]	3	2970 RL	1787 RL	Systolic blood pressure less than 100 mmHg and systolic blood pressure of less than 80% baseline	9/19 (47%)	12/18 (67%)	No significant difference. Ephedrine and additional fluid not standardized
Husaini et al. 1998[11]	5	1000 RL	0	More than a 30% decrease in systolic blood pressure from baseline or a systolic blood pressure less than 90 mmHg	4/21 (19%)	7/19 (37%)	Prophylactic ephedrine infusion both groups. No significant difference. Spinal technique not controlled
Frölich 2001[14]	1	15 mL/kg RL immediately before ("traditional") or after ("late") spinal anesthesia	0	More than 20% decrease in mean arterial blood pressure from baseline	13/16 (81%) "Traditional fluid loading" group 12/16 (75%) "late fluid load group"	11/16 (69%)	Three group trial ("traditional, late and no fluid loading"). Blood pressure data collected for only 10 min after spinal placement. Plasma atrial natriuretic peptide levels were the primary outcome. No significant difference
Tercanli et al. 2002[19]	3	15 mL/kg RL	150 RL	Decrease in systolic pressure to 80% baseline	3/11 (27%)	7/11 (63%)	No significant difference

Total number of patients: preload N = 355, control = 248.
* Control group, lower fluid volume or no preload.
D5RL, 5% dextrose in Ringer's lactate; PL, plasmalyte; RL, Ringer's lactate.

Three studies demonstrated that fluid preloading decreased the incidence of hypotension,[2,10,18] whereas the remaining eight studies did not find a significant difference between low and higher volume groups.[11–17,19]

With respect to side-effects related to maternal hypotension, only two studies reported the incidence of nausea and vomiting and found no significant difference between groups.[11,13] With the exception of the earliest paper by Marx et al.,[2] neonatal outcome as measured by fetal acid–base status did not differ between groups.[11,12,18]

Researchers have postulated that the amount of fluid and the rapidity of infusion might have a role in the lack of preload effectiveness demonstrated in the literature. This fact has led to the use of large volumes of fluid as a preload. The administration of such volumes may cause harm. Hemodilution can occur with subsequent decrease in oxygen carrying capacity. The parturient, by virtue of the reduction in plasma oncotic pressure, may be at higher risk for pulmonary edema with massive fluid boluses.[20] Rout et al.[17] demonstrated unacceptably high central venous pressure readings with volume preloading prior to spinal anesthesia.

Two systematic reviews of the literature demonstrated that the administration of an intravenous crystalloid preload was inconsistent in the prevention of hypotension.[21,22] Varying endpoints and definitions make it difficult to compare the outcomes of these studies statistically.

Reasons for the lack of efficacy of prophylactic fluid boluses to prevent spinal-induced hypotension may involve the relatively short intravascular half-life of the crystalloid solution or the effect of atrial natriuretic peptide (ANP). It has been postulated that with rapid increases in preload and subsequent increases in right atrial pressure, ANP is released and in turn causes vasodilatation through the relaxation of vascular smooth muscle.[14,23] Vasodilation then leads to a fall in blood pressure and may account for the lack of effect of intravenous crystalloid preloading. Pouta et al.[23] noted an increase in the plasma ANP levels during crystalloid infusion prior to spinal anesthesia for cesarean section. In another study, similar findings were demonstrated in that ANP increased in patients receiving an intravenous crystalloid preload as compared to a control group who did not receive a fluid preload.[14] However, there was no significant correlation between ANP levels and blood pressure or ephedrine requirements. ANP acted as a potent endogenous diuretic in the parturient.

Increasing central blood volume using colloid solutions

Ten studies met the inclusion criteria with sample sizes ranging from 22 to 160 subjects (Table 9.2).[23–32] There were a total of 290 subjects in the no preload or crystalloid preload versus 339 in the colloid group. All studies were randomized but only four indicated that allocation was concealed.[24,25,28,30] Only one study included a sample size calculation.[28]

Types of colloid solutions included albumin, 6% hetastarch (HES), dextran and modified gelatin. In all studies, the incidence of hypotension was reduced in patients who received colloid compared with those who received crystalloid (Table 9.2). This difference was statistically significant in seven studies.[24,26,28–32] Of the four studies that reported on the incidence of nausea and vomiting, two found no difference[26,29] and two noted a significantly lower incidence in the colloid group.[28,30] Four studies reported no significant differences in neonatal outcomes between groups.[28–30,33]

Ueyama et al.[31] demonstrated that only 28% of Ringer's lactate given as a preload remained in the intravascular space as compared with 100% of the HES. These findings occurred 30 min after administration. Although the efficacy of colloids are apparent, their side-effects profile cannot be overlooked. The use of human serum albumin is limited because of the risk of disease transmission. The risk of anaphylaxis to starch has been well documented with incidence of allergic reactions cited as: gelatin 0.115%, dextran 0.32%, HES 0.085%.[34,35] Of all the colloid volume substitutes, pentastarch has the lowest incidence of allergic reactions.[36] It should be noted that there are too few patients included in this review to draw conclusions about these side-effects. Further, none of the studies included a cost analysis.

Because colloid solutions remain in the intravascular space longer than crystalloid solutions, they have been used for fluid preloading before spinal anesthesia. With the exception of one study,[33] the literature does support the efficacy of colloid versus crystalloid for the prevention of hypotension in the parturient (Table 9.2).

Table 9.2 Colloid preload and the incidence of hypotension.

Reference	Quality score	Fluid protocol Crystalloid group	Colloid group	Definition of hypotension	Incidence of hypotension n/N (%) Crystalloid group	Colloid group	Comments
Mathru et al. 1980[27]	2	D5RL 15 mL/kg (n = 21) D5RL 15 mL/kg + ephedrine 25 mg IM (n = 20)	5% albumin in D5RL 15 mL/kg 5% (n = 22) albumin in D5RL 15 mL/kg + 25 mg ephedrine IM (n = 24)	Systolic blood pressure less than 100 mmHg or mean arterial pressure less than 85 mmHg	7/21 (33%) D5RL 5/20 (25%) D5RL + ephedrine	0/22 (0%) 5% albumin 0/24 (0%) 5% albumin + ephedrine	4-group comparison: **1** Crystalloid **2** Crystalloid + ephedrine **3** Colloid **4** Colloid + ephedrine Statistically significant decrease in the incidence of hypotension in the albumin groups Statistically significant decrease in heart rate, increase in mean arterial pressure in albumin groups
Karinen et al. 1995[25]	3	RL 1000 mL	6% HES 500 mL	Systolic blood pressure less than 90 mmHg *and* less than 80% baseline	8/13 (62%)	5/13 (38%)	No statistical difference in incidence of hypotension
Riley et al. 1995[29]	4	RL 1000 mL	6% HES 500 mL	Systolic blood pressure less than 100 mmHg *and* less than 80% of baseline	17/20 (85%)	9/20 (45%)	Statistically significant difference in incidence of hypotension favoring colloid All patients received 10 mg ephedrine IV
Vercauteren et al. 1996[32]	3	3-group comparison All groups received colloid Group 1 = RL 1000 + gelatin Group 2 = RL 1000 + HES Group 3 = 500 mL 6% HES		Systolic blood pressure less than 100 mmHg	Group 1 18/30 (60%) Group 2 8/30 (27%) Group 3 16/30 (53%)		Initial volume given on ward, 2nd volume in operating room No difference in volumes of colloid between groups Significantly less hypotension and less ephedrine use in RL–HES group

Study		Crystalloid	Colloid	Definition of hypotension	Crystalloid incidence	Colloid incidence	Comments
Pouta et al. 1996[23]	2	RL 2000 mL	6% HES 500 mL	Systolic blood pressure less than 90 mmHg or less than 80% baseline	—	—	Incidence of hypotension not reported. No significant differences in blood pressure noted between groups. No patient required ephedrine
Ueyama et al. 1999[31]	2	Group 1 RL 1500 mL	Group 2 6% HES 500 mL Group 3 6% HES 1000 mL	Systolic blood pressure less than 100 mmHg *and* less than 80% baseline	9/12 (75%)	Group 2 7/12 (58%) Group 3 2/12 (17%)	3-group comparison: Significantly less hypotension, higher systolic blood pressure, cardiac output and blood volume in 1000 mL HES group
French et al. 1999[24]	5	15 mL/kg Hartmann's Solution	15 mL/kg 10% pentastarch	Systolic blood pressure less than 90 mmHg or less than 70% baseline	38/80 (48%)	14/80 (17%)	Significantly less hypotension and ephedrine use in pentastarch group
Lin et al. 1999[26]	3	RL 1000 mL	10% dextran 40 500 mL	Systolic blood pressure less than 70% baseline	16/30 (53%)	8/30 (27%)	Significantly less hypotension and ephedrine use in dextran group
Ngan Kee et al. 2001[28]	5	No preload	Gelofusine 15 mL/kg	Systolic blood pressure less than 90% baseline Incidence of hypotension reported as more than a 20% fall in systolic blood pressure	21/33 (64%)	11/35 (27%)	Metaraminol infused for a fall in blood pressure Significant difference in incidence of hypotension in colloid group
Siddik et al. 2000[30]	4	RL 1000 mL	10% HES 500 mL	Systolic blood pressure less than 80% baseline and less than 100 mmHg	16/20 (80%)	8/20 (40%)	Significant difference between groups favoring colloid

Total number of patients: 290 crystalloid, 339 colloid.
D5RL, 5% dextrose in Ringer's lactate; HES, hetastarch; IM, intramuscular; IV, intravenous; RL, Ringer's lactate.

As can be seen in Table 9.2, there are a number of methodologic differences among studies. In one study,[32] there was no crystalloid group but a comparison of different colloid regimens.

The use of colloid to prevent spinal induced hypotension in the obstetric population has merit but its use must be weighed against the additional cost and risk of an anaphylactic reaction.[37] As was demonstrated in the crystalloid studies, the use of colloid does not eliminate hypotension with spinal anesthesia so therapeutic interventions still may be necessary.

Increasing central blood volume using mechanical interventions

Thirteen studies have examined different mechanical interventions with sample sizes ranging from 12 to 51 subjects per intervention (Table 9.3).[38–49,54] One of these did not report the incidence of hypotension and was therefore excluded.[41] In total, there were 735 patients, 406 patients receiving some method of mechanical intervention and the remaining 329 patients acting as "controls" with sample sizes ranging from 24 to 100. Eleven studies were reported as randomized trials[38,39,42–49,54] and one was quasi-randomized by alternate treatments. Three of the studies described the allocation concealment.[38,42,49] Two studies performed sample size calculations[42,49] based on a difference in the incidence of hypotension between groups.

Four studies examined the differences in hypotension when different positions were adopted during the induction of spinal anesthesia. Russell[47] compared the induction of spinal anesthesia in either the right or left lateral position and found no difference in the incidence of hypotension, although the author did not report his definition of hypotension. Køhler et al.[42] compared the immediate supine position following the administration of the spinal drugs with the maintenance of the sitting position for 3 min. There was no difference in the incidence of hypotension in this study. Positioning the operating room table in either the head up or head down position following administration of hyperbaric spinal anesthesia did not significantly affect the hypotension incidence when compared with having the table horizontal.[44,49] The sensory block was significantly higher, however, in the patients who had the operating room table maintained in the neutral position as compared to a 10° head up tilt.[49]

The remaining eight studies examined various methods of increasing venous return including leg elevation, leg wrapping, thromboembolic (TED) stockings and automated devices. Theoretically, compression of the lower limbs using Esmarch bandages or inflatable devices seems of potential benefit in the prevention of spinal-induced hypotension. An auto-transfusion of up to 700 mL has been demonstrated in orthopedic patients with lower limb tourniquet use.[50] Graduated compression stockings that produce approximately 20 mmHg pressure result in compression of the cutaneous veins and prevent spinal hypotension in non-pregnant patients but were shown to be ineffective in parturients undergoing cesarean section.[51,52] Iwama et al.[53] have suggested that extra strong graduated compression stockings which produce 50–60 mmHg may be more effective in the parturient because the deep venous system is also compressed. This may overcome the effects of the gravid uterus.

All studies involving leg wrapping demonstrated a decrease in spinal induced hypotension.[39,45,54] Less convincing results were seen in the two studies using TED stockings. While both studies showed a reduction in the incidence of hypotension with TED stockings, the difference was not statistically significant (Table 9.3).[46,48]

None of the studies that examined neonatal outcomes demonstrated any differences.[42,45,46,49] Raising the legs after induction of anesthesia was not effective.[45,54]

Positioning, leg wrapping, leg elevation and TED stockings have all been used to decrease the incidence of spinal-induced hypotension. Positioning alone is not effective in reducing the incidence of hypotension. The advantage of the other techniques includes the relative ease of the intervention, the lack of serious side-effects and the fact that the intervention is non-invasive in nature. However, the process may be time consuming and unacceptable for some parturients.

Conclusions

Although crystalloid preload is commonly administered before spinal anesthesia for cesarean section, the effect on the incidence of hypotension is not consistent. The use of colloid solutions is more efficacious but the potential for disease transmission (for human albumin), anaphylaxis and additional costs must be

Table 9.3 Mechanical and positioning interventions and the incidence of hypotension.

Reference	Quality score	Protocol Intervention	Protocol Control	Definition of hypotension	Incidence of hypotension n/N (%) Intervention	Incidence of hypotension n/N (%) Control	Comments
van Bogaert 1998[54]	3	*Group 1:* Leg wrapping *Group 2:* Leg elevation *Group 3:* Leg wrapping and elevation	No leg wrapping or elevation	Severe hypotension defined as decrease in systolic blood pressure > 20% or absolute blood pressure < 100 mmHg	*Group 1:* 3/19 (16%) *Group 2:* 10/22 (45%) *Group 3:* 3/19 (16%)	12/22 (55%)	Trial stopped early for logistic reasons Statistically significant difference in "severe" hypotension between groups 1 and control favoring leg wrapping compared to 2 and 3 Leg wrapping was better than no treatment or leg elevation
Rout et al. 1993[45]	2	*Group 1:* Leg elevation *Group 2:* Leg wrapping and elevation	No leg wrapping or elevation	Systolic blood pressure of 100 mmHg and < 80% baseline	*Group 1:* 12/31 (39%) *Group 2:* 6/34 (18%)	17/32 (53%)	Significantly less hypotension in leg wrapping group Leg elevation alone did not reduce incidence of hypotension
Goudie et al. 1988[40]	0	Splints	No splints	2 consecutive systolic readings < 100 mmHg or < 80% control	11/23 (48%)	19/23 (83%)	% fall in blood pressure significantly lower in control than splint group
Bhagwanjee et al. 1990[39]	2	Legs elevated, then wrapped	No leg elevation or wrapping	Fall in systolic blood pressure > 20% and an absolute value < 100 mmHg	2/12 (17%)	10/12 (83%)	Leg wrapping significantly decreased incidence of hypotension No patient developed hypotension when legs unwrapped
James & Greiss 1973[43]	1	Legs elevated, then inflatable boots	No leg elevation or inflatable boots	Systolic blood pressure < 100 mmHg	25/41 (61%)	23/38 (61%)	Left uterine displacement if patient hypotensive Incidence of "requiring" left uterine displacement: 13% (boots) vs 26% (control)
Sutherland et al. 2001[46]	2	Thromboembolic stockings + sequential compression device	No stockings or compression device	Systolic blood pressure < 100 mmHg and < 20% baseline	38/51 (65%)	39/49 (80%)	Excluded women with a thigh circumference > 64 cm Violations in protocol re. administration of ephedrine (2.3%, evenly divided between groups) No significant difference in incidence of hypotension

Continued

Table 9.3 (*continued*)

Reference	Quality score	Protocol Intervention	Control	Definition of hypotension	Incidence of hypotension n/N (%) Intervention	Control	Comments
Sood et al. 1996[48]	2	Thromboembolic stockings	No stockings	Systolic blood pressure of 90 mmHg or > 20% fall in baseline	5/25 (20%)	11/25 (44%)	Baseline blood pressure higher in control group Gave all patients who were hypotensive 3-mg ephedrine increments
Miyabe & Sato 1997[44]	2	Bed tilted head down 10°	Bed horizontal	Systolic blood pressure < 100 mmHg	14/17 (82%)	15/17 (88%)	No significant differences in hypotension
Russell 1987[47]	1	Right lateral position for spinal	Left lateral position for spinal	Not defined	8/17 (50%)	9/18 (50%)	Some patients received RL and some received RL and Haemaccel® and RL
Loke et al. 2002[49]	3	Bed tilted head up 10°	Bed horizontal	Systolic blood pressure < 90 mmHg	12/20 (60%)	17/20 (85%)	Spinal blocks were performed by one operator who did not take part in subsequent measurements Sensory block statistically higher in control group
Køhler et al. 2002[42]	2	Patient remained sitting for 3 min after placement of the spinal	Patient placed supine immediately (with left uterine displacement)	Systolic blood pressure < 100 mmHg or < 70% baseline	24/43 (52%)	35/52 (67%)	Fluid bolus standardized Higher sensory level in control group No significant differences in hypotension
Adsumelli et al. 2003[38]	2	Sequential compression device		Decrease in any mean arterial pressure to less than 80% baseline	13/25 (52%)	23/25 (92%)	Statistically significant difference in 20% decrease in mean arterial pressure between groups No statistical difference in systolic blood pressure

Total number of patients: mechanical maneuvers N = 406, control = 329.
RL, Ringer's lactate.

considered. Simple mechanical measures such as leg wrapping have been shown to be efficacious but are also time consuming and unacceptable for some parturients. Of interest, while this may be among the most effective treatments, it has not come into widespread use. In all studies, the hypotension that occurred was of short duration and had no measurable effect on the neonate. However, only a few of the studies reported the incidence of troubling side-effects such as dizziness, nausea and vomiting in the mother. These important endpoints should be considered in future studies.

References

1 Rout CC, Rocke DA. Prevention of hypotension following spinal anesthesia for cesarean section. *Int Anesthesiol Clin* 1994;**32**:117–35.

2 Marx GF, Cosmi EV, Wollman SB. Biochemical status and clinical condition of mother and infant at cesarean section. *Anesth Analg* 1969;**48**:986–94.

3 Chamberlain DP, Chamberlain BD. Changes in the skin temperature of the trunk and their relationship to sympathetic blockade during spinal anesthesia. *Anesthesiology* 1986;**65**:139–43.

4 Greene NM. The area of differential block during spinal anesthesia with hyperbaric tetracaine. *Anesthesiology* 1958; **19**:45–50.

5 Shen C-L, Ho Y-Y, Hung Y-C, Chen P-L. Arrhythmias during spinal anaesthesia for cesarean section. *Can J Anesth* 2000;**47**:393–7.

6 Datta S, Brown WU, Ostheimer GW, Weiss JB, Alper MH. Epidural anesthesia for cesarean section in diabetic parturients: maternal and neonatal acid–base status and bupivacaine concentration. *Anesth Analg* 1981;**60**:574–80.

7 Datta S, Kitzmiller JL, Naulty JS, Ostheimer GW, Weiss JB. Acid–base status of diabetic mothers and their infants following spinal anesthesia for cesarean section. *Anesth Analg* 1982;**61**:662–5.

8 Burns S, Cowan C, Wilkes R. Prevention and management of hypotension during anaesthesia for elective caesarean section: a survey of practice. *Anaesthesia* 2001;**56**:777–98.

9 Altman DG, Schulz KF, Moher D, et al. The revised CONSORT statement for reporting randomized trials: explanation and elaboration. *Ann Intern Med* 2001;**134**:663–94.

10 Clark RB, Thompson DS, Thompson CH. Prevention of spinal hypotension associated with cesarean section. *Anesthesiology* 1976;**45**:670–4.

11 Husaini SW, Russell IF. Volume preload: lack of effect in the prevention of spinal-induced hypotension at cesarean section. *Int J Obstet Anesth* 1998;**7**:76–81.

12 Jackson R, Reid JA, Thorburn J. Volume preloading is not essential to prevent spinal-induced hypotension at caesarean section. *Br J Anaesth* 1995;**75**:262–5.

13 Kangas-Saarela T, Hollmén AI, Tolonen U, et al. Does ephedrine influence newborn neurobehavioural responses and spectral EEG when used to prevent maternal hypotension during caesarean section? *Acta Anaesthesiol Scand* 1990;**34**:8–16.

14 Frölich MA. Role of the atrial natriuretic factor in obstetric spinal hypotension. *Anesthesiology* 2001;**95**:371–6.

15 Olsen K, Feiblerg V, Hansen C, Rudkjøbing O, Pedersen T. Prevention of hypotension during spinal anesthesia for cesarean section. *Int J Obstet Anesth* 1994;**3**:20–4.

16 Park G, Hauch M, Curlin F, Datta S, Bader A. The effects of varying volumes of crystalloid administration before cesarean delivery on maternal hemodynamics and colloid osmotic pressure. *Anesth Analg* 1996;**83**:299–303.

17 Rout CC, Akoojee SS, Rocke DA, Gouws E. Rapid administration of crystalloid preload does not decrease the incidence of hypotension after spinal anaesthesia for elective caesarean section. *Br J Anaesth* 1992;**68**:394–7.

18 Rout CC, Rocke DA, Levin J, Gouws E, Reddy D. A reevaluation of the role of crystalloid preload in the prevention of hypotension associated with spinal anesthesia for elective cesarean section. *Anesthesiology* 1993;**79**:262–9.

19 Tercanli S, Schneider M, Visac E, et al. Influence of volume preloading on uteroplacental and fetal circulation during spinal anesthesia for cesarean section in uncomplicated singleton pregnancies. *Fetal Diagn Ther* 2002;**17**:142–6.

20 MacLennan FM, Macdonald AF, Campbell DM. Lung water during the puerperium. *Anaesthesia* 1987;**42**:141–7.

21 Morgan PJ, Halpern S, Tarshis J. The effects of an increase of central blood volume before spinal anesthesia for cesarean delivery: a qualitative systematic review. *Anesth Analg* 2001;**92**:997–1005.

22 Emmett RS, Cyna AM, Andrew M, Simmons SW. Techniques for preventing hypotension during spinal anesthesia for caesarean section (Cochrane Review). The Cochrane Library. *Oxford: Update Software*, 2003.

23 Pouta AM, Karinen J, Vuolteenaho LJ, Laatkainen TJ. Effect of intravenous fluid preload on vasoactive peptide secretion during caesarean section under spinal anaesthesia. *Anaesthesia* 1996;**51**:128–32.

24 French GWG, White JB, Howell SJ, Popat M. Comparison of pentastarch and Hartmann's solution for volume preloading in spinal anaesthesia for elective caesarean section. *Br J Anaesth* 1999;**83**:475–7.

25 Karinen J, Rasanen J, Alahuhta S, Jouppila R, Jouppila P. Effect of crystalloid and colloid preloading on uteroplacental and maternal haemodynamic state during spinal anaesthesia for caesarean section. *Br J Anaesth* 1995;**75**:531–5.

26 Lin C-S, Lin T-Y, Huang C-H, et al. Prevention of hypotension after spinal anesthesia for cesarean section: dextran 40 versus lactated Ringer's solution. *Acta Anaesthesiol Sin* 1999;**37**:55–9.

27 Mathru M, Rao TLK, Kartha RK, Shanmugham M, Jacobs HK. Intravenous albumin administration for prevention of spinal hypotension during cesarean section. *Anesth Analg* 1980;**59**:655–8.

28 Ngan Kee WD, Khaw KS, Lee BB, Ng FF, Wong MMS.

Randomized controlled study of colloid preload before spinal anaesthesia for caesarean section. *Br J Anaesth* 2001;**87**:772–4.

29 Riley ET, Cohen SE, Rubenstein AJ, Flanagan B. Prevention of hypotension after spinal anesthesia for cesarean section: 6% hetastarch versus lactated Ringer's solution. *Anesth Analg* 1995;**81**:838–42.

30 Siddik SM, Aouad MT, Kai GE, Sfeir MM, Baraka AS. Hydroxyethylstarch 10% is superior to Ringer's solution for preloading before spinal anaesthesia for caesarean section. *Can J Anesth* 2000;**47**:616–21.

31 Ueyama H, Le H, Tanigami H, Mashimo T, Yoshiya I. Effects of crystalloid and colloid preload on blood volume in the parturient undergoing spinal anesthesia for elective cesarean section. *Anesthesiology* 1999;**91**:1571–6.

32 Vercauteren MP, Hoffmann V, Steenberge ALV, Adriaensen HA. Hydroxyethylstarch compared with modified gelatin as volume preload before spinal anaesthesia for caesarean section. *Br J Anaesth* 1996;**76**:731–3.

33 Karinen J, Rasanen J, Alahuhta S, Jouppila R, Jouppila P. Maternal and uteroplacental haemodynamic state in preeclamptic patients during spinal anaesthesia for caesarean section. *Br J Anaesth* 1996;**76**:616–20.

34 Morgan PJ. Allergic reactions. In: Birnbach D, Gatt S, Datta S, eds. *Textbook of Obstetric Anaesthesia*. New York: Churchill Livingstone, 2000: 475–86.

35 Ring J, Messmer K. Incidence and severity of anaphylactoid reactions to colloid volume substitutes. *Lancet* 1977;**1**:466–9.

36 McHugh GJ. Anaphylactoid reaction to pentastarch. *Can J Anaesth* 1998;**45**:270–2.

37 Weeks S. Reflections on hypotension during cesarean section under spinal anesthesia: do we need to use colloid? *Can J Anesth* 2000;**47**:607–10.

38 Adsumelli RSN, Steinberg ES, Schabel JE, Saunders TA, Poppers PJ. Sequential compression device with thigh-high sleeves supports mean arterial pressure during caesarean section under spinal anaesthesia. *Br J Anaesth* 2003;**91**:695–8.

39 Bhagwanjee S, Rocke DA, Rout CC, Koovarjee RV, Brijball R. Prevention of hypotension following spinal anaesthesia for elective caesarean section by wrapping of the legs. *Br J Anaesth* 1990;**65**:819–22.

40 Goudie TA, Winter AW, Ferguson DJM. Lower limb compression using inflatable splints to prevent hypotension during spinal anaesthesia for caesarean section. *Acta Anaesthesiol Scand* 1988;**32**:541–4.

41 Inglis A, McGrady E. Maternal position during induction of spinal anaesthesia for caesarean section. *Anaesthesia* 1994;**50**:363–5.

42 Køhler F, Sørensen JF, Helbo-Hansen HS. Effect of delayed supine positioning after induction of spinal anesthesia for caesarean section. *Acta Anaesthesiol Scand* 2002;**46**:441–6.

43 James FM, Greiss FCJ. The use of inflatable boots to prevent hypotension during spinal anesthesia for cesarean section. *Anesth Analg* 1973;**52**:246–51.

44 Miyabe M, Sato S. The effect of head down tilt position on arterial blood pressure after spinal anesthesia for cesarean delivery. *Reg Anesth* 1997;**22**:239–42.

45 Rout CC, Rocke DA, Gouws E. Leg elevation and wrapping in the prevention of hypotension following spinal anaesthesia for elective caesarean section. *Anaesthesia* 1993;**48**:304–8.

46 Sutherland OD, Wee MYK, Weston-Smith T, Thomas P. The use of thromboembolic deterrent stockings and a sequential compression device to prevent spinal hypotension during cesarean section. *Int J Obstet Anesth* 2001;**10**:97–102.

47 Russell IF. Effect of posture during the induction of subarachnoid analgesia for caesarean section. *Br J Anaesth* 1987;**59**:342–6.

48 Sood PK, Cooper PJF, Michel MZ, Wee MYK, Pickering RM. Thromboembolic deterrent stockings fail to prevent hypotension associated with spinal anesthesia for elective cesarean section. *Int J Obstet Anesth* 1996;**5**:172–5.

49 Loke GPY, Chan EHY, Sia ATH. The effect of 10° head-up tilt in the right lateral position on the systemic blood pressure after subarachnoid block for caesarean section. *Anaesthesia* 2002;**57**:169–72.

50 Bradford E. Haemodynamic changes associated with lower limb tourniquets. *Anaesthesia* 1969;**24**:190–7.

51 Iwama H. Graduated compression stocking prevents hypotension during spinal anaesthesia. *Can J Anaesth* 1996;**43**:984–5.

52 Iwama H, Furuta S, Tanigawa S, Ohmizo H, Ohmori S, Kaneko T. Extra-strong graduated compression stocking reduces usage of vasopressor agents during spinal anesthesia for cesarean section. *Arch Gynecol Obstet* 2001;**265**:60–3.

53 Iwama H, Ohmizo H, Furuta S, Ohmori S, Watanabe K, Kaneko T. Spinal anesthesia hypotension in elective cesarean section in parturients wearing extra-strong compression stockings. *Arch Gynecol Obstet* 2002;**267**:85–9.

54 van Bogaert LJ. Prevention of post-spinal hypotension at elective cesarean section by wrapping of the lower limbs. *Int J Gynaecol Obstet* 1998;**61**:233–8.

The use of vasopressors for the prevention and treatment of hypotension secondary to regional anesthesia for cesarean section

Stephen H. Halpern & Michelle Chochinov

Introduction

Spinal and epidural anesthesia are the most common techniques of anesthesia for cesarean section. A common, potentially severe side-effect is maternal hypotension, secondary to the rapid onset of a dense sympathetic blockade. While fluid preload (see Chapter 9) and left uterine displacement are often employed in an attempt to prevent this complication, a vasopressor is often required.

Ephedrine, an indirect-acting vasopressor with primarily β-adrenergic agonist activity, has been recommended as the vasopressor of choice for the hypotensive obstetric patient. A recent British survey has shown that more than 95% of anesthesiologists use ephedrine exclusively to correct hypotension caused by spinal anesthesia in elective cesarean sections.[1] In classic sheep studies, both ephedrine and α-adrenergic agonists were effective in restoring blood pressure after hypotension induced by spinal anesthesia. However, ephedrine was superior to the α-agonists in restoring uterine blood flow and improving fetal oxygenation and acid–base balance.[2–5]

There are many clinical situations in which side-effects associated with β-adrenergic agonist activity – especially tachycardia – are undesirable. Over the last 15 years there has been a considerable experience, in humans, with phenylephrine and other α-agonists to correct hypotension after regional anesthesia. These do not seem to corroborate the fetal effects seen in earlier animal studies.

Many studies have compared ephedrine with phenylephrine (or other α-adrenergic agonists) in patients who underwent cesarean section under regional anesthesia. The main outcomes for these studies were indices of fetal well being (umbilical cord gases, Apgar scores) and the effects on the mother (incidence of hypotension, nausea and bradycardia). Some of the studies included measures of uterine and umbilical artery blood flow. In this chapter we systematically review studies that compare ephedrine with phenylephrine or other α-adrenergic agonists in patients who have received regional anesthesia for cesarean section.

The data for this chapter come from randomized controlled trials (RCTs). We reviewed MEDLINE®, EMBASE®, Science Citation Index® and the Cochrane Library for studies comparing α-adrenergic agonists (phenylephrine, metaraminol or methoxamine) or angiotensin II with ephedrine in patients undergoing epidural or spinal anesthesia for cesarean section. These databases were last consulted in February 2004. Each RCT was given a quality score[6] based on their description of appropriate randomization, blinding and reporting of attrition (see Appendix for a description of the scale). In total, there were nine RCTs that met the search criteria and compared phenylephrine with ephedrine. There were four RCTs that compared other α-adrenergic agonists with ephedrine. All studies were in healthy patients, not in labor, who received spinal anesthesia and vasopressors. There was one comparative study involving only hypotensive patients

Table 10.1 Description of studies.

Study	Quality (0–5)	Ephedrine (N)	α-agonists (N)	Preparation and anesthesia	Intervention	Comments
Ephedrine vs phenylephrine						
Moran et al.[21]	4	29	31	2000 mL preload Spinal anesthesia with hyperbaric bupivacaine 7.5–15 mg	Ephedrine 10 mg IV boluses or phenylephrine 80 µg IV bolus initially. 5–10 mg ephedrine or 40–80 µg phenylephrine to maintain systolic blood pressure > 100	One patient in the ephedrine group became hypotensive for more than 5 min. Data from that patient was eliminated from the neonatal data
Alahuhta et al.[17]	2	9	8	20 mL/kg preload Spinal anesthesia with hyperbaric bupivacaine 11–13 mg	Ephedrine 5 mg bolus + infusion + 5 mg rescue as needed Phenylephrine 100 µg IV bolus + infusion + 100 µg rescue as needed	One patient eliminated because of maternal bradycardia (?group) Primary outcomes were maternal and fetal Doppler measures of blood flow
Hall et al.[18]	3	19	10	20 mL/kg preload Spinal anesthesia with hyperbaric bupivacaine 12.5–15 mg	Ephedrine 6 mg bolus and 1 or 2 mg/min Rescue 6 mg bolus Phenylephrine 20 µg bolus then 10 µg/min Rescue 20 µg bolus	3-group comparison (two different ephedrine infusion rates) Blinding unclear
Pierce et al.[20]	2	13	13	2000 mL preload Spinal anesthesia with hyperbaric bupivacaine 7.5–15 mg + 10 µg fentanyl	Ephedrine 5–10 mg boluses to maintain systolic blood pressure > 100 Phenylephrine 40–80 µg boluses to maintain systolic blood pressure > 100	Data from 3 patients in the ephedrine group and one in the phenylephrine group were eliminated because the neonatal pH was < 7.25 Primary outcome was the concentration of atrial natriuretic peptides
LaPorta et al.[19]	2	20	20	1500–2000 mL preload Spinal anesthesia with hyperbaric bupivacaine 7.5–15 mg	Ephedrine 5–10 mg boluses to maintain systolic blood pressure > 100 Phenylephrine 40–80 µg boluses to maintain systolic blood pressure > 100	Primary outcome was neonatal catecholamine levels as well as Apgar scores
Thomas et al.[12]	5	19	19	1500 mL preload Spinal anesthesia with hyperbaric bupivacaine 12.5 mg	Ephedrine 5 mg boluses to maintain systolic blood pressure at 90% preoperative values Phenylephrine 100 µg boluses to maintain systolic blood pressure at 90% preoperative values	2 patients (1 from each group) eliminated because of poor Doppler wave forms
Mercier et al.[9]	5	19	20	15 mL/kg preload Spinal anesthesia with hyperbaric bupivacaine 11 mg + sufentanil 2.5 µg + morphine 0.1 mg	Ephedrine 60 mg in 20 mL normal saline at 40 cc/h Ephedrine 60 mg + phenylephrine 300 µg in 20 mL normal saline at 40 cc/h	Primary outcome was the incidence of hypotension Both groups exposed to ephedrine

Study				Method	Treatment	Comments
Ayorinde et al.[10]	4	27	54	500 mL preload Spinal anesthesia with hyperbaric bupivacaine 11 mg + 20 µg fentanyl	Ephedrine 45 mg IM prespinal anesthesia Phenylephrine 2 or 4 mg IM prespinal anesthesia IV ephedrine rescue for both groups	A placebo group was included There were 2 groups that received different doses of prophylactic phenylephrine
Cooper et al.[11]	5	50	48	10 mL/kg preload Spinal technique–one of 4 techniques using either hyperbaric bupivacaine or levobupivacaine	Ephedrine 12 mg/min by infusion, adjusted to maintain systolic blood pressure at baseline Phenylephrine 150 µg/min by infusion adjusted to maintain systolic blood pressure at baseline	3rd group included ephedrine 6 mg/min and phenylephrine 75 µg/min
Ephedrine vs other vasopressors						
Wright et al.[14]	2	17	15	10 mL/kg preload Epidural with 20 mL 2% lidocaine	Ephedrine 12 mg IV followed by 3 mg IV as needed to maintain systolic blood pressure > 90 Methoxamine 2 mg IV followed by 0.5 mg IV as needed to maintain systolic blood pressure > 90	Only patients who became hypotensive after randomization were treated Effects on uterine and umbilical artery blood flow were the main outcomes
Vincent et al.[16]	3	25	27	15 mL/kg preload Spinal anesthesia with hyperbaric bupivacaine 10.5–13.5 mg + 25 µg fentanyl + 0.2 mg morphine	Prophylactic ephedrine infusion adjusted by the anesthesiologist to maintain systolic blood pressure at 90–100% baseline Prophylactic angiotensin II infusion adjusted by the anesthesiologist to maintain systolic blood pressure at 90–100% baseline	Concealment of allocation by opaque numbered envelopes Blinding of study group is not mentioned Sample size calculation based on umbilical artery pH
Ramin et al.[15]	2	10	10	Prophylactic ephedrine or angiotensin II titrated to diastolic blood pressure 0–10 mmHg above baseline 2000 mL 5% dextrose preload Spinal anesthesia with 8–9 mg of hyperbaric tetracaine	No further therapy after prophylactic infusion	Included a control group that received no prophylaxis (N = 10) Blinding of study group not mentioned Randomized the night before surgery – 2 women excluded
Ngan Kee et al.[13]	4	25	25	20 mL/kg preload Spinal anesthesia with 10 mg hyperbaric bupivacaine, and 15 µg fentanyl	10 mg ephedrine given if the systolic blood pressure < 90% control followed by 5 mg/min infusion 0.5 mg metaraminol given if the systolic blood pressure < 90% control followed by 0.25 mg/min Infusions adjusted to maintain systolic blood pressure between 80% and 100% baseline	Randomization by shuffled envelopes Sample size based on the difference between umbilical cord pH

IM, intramuscular; IV, intravenous.

under epidural anesthesia, but it was not randomized.[7] Finally, there was one retrospective cohort study.[8]

The RCTs are presented in Table 10.1. There were 205 patients who received ephedrine and 223 who received phenylephrine in those undergoing spinal anesthesia in the nine RCTs. In two of the trials, both groups were exposed to ephedrine, either because it was co-administered with the phenylephrine[9] or was used for rescue medication in both groups.[10] One study incorporated a third group who received 50% ephedrine and 50% phenylephrine.[11] Most of the RCTs were of high quality.

Four studies reported how the allocation to group was concealed and how the sample sizes were determined.[9–12] Four studies compared metaraminol,[13] methoxamine[14] or angiotensin II[15,16] with ephedrine. In these studies, 77 patients received ephedrine and 77 received one of the other vasopressors. Spinal anesthesia was used in all but one of these studies.[14] All of these studies were small and two did not report whether or not the investigators were blinded to treatment group.[15,16] The primary outcome of two of the studies was the difference in umbilical cord pH and the sample size was based on this.[13,16]

Neonatal outcomes

Twelve of the 13 studies recorded umbilical artery cord pH. The mean pH was lower in the ephedrine group compared with the other vasopressors in all studies (Fig. 10.1). The difference was statistically significant in eight of these.[9,11,13,15,17–20] One study reported that

the pH gradient between the maternal artery and umbilical vein was similar between patients who received methoxamine and those who receive ephedrine.[14]

Five clinical trials reported the incidence of fetal acidosis (umbilical artery cord pH < 7.20).[9,11,12,15,17] This incidence varied widely between studies. Mercier et al.[9] found that the incidence of fetal acidosis was reduced when phenylephrine was added to ephedrine compared with ephedrine alone (6/19 vs 13/20, $P = 0.09$). Similarly, Carpenter and Cooper[8] noted that the incidence of fetal acidosis was very low in neonates exposed to phenylephrine (1/48) or a combination of phenylephrine and ephedrine (1/47) compared with ephedrine alone (10/48). The difference was statistically significant ($P < 0.001$). Ramin et al.[15] reported the incidence of fetal acidosis was 4/10 in parturients who received ephedrine compared with 0/10 in patients who received no vasopressor and 0/10 in patients who received angiotensin II. The two other studies that reported fetal acidosis only had one patient in each group[17] or one patient in the ephedrine group (none in the phenylephrine group)[12] who met the criteria. One study excluded more patients exposed to ephedrine (3/16) compared with phenylephrine (1/14) because the umbilical artery pH was less than 7.25.[20]

The incidence of an Apgar score of less than 7 at 1 and 5 min after delivery was extremely low. In total, there were only three patients exposed to ephedrine and four exposed to other vasopressors who had a 1-min Apgar score less than 7.[13,16] Only one patient, exposed to angiotensin II, had a 5-min Apgar score of less than 7.[16]

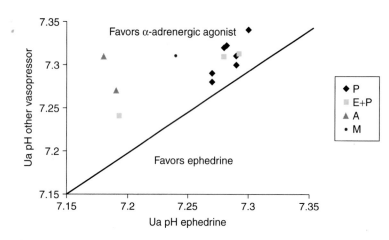

Fig. 10.1 L'Abbé plot showing the umbilical artery (Ua) pH in the ephedrine group (x-axis) and the umbilical artery pH in the other vasopressors (y-axis). Each symbol represents a study. In all studies, the umbilical artery pH was lower in the ephedrine group. A, angiotensin II; E, ephedrine; M, metaraminol; P, phenylephrine.

Maternal outcomes

Important maternal outcomes include the incidence of hypotension, nausea and vomiting, and cardiac arrhythmias. The RCTs that reported the results of studies which compared phenylephrine with ephedrine[12,19–21] were recently combined in a meta-analysis.[22] In these trials, there was no difference between groups in the incidence of maternal hypotension (risk ratio = 1.0; 95% confidence interval, 0.96–1.06). The risk of hypotension in patients exposed to other vasopressors was similar to that of ephedrine.[13,16] There was a statistically significant difference in incidence of hypotension when 4 mg phenylephrine was used prophylactically compared with 2 mg ($P = 0.03$).[10] Hypertension from prophylactic ephedrine or phenylephrine was extremely uncommon and the risk was similar for both drugs[22] (risk ratio = 0.65; 95% confidence interval, 0.08–5.13).

The incidence of nausea and vomiting was reported in five studies.[9,11,13,14,16] One study showed a statistically significant reduction in the incidence of nausea when phenylephrine was used compared with ephedrine or a combination of both drugs.[11] A second study demonstrated an increase in nausea score when ephedrine alone was used compared with a combination of ephedrine and phenylephrine.[9] None of the other studies showed a statistically significant difference between groups.

Maternal bradycardia may be an important side-effect of vasopressor therapy. One investigator, who defined bradycardia as a heart rate less than 60 b/min, treated 11/19 patients in the phenylephrine group and 2/19 patients in the ephedrine group with atropine.[12] Another, using the same criteria found no bradycardia, even though the sample size was larger.[10] The difference may have been because of the route of administration – in the first study, the drugs were given intravenously, in the second intramuscularly. While Lee et al.[22] concluded that the incidence of bradycardia was higher in patients exposed to phenylephrine, a recent study, not included in their meta-analysis, showed an increased incidence of bradycardia in the ephedrine group (10% vs 2%, $P = 0.1$),[11] reducing the reliability of this conclusion.

There was no difference in the incidence of maternal tachycardia in patients exposed to ephedrine, although the pooled heart rate tended to be higher in that group than in the comparison vasopressor.[9,11,13,14,16,21] There were a few patients in each group who suffered from both tachyarrhythmias and bradyarrhythmias.[11,17,18]

Uterine and umbilical blood flow

Four studies measured the pulsatiliy index (PI) of the uterine arteries using Doppler ultrasound.[12–14,17] The PI is calculated as the difference between systolic and diastolic blood flow divided by the mean blood flow. An increase in PI implies an increase in resistance in the artery and therefore indirectly measures a reduction in blood flow.[23] In one of the studies, the PI of the uterine arteries increased significantly after treatment with phenylephrine, but not with ephedrine.[17] None of the other studies showed a significant effect for ephedrine,[12–14] metaraminol[13] or methoxamine.[14] Interestingly, hypotension at the time of measurement also caused an increase in the PI.[14]

There was little change in the fetal circulation with either ephedrine or other vasopressors. None of the studies demonstrated changes in the PI in the umbilical arteries. Maternal hypotension was associated with a small, statistically insignificant increase in the PI.[14] One study demonstrated a decrease in the PI in the fetal middle cerebral and renal arteries in patients who received either ephedrine or phenylephrine. This was statistically significant for the renal arteries.[17]

Conclusions

Traditionally, ephedrine has been used almost exclusively to prevent or treat hypotension caused by regional anesthesia for cesarean section. This review demonstrates that α-adrenergic agents such as phenylephrine do not compromise blood flow to the fetus. There was no difference in the Apgar scores or the incidence of low Apgar scores in any of the RCTs. Surprisingly, the umbilical artery cord pH was consistently lower in neonates exposed to ephedrine compared with those exposed to other α-adrenergic agents. This finding further reduces the likelihood that drugs such as phenylephrine cause harm.

There does not appear to be a considerable difference in the change in uterine blood flow caused by ephedrine or the other α-adrenergic agonists. Hypotension has a greater effect and therefore should be treated promptly. There was no evidence in any of the studies of detrimental effects of either class of drug on umbilical blood flow.

The cause for lower pH in umbilical artery blood in patients receiving ephedrine is unknown. None of the evidence above supports the concept that it is caused by a reduction in blood flow to the fetus. Some authors have speculated that the transplacental diffusion of ephedrine causes β-sympathomimetic stimulation in the fetus, resulting in an increase in metabolism and lower pH.[11] This does not seem to have any other measurable effect on the neonate.

Ephedrine and α-adrenergic agonists appear to be equally efficacious in maintaining maternal blood pressure and reducing symptoms caused by hypotension such as nausea and vomiting. The efficacy depends on the drug dose, mode of administration and the conduct of regional anesthesia rather than class of drug.

Provided that hypotension is treated promptly, the evidence supports the use of either phenylephrine or ephedrine in patients undergoing cesarean section. There is less evidence that angiotensin II, metaraminol or methoxamine are safe and effective, but some centers may have extensive unpublished experience with these drugs. It should be noted that all the patients recruited to the RCTs in the current review were healthy and their fetuses were normal. There is no evidence in the current literature that allows us to recommend a vasopressor in patients in whom the uterine circulation is already compromised.

References

1 Burns SM, Cowan CM, Wilkes RG. Prevention and management of hypotension during spinal anaesthesia for elective caesarean section: a survey of practice. *Anaesthesia* 2001;**56**:777–98.

2 Ralson DH, Shnider SM, deLorimier AA. Effects of equipotent ephedrine, metaraminol, mephentermine, and methoxamine on uterine blood flow in the pregnant ewe. *Anesthesiology* 1974;**40**:354–70.

3 Shnider SM, deLorimier AA, Asling JH, Morishima HO. Vasopressors in obstetrics. II. Fetal hazards of methoxamine administration during spinal anesthesia. *Am J Obstet Gynecol* 1970;**106**:680–6.

4 Shnider SM, deLorimier AA, Steffenson JL. Vasopressors in obstetrics. III. Fetal effects of metaraminol infusion during obstetric spinal hypotension. *Am J Obstet Gynecol* 1970;**106**:1017–22.

5 Sipes SL, Chestnut DH, Vincent-RD J, DeBruyn CS, Bleuer SA, Chatterjee P. Which vasopressor should be used to treat hypotension during magnesium sulfate infusion and epidural anesthesia? *Anesthesiology* 1992;**77**:101–8.

6 Jadad AR, Moore RA, Carroll D, *et al.* Assessing the quality of reports of randomized clinical trials: is blinding necessary? *Control Clin Trials* 1996;**17**:1–12.

7 Ramanathan S, Grant GJ. Vasopressor therapy for hypotension due to epidural anesthesia for cesarean section. *Acta Anaesthesiol Scand* 1988;**32**:559–65.

8 Carpenter MR, Cooper DW. Fetal acidosis, spinal anaesthesia and phenylephrine. *Anaesthesia* 2001;**56**:920–1.

9 Mercier FJ, Riley ET, Frederickson WL, Roger-Christoph S, Benhamou D, Cohen SE. Phenylephrine added to prophylactic ephedrine infusion during spinal anesthesia for elective cesarean section. *Anesthesiology* 2001;**95**:668–74.

10 Ayorinde BT, Buczkowski P, Brown J, Shah J, Buggy DJ. Evaluation of pre-emptive intramuscular phenylephrine and ephedrine for reduction of spinal anaesthesia-induced hypotension during caesarean section. *Br J Anaesth* 2001;**86**:372–6.

11 Cooper DW, Carpenter M, Mowbray P, Desira WR, Ryall DM, Kokri MS. Fetal and maternal effects of phenylephrine and ephedrine during spinal anesthesia for cesarean delivery. *Anesthesiology* 2002;**97**:1582–90.

12 Thomas DG, Robson SC, Redfern N, Hughes D, Boys RJ. Randomized trial of bolus phenylephrine or ephedrine for maintenance of arterial pressure during spinal anaesthesia for caesarean section. *Br J Anaesth* 1996;**76**:61–5.

13 Ngan Kee WD, Lau TK, Khaw KS, Lee BB. Comparison of metaraminol and ephedrine infusions for maintaining arterial pressure during spinal anaesthesia for elective cesarean section. *Anesthesiology* 2001;**95**:307–13.

14 Wright PMC, Iftikhar M, Fitzpatrick KT, Moore J, Thompson W. Vasopressor therapy for hypotension during epidural anesthesia for cesarean section: effects on maternal and fetal flow velocities. *Anesth Analg* 1992;**75**:56–63.

15 Ramin SM, Ramin KD, Cox K, Shearer RR, Grant VE, Gant NF. Comparison of prophylactic angiotensin II versus ephedrine infusion for prevention of maternal hypotension during spinal anesthesia. *Am J Obstet Gynecol* 1994;**171**:734–9.

16 Vincent RD Jr, Werhan CF, Norman PF, *et al.* Prophylactic angiotensin II infusion during spinal anesthesia for elective cesarean delivery. *Anesthesiology* 1998;**88**:1475–9.

17 Alahuhta S, Räsanen J, Jouppila P, Jouppila R, Hollmén AI. Ephedrine and phenylephrine for avoiding maternal hypotension due to spinal anesthesia for cesarean section. *Int J Obstet Anesth* 1992;**1**:129–34.

18 Hall PA, Bennett A, Wilkes MP, Lewis M. Spinal anaesthesia for caesarean section: comparison of infusions of phenylephrine and ephedrine. *Br J Anaesth* 1994;**73**:471–4.

19 LaPorta RF, Arthur GR, Datta S. Phenylephrine in treating maternal hypotension due to spinal anaesthesia for caesarean delivery: effects on neonatal catecholamine concentrations, acid–base status and Apgar scores. *Acta Anaesthesiol Scand* 1995;**39**:901–5.

20 Pierce ET, Carr DB, Datta S. Effects of ephedrine and phenylephrine on maternal and fetal atrial natriuretic peptide

levels during elective cesarean section. *Acta Anaesthesiol Scand* 1994;**38**:48–51.

21 Moran DH, Perillo M, LaPorta RF, Bader AM, Datta S. Phenylephrine in the prevention of hypotension following spinal anesthesia for cesarean delivery. *J Clin Anesth* 1991;**3**:301–5.

22 Lee A, Ngan Kee WD, Gin T. A quantitative, systematic review of randomized controlled trials of ephedrine versus phenylephrine for the management of hypotension during spinal anesthesia for cesarean delivery. *Anesth Analg* 2002;**94**:920–6.

23 Trudinger B. Doppler ultrasound assessment of blood flow. In: Creasy RK, Resnik R, eds. *Maternal Fetal Medicine*. Philadelphia: Saunders, 1999: 216–29.

CHAPTER 11

Is regional anesthesia safer than general anesthesia for cesarean section?

Yehuda Ginosar, Ian F. Russell & Stephen H. Halpern

Introduction

The anesthetic techniques currently available for cesarean delivery are general and regional anesthesia; including spinal, epidural and combined spinal epidural (CSE). Each technique has its advantages and disadvantages; the relative clinical significance of these varies with the clinical situation and the perspectives of individual patients and practitioners.

Current teaching is that regional anesthesia is safer than general anesthesia (GA). Authors cite pulmonary aspiration of gastric contents and difficult endotracheal intubation as major causes of maternal mortality and morbidity associated with GA that can be avoided using regional anesthesia.[1] However, as discussed in Chapters 15 and 19, the incidence of these problems may not be as high as previously thought. In addition, there are strategies available to further reduce their impact. In the absence of specific risk factors, authors infrequently cite total spinal anesthesia, asystole and epidural hematoma as potential problems that can be avoided using GA.[1]

To answer the question as to what type of anesthesia is safer one must decide on the markers that can be used to define safety for mother and neonate (Table 11.1). Maternal and neonatal mortality are probably the most important markers and have the advantage of being unambiguous. Fortunately, the incidence of both is very low and therefore the most appropriate data come from population-based cohort studies. Population-based cohort data are also suitable to assess severe maternal morbidity although the incidence of such complications as maternal hemorrhage requiring transfusion, hypoxic brain injury and intensive care unit admission may be under-reported.[2] It should be noted that each population is unique and results obtained from one population may not apply to others. Further, there are frequently limitations concerning the accuracy and completeness of the databases.

While maternal mortality and severe morbidity are important, there are other adverse outcomes that may affect maternal and neonatal well being. These include estimated maternal blood loss, adverse effects on breastfeeding, neonatal Apgar scores, cord pH and

Maternal	Neonatal
Mortality	Mortality
Morbidity	Morbidity
Total blood loss	Low Apgar scores
Transfusion requirement	Abnormal fetal acid–base status
Hypoxemia	Changes in neurobehavior at birth
Hemodynamic instability	Breastfeeding behavior
Postoperative pain	
Postoperative chronic pain	

Table 11.1 Factors to define the safety of type of anesthesia.

neurologic assessments at birth. Some of these, particularly the neonatal outcomes, may be surrogate outcomes for more serious (but less common) morbidity.

This chapter is divided into two parts. In the first part, the issue of maternal mortality is discussed in full. The data are derived primarily from the Centers for Disease Control (CDC) in the USA and the Triennial Report on Confidential Enquiries into Maternal Deaths in the UK. The methodology and results of these are compared briefly. The data that describe neonatal mortality are taken from the Confidential Inquiry into Stillbirths and Deaths in Infancy in the UK. The second part of the chapter deals with other markers of maternal and neonatal morbidity. The data for this section are derived from a systematic review described below.

Maternal mortality

There is a widely held belief that regional anesthesia is safer for the mother and baby. A recent review[3] made the following claims:

> Maternal death due to anesthesia is the sixth leading cause of pregnancy-related death in the United States. Most anesthesia-related deaths occur during general anesthesia for cesarean delivery. The risk of maternal death from complications of general anesthesia is 17 times as high as that associated with regional anesthesia. Recognition of the risks to the mother associated with general anesthesia has led to an increased use of spinal and epidural anesthesia for both elective and emergency cesarean deliveries. This shift may be the most important reason for a decrease in anesthesia-associated maternal mortality from 4.3 to 1.7 per 1 million live births in the United States.

This review cites an important nationwide survey of anesthesia-related peripartum maternal death in the USA, from Hawkins et al.[4] working together with the CDC, for the years 1979–1984 and 1985–1990. The summary results from the original article are quoted below:

> The anesthesia-related maternal mortality rate decreased from 4.3 per million live births in the first triennium (1979–1981) to 1.7 per million in

the last (1988–1990). The number of deaths involving general anesthesia have remained stable, but the number of regional anesthesia-related deaths have decreased since 1984. The case–fatality risk ratio for general anesthesia was 2.3 (95% confidence interval, 1.9–2.9) times that for regional anesthesia before 1985, increasing to 16.7 (95% CI, 12.9–21.8) times that after 1985.

The authors calculated case–fatality rates for cesarean section conducted under both GA and regional anesthesia using a number of assumptions and approximations and then compared them using a risk ratio. The details of these calculations are outlined below.

The case–fatality rate for GA was calculated by dividing the number of maternal deaths (fatalities) under GA by the total number of cesarean sections performed under GA (cases). Similarly, the case–fatality rate for regional anesthesia was obtained by dividing the number of maternal deaths under regional anesthesia by the number of cesarean deliveries performed under regional anesthesia. The ratio of these two rates was taken to provide a risk ratio. Therefore it is important to identify factors that may lead to errors in the estimation of the number of maternal mortalities, the number of cesarean sections and the type of anesthesia used for each cesarean section. Further, it would be helpful to compare the incidence of known preanesthetic risk factors for death in the two groups.

In their study, Hawkins et al.[4] used data from the National Pregnancy Mortality Surveillance System, based on information from death certificates, to identify all maternal deaths that occurred in the USA 1979–1990. Of note, it was not possible for the authors to inspect the medical records of any of the cases. Of the 4097 cases of "pregnancy-related death," 155 cases were categorized as anesthesia-related. After eliminating early abortions and ectopic pregnancies, 129 cases remained.

There were several sources of uncertainty in the estimated incidence of maternal death. First, it is likely that the incidence of maternal death was underestimated, possibly by as much as 37%.[4] Second, because the personnel who filled out the death certificates were unlikely to have anesthetic training, the incidence of anesthesia-related mortality may also have been underestimated or misclassified. The magnitude of this source of error is unknown. The information on death certificates is often incomplete. For example, in 17 of the 129 cases, the mode of delivery was unknown. In 25 cases, the type of anesthesia was unknown. Six of the fatalities occurred during vaginal delivery, even though the "cases" were estimated from the number of cesarean sections. Finally, the authors apportioned these deaths to the anesthetic technique chosen for delivery. It should be noted that an unknown number of regional anesthetics requiring conversion to GA were considered for analysis as patients receiving GA (J.L. Hawkins, personal communication).

The total number of cases in the time period was also based on a number of estimates and assumptions. First, the number of live births nationally for each year during the period 1979–1990 was obtained from the natality files of the National Center for Health Statistics. The authors applied national cesarean delivery rates for each year, derived from National Hospital Discharge Survey data, to the number of live births, and then calculated the number of cesarean deliveries for each of the two periods 1979–1984 and 1985–1990. The absolute number of cesarean deliveries under regional anesthesia and GA for each of the two time periods was estimated based upon the proportions of each technique reported in a written survey which was sent to every hospital for each of the time periods. This survey had a response rate of approximately 50%, which covered 30% and 56% of the births for the two 6-year periods, respectively.

Chestnut[5] identified three major sources of error in the estimate of how many parturients received which type of anesthesia. First, the proportion of patients who received GA and regional anesthesia was extrapolated from the sample of institutions that responded to the questionnaire. This sample may not be representative of practice in the USA. Second, the data from the survey were not checked for accuracy, meaning that the data supplied by the individual respondents may have been unreliable. Third, the incidence of GA may have been understated for the second time period (1985–1990), leading to an erroneously high case–fatality rate during that time. This was, to some extent, confirmed by the steep reduction in fatalities under GA, from 32.3 per million to 16.8 per million, recorded from 1991 to 1996.[6]

While the exact number of cases and fatalities may be debated, it is likely that the case–fatality rate is higher in parturients who receive GA compared with regional anesthesia. However, it is probable that factors other than type of anesthesia were the cause of this difference. Chestnut[5] identified four demographic and personal characteristics that are associated with maternal death (non-Caucasian ethnicity, poor socioeconomic status, obesity and advanced maternal age). To this list, other factors such as emergency surgery,[7] pre-eclampsia/eclampsia,[7] bleeding diathesis and failed regional anesthesia may have been more prevalent in the GA group. Therefore, a causal link between the type of anesthesia and death rate cannot be established for these data and it is inappropriate to suggest that "general anesthesia is riskier than regional anesthesia in the obstetric patient."[8]

Similar data are observed in the Triennial Confidential Inquiries into Maternal Deaths in the UK, although the method of obtaining the data is different. In England and Wales, when a maternal death is identified, a statement is obtained from all medical and midwifery personnel involved in her care. These statements, with identifying data removed, together with the medical record are passed on to a regional assessor for midwifery care, obstetric care and anesthetic care. These regional assessors then independently comment on their respective aspects of care and provide independent opinions on their speciality's care. Following this, the data are passed on to national assessors in midwifery, obstetrics, anesthesia and pathology. The process is similar in Scotland and Northern Ireland, except that there are no regional assessors. Finally, an editorial board, consisting of clinicians, statisticians and representatives from the Department of Health considers all that has been documented and is responsible for the final classification of the cause of death. Therefore, in contrast to the CDC data, both clinical and pathologic notes are available when assigning cause of death. The latest report is available at: http://www.cemach.org.uk/publications/CEMDreports/cemdrpt.pdf (last accessed July 13, 2004). There has been a steady reduction in the absolute numbers of maternal deaths directly related to anesthesia from 37 in 1970–1972 to a single death in 1994–1996 and three deaths in 1997–1999 (Fig. 11.1). This improvement has been paralleled by a reduction in the proportion of cesarean sections being conducted under GA over a strikingly similar time course[9–11] (Fig. 11.2). In a series of surveys in the UK, Russell et al. demonstrated that the percentage of cesarean deliveries performed under

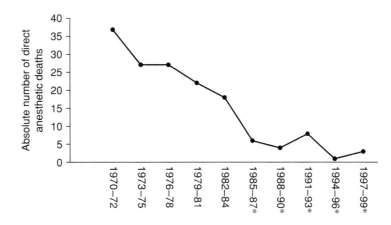

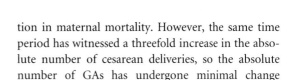

Fig. 11.1 Reduction in anesthesia-related maternal mortality in the UK (1970–1999) from Triennial Confidential Inquiries into Maternal Deaths in the UK.

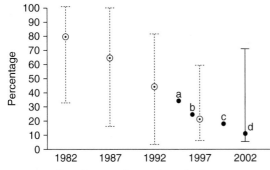

Fig. 11.2 Changing use of general anesthesia 1982–2002. Adapted from reference 11. Median incidence (⊙) and range (dotted line) of the use of general anesthesia shown for institutions in the UK surveyed. Comparison data (points a, b, c and d) are derived from NHS maternity statistics. (http://www.publications.doh.gov.uk/public/work_health_care.htm#cat-hosp.)

regional anesthesia rose from 23% in 1982 to 56% in 1992, and 75% in 1997.[11,12] Data from the Royal College of Obstetrician and Gynaecologists' National Caesarean Section Audit showed that 77% of emergency sections and 91% of elective sections were performed with a regional anesthetic technique.[10]

It might be tempting to suggest that the two phenomena are causally related; namely that it is the reduction in the proportion of cesarean deliveries being performed under GA that has caused this reduc-

tion in maternal mortality. However, the same time period has witnessed a threefold increase in the absolute number of cesarean deliveries, so the absolute number of GAs has undergone minimal change (Fig. 11.3).

Neonatal mortality

There are limited data available to assess whether neonatal death is affected by the choice of anesthesia for cesarean delivery. The incidence of unexpected neonatal death following cesarean section is highlighted in the Confidential Inquiry into Stillbirths and Deaths in Infancy in the UK (http://www.cemach.org.uk/publications.htm – last accessed July 13, 2004).

For the years 1994–1995, 873 infants over 1.5 kg died unexpectedly; in 25 of these 873 deaths, anesthesia was the direct cause or made a significant contribution to the infant death. In four cases the problem was "directly related" to the giving of the anesthetic – all GAs, two of which were for elective cesarean section. Importantly, there were 21 cases, all emergencies (15 GA, three spinal, three epidural), where deficiencies in anesthesia care were judged to have made a "significant contribution" to neonatal death. Although 15 of these 21 cases ultimately received GA, 10 cases involved prolonged attempted regional anesthesia, where technical problems in identifying the target

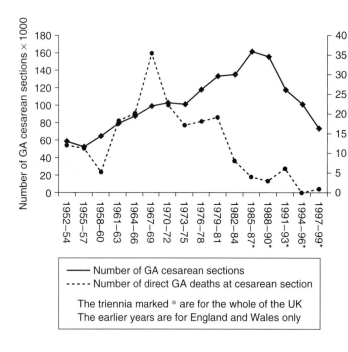

Fig. 11.3 The number of cesarean sections under general anesthesia and the number of direct maternal deaths under general anesthesia 1952–1999. Data from Thomas and Paranjothy.[10]

space led to delay in establishing anesthesia after the anesthesiologist was present. The remaining 11 cases resulted from delay in obtaining appropriate anesthesia staff.

Conclusions

The data from investigations in the USA and UK show a very low risk of maternal and neonatal death associated with anesthesia for cesarean section. It is inappropriate to compare the case–fatality rates (using risk ratios) of general versus regional anesthesia because the populations that received the two types of anesthesia are different in important demographic risk factors. An increase in neonatal deaths does not appear to be associated with the type of anesthesia but with individual logistic and judgment issues. It is therefore not possible to state that one type of anesthesia is safer for mother or neonate without considering the complete clinical scenario.

Maternal and neonatal morbidity

In order to assess whether anesthetic technique increases the risk of maternal or neonatal morbidity, studies have examined other outcome variables that occur more frequently than death. Important maternal outcomes include measures of intraoperative

blood loss such as estimated maternal blood loss or fall in hematocrit, incidence of desaturation, hemodynamic instability and acute or chronic postoperative pain. Neonatal outcomes include abnormal fetal acid–base status and low Apgar scores. Some outcomes such as anesthesia–incision time, transfusion requirement, length or cost of hospital admission for mother or neonate are dependent upon local medical practices and the results may not be applicable to all settings.

In order to compare the incidence of these outcomes in patients who received GA or regional anesthesia, we conducted a systematic literature search using the following databases: MEDLINE® (1966–2004), EMBASE® (1980–2004) and the Cochrane Central Register of Clinical Trials. In addition, all the volumes of the *International Journal of Obstetric Anesthesia* were hand searched. The search strategy used the following text and key words: [cesarean or caesarean], [anesth* or anaesth*] and [general] and [regional or epidural or spinal or extradural or peridural or neuraxial]. We included all human studies, regardless of study design and without language restriction, that compared GA with regional anesthesia and reported at least one outcome of interest. The search was performed by two individuals independently (YG and SH). The search was last updated to April 30, 2004.

We identified 627 studies. We eliminated studies

that did not meet inclusion criteria and those that compared archaic anesthetic techniques. We arbitrarily took the year 1989 as the earliest publication date for our review; this allows a 15-year perspective and coincides with major changes in current anesthesia practice (the introduction of pulse oximetry, capnography and the avoidance of 0.75% epidural bupivacaine).

There were 28 studies[13-41] that met the inclusion criteria. Of these, eight were randomized controlled trials,[13-16,18-21] six were prospective non-randomized trials[22-27] and 14 were retrospective reviews.[28-41] The details of these studies, including the Jadad score for quality (see Appendix for a description of this score), patient population and sample size can be seen in Table 11.2.

Maternal outcomes

Fifteen of the studies reported one or more maternal outcomes.[13,14,16,18-20,24,25,30,31,35,37-39,41] Changes in blood pressure and blood loss were the most commonly reported outcomes. The results for these studies are shown in Table 11.3.

Blood pressure

Six of the studies reported changes in blood pressure at various points during surgery[13,14,18,20,25,30] but this was not the primary outcome for any study. As expected, the incidence of hypotension was increased in the regional anesthesia group and the incidence of hypertension was higher in the GA group (Table 11.3).

Blood loss

Blood loss is difficult to measure accurately in cesarean delivery owing to the spillage of copious quantities of amniotic fluid into the surgical field. Similarly, studies that interpret changes in maternal hematocrit, hemoglobin and plasma volume as surrogate markers for blood loss are complicated by the parallel changes that occur in plasma volume during and after cesarean delivery.

Out of eight studies in our systematic review that addressed the issue of maternal blood loss, seven found a significant increase in blood loss in patients who received GA (Table 11.3). The study that did not find statistical significance was a retrospective study of 121 patients. No study found data to suggest that

regional anesthesia was associated with greater bleeding than GA.

Other maternal outcomes

Acute and chronic post-cesarean section pain

The clinical impression of the authors is that regional anesthesia provides better in-hospital pain relief than GA. Multiple studies have compared different techniques of postoperative pain relief but few have compared regional anesthesia with GA in this regard. Only two of the studies in our review assessed pain following cesarean section: one study reported first day postoperative analgesia requirements (amongst several secondary endpoints) and one study assessed chronic pain.[20,38] In a small, prospective, randomized controlled trial, Hong et al.[20] demonstrated that 11/12 patients in the GA group required postoperative analgesia, as compared with 3/13 in the regional anesthesia group ($P = 0.0007$).

Nikolajsen et al.[38] conducted a written postal survey of 220 responders (out of 244 surveys that were mailed) who had undergone cesarean section. Of these patients, 18.6% continued to have pain 3 months following surgery and 12.3% still had pain by 10 months; 5.9% reported daily (or almost daily) pain. Patients who had undergone GA had a higher incidence of chronic pain (10/27) than those who received regional anesthesia (33/193) ($P < 0.02$). The reasons for GA in this sample were not known, so it is unclear whether these differences are because of the prevention of nociceptive bombardment of the spinal cord as the authors speculate, or whether the underlying condition (such as emergency or more extensive surgery) may be the more relevant factor.

Breastfeeding

Although none of the studies in our systematic review assessed breastfeeding ability following cesarean section, this was examined in a small retrospective study published in 1988, 1 year prior to the period of our review.[42] The authors studied 88 patients, from which 56 patients were selected for analysis (no data were presented to explain the selective population reduction). Breastfeeding started earlier and persisted longer following regional anesthesia, such that by 6 months 71% were still breastfeeding in the epidural group and only 39% in the GA group ($P < 0.025$).

Table 11.2 Studies described by design.

Author and date	Type of study	Quality (Jadad)	Population	General anesthesia (GA)		Regional anesthesia (RA)		Comments
				N	Anesthetic management	N	Anesthetic management	
Dyer et al. 2003[13]	RCT	5	Severe pre-eclampsia with fetal distress	35	Thiopental, suxamethonium, N₂O, isoflurane, morphine	35	Spinal anesthesia. 9 mg bupivacaine, 10 μg fentanyl	Blinded allocation (sealed envelopes) Sample size calculation based on hypothesized base deficit increase in spinal group Identical fluid management between groups (< 750 mL Ringer's lactate) GA group but not RA group received IV magnesium Controlled relative hypercarbia for pregnancy in GA group (P_{aCO_2} 32.4 mmHg compared with 28.9 mmHg for RA)
Sener et al. 2003[14]	RCT	3	Healthy (both elective and obstructed labor)	15	Thiopental, suxamethonium, N₂O, isoflurane	15	Epidural anesthesia. 20 mL 0.375% bupivacaine	No blinded allocation or sample size calculation reported
Hong et al. 2003[20]	RCT	3	Elective Placenta previa totalis	12	Thiopental, suxamethonium, enflurane–N₂O	13	Epidural lidocaine 2%, 23 mL + epidural morphine	25 consecutive placenta previa patients identified out of 5510 deliveries. All were enrolled in the RCT No sample size calculation No mention of randomization technique or whether there was a blinded allocation
Kavak et al. 2001[15]	RCT	1	Elective repeat Healthy	38	Non-specified technique	46	Spinal anesthesia: Non-specified technique	No blinded allocation or sample size calculation reported 1500 mL crystalloid administered to spinal group only
Lertakyamanee et al. 1999[16]	RCT	NA	Elective Healthy	103	Non-specified technique	120 / 118	Epidural: non-specified technique Spinal: non-specified technique	19 patients excluded for incomplete data: only 5 patients missing umbilical artery pH, remainder missing only cortisol, creatinine kinase or bicarbonate; the umbilical artery data were not presented in these patients Abstract. Maternal outcomes reported

Continued

Study	Design		Patients	n	GA technique	n	RA technique	Comments
Kolatat et al. 1999[17]	RCT	NA	Elective Healthy	103	Non-specified technique	120 / 118	Epidural: non-specified technique / Spinal: non-specified technique	Abstract (data identical to Ref. 16). Neonatal outcomes reported
Mahajan et al. 1992[18]	RCT	5	Elective Healthy	30	Thiopental, suxamethonium, halothane–N_2O	30	Epidural: 12–20 mL bupivacaine 0.5% / Spinal: bupivacaine 12–15 mg	No blinded allocation or sample size calculation reported. Ephedrine used to treat hypotension. Fluid bolus of 750–1000 mL in RA groups only
Wallace et al. 1995[19]	RCT	3	Severe pre-eclampsia	26	Anesthetic drugs not specified. IV hydralazine, nitroglycerin and lidocaine given prior to induction in GA group only	27 / 27	Epidural: lidocaine 2% or chlorprocaine 3% to T4 / CSE: 11.25 mg heavy bupivacaine	No sample size calculation. Study not blinded Patients with less than 100,000 platelets or fetal distress were excluded 1000 mL fluid bolus in RA groups only
Yegin et al. 2003[21]	RCT	2	Elective Healthy	31	Thiopental, suxamethonium, isoflurane–N_2O	31	Epidural: bupivacaine 0.5% 18 mL	No blinded allocation or sample size calculation reported, no mention of the type of randomization or physician blinding
Gambling et al. 1995[22]	Prospective non-randomized	NA	Healthy Elective	28 / 27	Group 1: Thiopental, suxamethonium, sevoflurane / Group 2: Thiopental, suxamethonium, isoflurane	20	Spinal (11.25 mg heavy bupivacaine, 10 µg fentanyl)	Spinal vs GA by patient choice; two GA groups randomized. 1500–2000 mL crystalloid in spinal group vs 500 mL in GA groups. No sample size calculation reported
Adams et al. 2003[23]	Prospective non-randomized	NA	Healthy Elective	21 / 21	Ketamine, methohexital / Sevoflurane, methohexital	22	Spinal (13–15 mg plain bupivacaine)	Spinal vs GA by patient choice; two GA groups randomized
Afolabi et al. 2003[24]	Prospective case controlled study	NA	Elective and emergency	39	Thiopental or ketamine, suxamethonium, volatile agent–N_2O	39	Spinal: bupivacaine 12.5–15 mg	Incomplete sample size calculation (based on Apgar, but not stating what difference expected)
Ramanathan et al. 1991[25]	Prospective non-randomized	NA	Severe pre-eclampsia	10	Non-specified technique	11	Epidural: lidocaine 2% to T4	Randomization refused by Institutional Board Review. No comment on blinding, patient selection or sample size calculation
Kangas-Saarela et al. 1989[26]	Prospective non-randomized	NA	Elective Repeat or "fetopelvic disproportion"	13	Thiopental, suxamethonium, halothane–N_2O	18	Epidural: bupivacaine 0.5% to T6	Epidural vs GA by patient choice 1500 mL bolus of crystalloid in epidural group only No comment on vasopressors

Table 11.2 (*continued*)

Author and date	Type of study	Quality (Jadad)	Population	General anesthesia (GA)		Regional anesthesia (RA)		Comments
				N	Anesthetic management	N	Anesthetic management	
Hodgson & Wauchob 1994[27]	Prospective non-randomized	NA	Elective Healthy	74	Thiopental, suxamethonium, isoflurane–N_2O	63	Spinal: heavy bupivacaine 10–15 mL	Institutional Board Review approval not obtained. Spinal vs GA by patient choice. 2000 mL crystalloid bolus before spinal group only
Evans et al. 1989[28]	Retrospective review	NA	Healthy Elective	471	Non-specified technique	139	Epidural: non-specified technique	Only 412 (GA) and 125 (RA) subjects analyzed due to incomplete cord gas data and exclusion of birth weight < 2500 g
Mueller et al. 1997[29]	Retrospective review	NA	Healthy term Elective	2649	Non-specified technique	2155 / 1002	Epidural: non-specified technique / Spinal: non-specified technique	5806 analyzed out of 40,858 cesarean sections in database (after excluding maternal–fetal risk factors, labor, inadequate cord pH data)
Moodley et al. 2001[30]	Retrospective review	NA	Conscious women after eclamptic seizure	27	Etomidate, magnesium, suxamethonium, isoflurane	37	Epidural: non-specified technique	66 patients analyzed out of 533 eclamptic patients in database. Patients with fetal distress, impaired consciousness, hemodynamic instability, coagulopathy or spinal anesthesia (n = 2) were excluded
Parekh et al. 2000[31]	Retrospective review	NA	Placenta previa Consecutive patients Emergency and elective	140	Non-specified technique	210	Non-specified technique	15 years recruiting period
Levy et al. 1998[32]	Retrospective review	NA	Intrauterine growth restriction	65	Non-specified technique	36	Spinal: non-specified technique	44–51 patients received epidurals but this group included both vaginal and cesarean deliveries; data were not presented to separate those patients who received epidurals for cesarean section, so this entire group has been removed from this assessment
Roberts et al. 1995[33]	Retrospective review	NA	Healthy Elective Repeat cesarean	371 / 54	Thiopental, suxamethonium, N_2O, isoflurane or enflurane / Failed RA requiring GA conversion	286 / 659 / 231	Epidural: non-specified technique / CSE: non-specified technique / Spinal: non-specified technique	No missing patients

Study	Design		Population	GA technique	n	RA technique	n	Comments
Rolbin et al. 1994[34]	Retrospective review	NA	Preterm delivery < 32 weeks	Non-specified technique	168	Epidural: non-specified technique. 1000–1500 mL fluid bolus in epidural group only	341	512 preterm cesarean deliveries out of 28,959 births. Data based on two separate independent prospective data bases (obstetric and neonatal). No data to explain reason for choice of anesthesia
Hood & Holubec 1990[35]	Retrospective review	NA	Elective Repeat	GA group 1: thiopental, suxamethonium, halothane–N_2O; GA group 2: thiopental, suxamethonium, no halothane	23; 14	Epidural: non-specified technique	84	
Petropoulos et al. 2003[36]	Retrospective review	NA	Elective Healthy	Non-specified technique		Epidural or CSE: non-specified technique		238 women assessed
Boyle 1993[40]	Retrospective review	NA	All cesarean sections	Non-specified technique	93	Epidural: non-specified technique; Spinal: non-specified technique	223; 5	
Lao et al. 1993[37]	Retrospective case control study	NA	Preterm (24 to 36 weeks' gestation)	Thiopental, suxamethonium, halothane–N_2O or enflurane–N_2O	30	Epidural: carbonated 2% lidocaine (& epinephrine) to T4	30	Of 233 patients over 4 years who had a cesarean section between 24 and 36 weeks, 58 had GA and 175 had RA. Out of these data, 30 matched pairs were created
Nikolajsen et al. 2004[38]	Retrospective questionnaire survey	NA	All cesarean sections	Non-specified technique	27	Spinal: non-specified technique	193	Survey conducted 8–18 months following surgery. 92% response rate. Survey questionnaire only asks for GA or spinal, even though some patients received epidural catheters
Vigil-De Gracia et al. 2001[39]	Retrospective cohort	NA	HELLP syndrome	Non-specified technique	9	Epidural: non-specified technique; Spinal: non-specified technique	58; 4	
Andrews et al. 1992[41]	Retrospective review	NA	Healthy Elective	Thiopental, suxamethonium, isoflurane–N_2O	42	Epidural: non-specified technique; Spinal: non-specified technique; CSE: non-specified technique	28; 2; 15	

CSE, combined spinal epidural; IV, intravenous; NA, not applicable; N_2O, nitrous oxide; RCT, randomized controlled trial.

Table 11.3 Maternal outcomes (for patient populations and study design, see Table 11.2).

Author and date	Maternal outcomes		Other maternal outcomes	Conclusions/comments
	Blood pressure	Blood loss		
Dyer et al. 2003[13]	Significantly lower in the spinal group at several time points	Blood loss was significantly higher in the GA group (446 mL ± 126) than the spinal group (393 mL ± 64, $P < 0.04$) No patient required transfusion	Significantly more ephedrine used in the spinal group (13.7 ± 17.5 compared to GA group (2.7 ± 8.9, $P = 0.002$)	Primary outcome neonatal (see Table 11.4)
Sener et al. 2003[14]	Incidence of hypotension: 0/15 in GA group vs 8/15 in RA group ($P = 0.001$)		*Shivering:* 8/15 in GA group 1/15 in RA group ($P = 0.007$) *Nausea:* 14/15 in GA group 9/15 in RA group ($P = 0.04$) *Vomiting:* 9/15 in GA group 2/15 in RA group ($P = 0.01$)	Primary outcomes neonatal (see Table 11.4) 4/15 patients in GA group had an "allergic reaction"
Moodley et al. 2001[30]	Incidence of hypotension 5/37 epidural 0/27 GA ($P = 0.06$)		1 late maternal death in the epidural group	Spinal anesthetics (n = 2) were excluded Small sample. Authors conclude that epidural anesthesia is justified in stable eclamptic patients
Hong et al. 2003[20]	Significant increase in systolic and diastolic pressure following intubation and extubation in the GA group ($P < 0.05$)	*Estimated blood loss (mL):* GA: 1623 ± 775; epidural: 1418 ± 996 (NS) *Postoperative blood transfusion (units):* GA: 1.08 ± 1.6; epidural: 0.38 ± 0.9 ($P < 0.05$) *Number of patients transfused:* GA: 5/12; epidural 2/13 ($P = 0.15$) *Immediate postoperative hematocrit < 30:* GA: 8/12 epidural 3/13 ($P = 0.04$)	*Ephedrine requirement (mg):* GA: 0; epidural: 5.4 ± 8.8 ($P < 0.05$) *Need for analgesia in 1st 24 h postoperative:* GA: 11/12; epidural 3/13 ($P = 0.0007$)	Patients in the GA group had a lower postoperative hematocrit and an increased transfusion requirement Postoperative analgesia was significantly better in the epidural group (with epidural morphine) No patient in the epidural group required conversion to GA
Afolabi et al. 2003[24]		*Estimated blood loss (mL):* GA: 539 ± 341; spinal: 405 ± 230 ($P < 0.005$) *Difference in hematocrit preoperative to 2nd postoperative day:* GA: -6.0% ± 4.1; spinal: -2.9 ± 3.8% ($P = 0.004$) *Need for transfusion:* 3/35 vs 0/35 (NS)		General anesthesia was associated with more blood loss than spinal anesthesia

Continued

Lertakyamanee et al. 1999[16]	GA: increased estimated blood loss, increased number of patients receiving transfusion and increased number of patients with postoperative hematocrit < 30; 50% of women in RA group became hypotensive	No difference in patient satisfaction scores	Blood pressure data from Ref. 17. No data on blood pressure in GA group
Ramanathan et al. 1991[25]	*Mean arterial pressure on intubation/skin incision:* GA: 143 ± 5 mmHg; epidural: 118 ± 5 mmHg (P < 0.004) *Mean arterial pressure postoperatively:* GA: 120 ± 4 mmHg; epidural: 99 ± 4 mmHg (P < 0.007)	Increase in maternal levels of ACTH, β-endorphin, epinephrine, norepinephrine, dopamine in the GA group. No change in these hormones in the epidural group, except for a reduction in norepinephrine following epidural anesthesia	
Wallace et al. 1995[19]		Ephedrine administered for hypotension GA: 0/26; epidural: 8/27; CSE: 6/27 (P = 0.002) when the regional groups are combined	Neither GA or RA is contraindicated in severe pre-eclampsia. Patients with fetal distress and thrombocytopenia were not studied
Parekh et al. 2000[31]	Mean blood loss (mL) GA: 756 ± 518; RA: 613 ± 367 (P = 0.006)		RA is appropriate for placenta previa
Hood & Holubec 1990[35]	*Hematocrit (baseline – 2 days postoperative) (NS)* GA (including halothane): 36.6% ± 2.5% to 32.7 ± 2.6% GA (with no halothane): 35.6% ± 2.3% to 31.9 ± 3.3% Epidural: 37.4% ± 2.8% to 34.0 ± 3.3%		3-group comparison (2 GA and 1 epidural) Note a 0% transfusion rate compared with 18% in a similar study from the same institution in 1987 (Gilstrap 1987). The earlier study examined both elective and emergency surgery
Nikolajsen et al. 2004[38]	Chronic pain higher following GA (10/27) than following spinal (33/193) (P < 0.02)		Authors speculate that inhibition of noxious stimulation of the cord during surgery may account for this observation, but accept that emergency surgery is more likely to lead to general anesthesia and the traumatic associations

Table 11.3 (*continued*)

| Author and date | Maternal outcomes | | | Conclusions/comments |
	Blood pressure	Blood loss	Other maternal outcomes	
Lao et al. 1993[37]		Number of patients with > 10% fall in hemoglobin following cesarean section: GA: 14/30; epidural: 6/30 ($P < 0.05$)		Authors conclude that GA is associated with an increased blood loss in CS, advised to avoid if possible in women with risk factors for excessive blood loss (NB Women with such risk factors were excluded from this analysis)
Mahajan et al. 1992[18]	Number of patients receiving ephedrine for hypotension (indication for intervention not defined): GA: 3/30; epidural: 7/30; spinal: 12/30		Maternal arterial blood gases GA: pH 7.36 ± 0.04, P_{CO_2} 34.5 ± 3 mmHg; epidural: pH 7.44 ± 0.06, P_{CO_2} 28.0 ± 0.3 mmHg Spinal: pH: 7.42 ± 0.03, P_{CO_2}: 30 ± 1.9 mmHg ($P < 0.01$)	In this study, GA patients were relatively hypoventilated
Andrews et al. 1992[41]		Hematocrit (baseline − 1 day postoperative) GA: 35.0 ± 0.6 − 32.6 ± 0.6 RA: 34.7 ± 0.3 − 33.3 ± 0.4 (NS) Number of patients with > 5 vol% fall in hematocrit following cesarean section: GA: 10/42; RA: 5/75 ($P = 0.018$)		Authors conclude that GA is associated with an increased blood loss in cesarean section (NB No patient in this study had blood transfused)
Vigil-De Gracia et al. 2001[39]			No epidural hematoma	The authors conclude that RA is safe in HELLP syndrome, based upon the lack of epidural hematoma in 62 patients. Because epidural hematoma is rare, one cannot draw reliable conclusions about safety

ACTH, adrenocorticotropic hormone; CSE, combined spinal epidural; GA, general anesthesia; NS, not significant; RA, regional anesthesia.

Neonatal outcomes

There were 21 studies that reported neonatal outcomes.[13–15,18–30,32–34,36,40] The most commonly reported outcomes were the Apgar score and cord blood gases. These and other outcomes are shown in detail in Table 11.4.

Apgar score

The 10-point Apgar score was introduced in 1952 and is the sum of ratings for five separate variables (heart rate, respiratory effort, muscle tone, reflex irritability, color), each variable receiving 0, 1 or 2 on the input ordinal scale. Attempts to use the Apgar score as a predictor of late neurologic impairment have aroused considerable controversy, as this is a use for which the score was not intended.[43] It should be stated, however, that the pressure to apply the Apgar score in this way arises from the lack of other clinical predictors for neurologic impairment that are comparable for simplicity, applicability and validity.

Of the 21 studies summarized in Table 11.4 that provide data on the Apgar score, 12 found that Apgar scores were significantly improved for regional anesthesia when compared with GA, eight found no significant difference and none found an improvement for GA. Of the 12 studies that found statistical significance, only six showed significance beyond 1 min. None of these were randomized controlled trials, nor were the assessors blinded to the type of anesthesia administered.

Fetal acid–base status

Umbilical arterial and venous blood sampling has been widely applied and different criteria have formed surrogate outcome measures in different studies. Of particular interest has been umbilical artery pH and base excess or deficit as an index of fetal acidemia and sustained asphyxia. The acids that potentially contribute to fetal acidemia are carbonic acid (the product of aerobic respiration) and lactic acid and β-hydroxybutyric acid (the products of anerobic respiration). Carbonic acid clearance is rapid and is affected to a large degree by maternal $Paco_2$ and maternal ventilation.[44] Thus, assessments of base deficit and excess are likely a better reflection of underlying anerobic metabolism and asphyxia than is the umbilical pH.

Of the 10 studies in our systematic review that assessed cord blood gas, four studies showed increased fetal acidemia in neonates delivered by regional anesthesia, six studies showed no significant difference while none showed increased fetal acidemia following GA. Of the studies demonstrating increased fetal acidemia, only one was a randomized controlled study,[13] which assessed pre-eclamptic pregnancies with non-reassuring fetal heart rate patterns. Both large retrospective studies[29,33] demonstrated strong relationships between regional anesthesia and a tendency to fetal acidemia.

A large retrospective review by Mueller et al.[29] from Switzerland analyzed 5806 healthy term pregnancies from a database of 40,858 elective cesarean deliveries over 10 years (1985–1994). Over the course of the study, the incidence of fetal acidemia (pH < 7.1) in the study population rose from 0.59% at the outset of the study period to 2.89% by the end, which paralleled an increase in spinal anesthesia from 1.2% to 47.5% ($P = 0.009$). Among the different groups, 46% underwent GA, 37% received epidural anesthesia and 17% received spinal anesthesia. The incidence of fetal acidemia was lower in the GA than in the regional anesthesia groups (Table 11.4). In contrast, the Apgar score in these patients was higher in the regional anesthesia groups than in the GA group. Notwithstanding, more neonates from the spinal group were transferred to neonatal intensive care than from other groups.

In a smaller retrospective study of 1600 elective repeat cesarean deliveries, Roberts et al.[33] reported similar findings, with odds ratio for fetal acidemia (pH < 7.1) for epidural, CSE and spinal of 3.7 (95% confidence interval [CI], 1.9–7.2), 6.1 (95% CI, 3.4–11.0) and 8.6 (95% CI, 4.6–16.2), respectively, when compared with GA.

Both investigators speculated that sympathectomy induced by regional anesthesia (and the consequent maternal hypotension) is the likely cause for this increased acidemia in the regional anesthesia groups, although neither study collected or presented hemodynamic data. These studies are retrospective analyses; the Mueller study in particular is open to the possibility for bias associated with a selective analysis of 14% of a retrospective sample. In addition, neither study presented data for base deficit or excess, although Roberts et al.[33] state that only one patient in the spinal group had evidence of metabolic acidemia.

Table 11.4 Neonatal outcomes (for patient populations and study designs, see Table 11.2).

Author/ date	Neonatal outcomes			
	Umbilical artery gases	Apgar scores	Other outcomes	Authors conclusions/comments
Dyer et al. 2003[13]	*Umbilical artery pH:* GA: 7.23 [range 7.05–7.4] Spinal: 7.20 [range 6.93–7.34] (P = 0.05) *Base deficit (mEq/L) (primary outcome):* GA: 4.68 ± 3.3 Spinal: 7.13 ± 4.0 (P = 0.02) *Bicarbonate (mEq/L):* GA: 20.4 ± 3.0 Spinal: 18.4 ± 3.0 (P < 0.05)	*Apgar (1 min):* GA: 7 [interquartile 4–8] Spinal: 8 [interquartile 6–9] (P < 0.05) *Apgar (5 min):* GA: 9 [interquartile range 9–10] Spinal: 9 [interquartile range 9–10] (P = 1.0)	Neonatal resuscitation 22/35 GA vs 15/35 spinal, P = 0.07	Spinal anesthesia for this high-risk population was associated with a higher mean base deficit and a lower median umbilical artery pH. The authors comment on the possibility that the low pH is associated with ephedrine use in the spinal anesthesia group
Sener et al. 2003[14]	*Umbilical artery pH:* GA: 7.26 ± 0.0 RA: 7.27 ± 0.0	*Apgar (1 min):* GA: 9 [4–9]; RA: 8 [8–10] (P < 0.001) *Apgar (5 min):* NS	*NACS:* *2 h* GA: 15.2 ± 0.5 RA: 19.1 ± 0.2 (P < 0.001) *24 h* GA: 18.0 ± 0.8 RA: 20.0 ± 0.0 (P < 0.001) *Delivery – 1st breast feed interval (min):* GA: 228 ± 23 RA: 107 ± 12 (P < 0.001)	Standard deviation for all outcomes appear to be too small. Statistical inference from them may be unreliable
Evans et al. 1989[28]		*Apgar (1 min):* (P < 0.0001) 1–3: GA: 29/467; RA: 0/139 4–7: GA: 72/467; RA: 6/139 *Apgar (5 min):* (P < 0.01) 1–3: GA: 8/467; RA: 0/139 4–7: GA: 19/467; RA: 0/139	Apgar (1 min), and cord pH Apgar < 7 and pH < 7.2 GA: 78/412; RA: 2/125 (P < 0.0001)	Greater neonatal depression associated with GA, increased fetal acidosis associated with RA. Ephedrine used as vasopressor No other significant differences in Apgar scores or cord pH

Study			Comments
Mueller et al. 1997[29]	Acidemia (%): GA: Spinal: Epidural pH < 7.0: 0.2%: 0.7%: 0.1% (Spinal: P = 0.002) pH < 7.1: 0.9%: 4.1%: 2.1% (Spinal & Epidural: P < 0.001) pH < 7.15: 2.3%: 6.7%: 5.5% (Spinal & Epidural: P < 0.001) pH < 7.2: 7.8%: 13.9%: 14.0% (Spinal & Epidural: P < 0.001)	Apgar (5 min): GA: 0–4: 0.5%; 5–7: 4.5% Spinal: 0–4: 0; 5–7: 2.2% (P = 0.002) Epidural: 0–4: 0.3%; 5–7: 2.9% (P = 0.005)	No data available on fluid/vasopressor management. "Routine" management includes IV ephedrine and fluid loading
Levy et al. 1998[32]	Apgar (1 min) < 7: GA: RA odds ratio = 3.5 (1.4, 8.9); P = 0.008 Apgar (5 min) < 7: GA: RA odds ratio = 6.2 (2.3, 16.9); (P < 0.001)	Need for neonatal endotracheal intubation: GA: RA odds ratio = 6.8 (2.4, 19.5); P < 0.001	Logistic regression modeling of multiple risk factors in intrauterine growth retardation. Among patients delivered by cesarean section, GA was a significant and an independent predictor of low Apgar scores at 1 and 5 min and need for neonatal resuscitation, when compared with RA
Roberts et al. 1995[33]	Umbilical artery pH: (P < 0.001) ≥ 7.2: GA: 358/371; GA (failed RA): 45/54; Epidural: 252/286; CSE: 539/659; Spinal: 176/231 7.1–7.19: GA: 13/371; GA (failed RA): 7/54; Epidural: 28/286; CSE: 97/659; Spinal: 44/231 7.1–7.19: GA: 0/371; GA (failed RA): 2/54; Epidural: 5/286; CSE: 17/659; Spinal: 9/231 < 7.0: GA: 0/371; GA (failed RA): 0/54; Epidural: 1/286; CSE: 6/659; Spinal: 2/231 Risk of fetal acidemia: GA: 1 (reference point) Epidural odds ratio = 3.7 (1.9, 7.2); CSE: odds ratio = 6.1 (3.4, 11.0); Spinal: odds ratio = 8.6 (4.6, 16.2)	Apgar (1 min) ≤ 3: (P < 0.001) GA: 5/371*; Epidural: 0/286; CSE: 0/659; Spinal: 1/231; Failed RA: 0/54 (*P < 0.001) No significant differences above Apgar 3 or for any Apgar score at 5 min Assisted ventilation at birth: GA: 31/371*; Epidural: 6/286; CSE: 8/659; Spinal: 3/231; Failed RA: 4/54 (*P < 0.001)	Greater neonatal depression associated with GA, increased fetal acidosis associated with RA. Among RA techniques, spinal has a higher association with fetal acidemia than epidural. Ephedrine used as vasopressor

Continued

Table 11.4 *(continued)*

Author/ date	Neonatal outcomes			Authors conclusions/comments
	Umbilical artery gases	Apgar scores	Other outcomes	
Gambling et al. 1995[22]	*Incidence of fetal acidemia:* (pH < 7.2): GA (sevoflurane): 0/28; GA (isoflurane): 1/27; Spinal: 2/20 (NS)	*Apgar (1 min) ≤ 7: (NS);* GA (sevoflurane): 5/28; GA (isoflurane): 5/27; Spinal: 2/20 *Apgar (5 min) ≤ 7: 0:* in all groups (NS)	*NACS (2 h): (NS)* GA (sevoflurane): 25 ± 6; GA (isoflurane): 26 ± 5; Spinal: 26 ± 4 *NACS (24 h): (NS)* GA (sevoflurane): 29 ± 6; GA (isoflurane): 30 ± 5; Spinal: 29 ± 6	No difference in neonatal depression. Increased fetal acidemia in RA; ephedrine used as vasopressor
Adams et al. 2003[23]	*Umbilical artery pH:* GA (ketamine): 7.29 (7.24–7.37); GA (sevoflurane): 7.29 (7.15–7.40); Spinal: 7.30 (7.20–7.40) (NS)	*Apgar (1 min):* GA (ketamine): 8.6 (7–9); GA (sevoflurane): 8.7 (7–10); Spinal: 8.6 (5–9) (NS) *Apgar (3 min):* GA (ketamine): 9.6 (9–10); GA (sevoflurane): 9.4 (8–10); Spinal: 9.7 (7–10) (NS) *Apgar (10 min):* GA (ketamine): 8.6 (7–9); GA (sevoflurane): 8.7 (7–10); Spinal: 8.6 (5–9) (NS)		
Moodley et al. 2001[30]		*Apgar (1 min) < 7:* GA: 17/27; Epidural: 12/37 (P = 0.03) *Apgar (5 min) < 7:* GA: 11/27; Epidural: 6/37 (P = 0.07)	Live fetus (discharged home) GA: 20/27; Epidural: 29/37 (P = 0.9)	Primary outcomes are maternal (see Table 11.2) RA is safe to use in hemodynamically stable women after eclamptic seizures
Ramanathan et al. 1991[25]	*Umbilical artery pH:* GA: 7.22 ± 0.01; Epidural: 7.29 ± 0.08 NS *Umbilical artery base deficit:* GA: 4.3 ± 0.69; Epidural: 2.44 ± 0.3 (P < 0.02)	*Apgar (1 min) < 7:* GA: 6/10; Epidural: 0/11 P < 0.05 *Apgar (5 min) < 7:* GA: 2/10; Epidural: 0/11		Primary outcome was maternal neuroendocrine changes (see Table 11.2)
Wallace et al. 1995[19]	*Umbilical artery pH:* GA: 7.30 ± 0.01; Epidural: 7.26 ± 0.01; CSE: 7.27 ± 0.01 (NS)	*Apgar (1 min) < 7:* GA: 5/26; Epidural: 3/31; CSE: 5/27 (NS) *Apgar (1 min) < 7:* GA: 2/26; Epidural: 0/31; CSE: 1/27 (NS)		

Study			
Kolatat 1999[17]	Significant worsening of Apgar scores at 1 min in the GA group, no difference at 5 min	No difference in NACS scores	Abstract
Rolbin et al. 1994[34]	*Apgar (1 min):* 0–3: GA: 78/168; Epidural: 75/341 Odds ratio = 2.92(1.99, 4.27) ($P < 0.0001$) 4–7: GA: 48/168; RA: 108/341 *Apgar (5 min):* 0–3: GA: 17/168; RA 13/341 4–7: GA: 108/168; RA: 42/341		
Hong et al. 2003[20]	*Apgar (1 min):* GA: 8 (4–9); epidural 8 (7–9) *Apgar (5 min):* GA: 10 (6–9); epidural 9 (9–10)		
Afolabi et al. 2003[24]	*Apgar (1 min):* GA: 5 ± 2.6; spinal: 7 ± 2.1 ($P = 0.002$) *Apgar (5 min):* GA: 8 ± 2.1; spinal: 9 ± 1.4 ($P = 0.01$)		
Kavak et al. 2001[15]	No difference in umbilical artery cord gases	No difference in Apgar scores at 1 and 5 min	No difference in neonatal intensive care unit admissions
Petropoulos et al. 2003[36]	*Umbilical artery pH:* GA: 7.29 ± 0.02 RA: 7.26 ± 0.06 ($P < 0.05$)	No difference in Apgar scores at 1 and 5 min	
Hodgson & Wauchob 1994[27]	*Apgar (1 min):* 0–3: GA: 3/74; spinal: 0/63 4–7: GA: 18/74; spinal: 3/63 8–10: GA: 52/74; spinal: 60/63 ($P < 0.002$): Wilcoxon unpaired rank sum test, $z = 3.07$ *Apgar (5 min):* 0–3: 0 patients 4–7: GA: 3/74; spinal 0/63 8–10: GA: 71/74; spinal 63/63 (NS)	*Umbilical vein pH:* *If uterine–delivery interval < 3 min:* GA ($n = 58$): 7.30 ± 0.05; Spinal ($n = 44$) 7.32 ± 0.04 ($P < 0.05$) *Incidence of pH < 7.28:* GA: 13/74; Spinal 3/63 ($P < 0.05$) *If uterine–delivery interval < 3 min:* GA ($n = 12$): 7.27 ± 0.09; Spinal 7.29 ± 0.07 (NS)	Umbilical venous pH reflects maternal acid–base changes, but these were not assessed in this study

Continued

Table 11.4 (*continued*)

Author/ date	Neonatal outcomes			Authors conclusions/comments
	Umbilical artery gases	Apgar scores	Other outcomes	
Mahajan *et al.* 1992[18]	*Umbilical artery pH: (NS)* GA: 7.28 ± 0.04 Epidural: 7.29 ± 0.07 Spinal: 7.28 ± 0.02 *Umbilical artery bade deficit: (NS)* GA: 4.31 ± 1.79 Epidural: 4.58 ± 1.99 Spinal: 4.53 ± 2.01	*Apgar (1 min):* < 7 GA: 27/30, epidural: 28/30, spinal: 28/30 *Apgar (5 min):* < 7 No patient in any group	*Time to sustained respiration (NS):* 61–90 s: GA: 1/30, epidural 1/30, spinal 0/30 20–60 s: GA: 2/30, epidural 4/30, spinal 2/30 All other patients < 20 s *NACS (15 min):* (*P* < 0.001) < 35 (low): GA: 18/30, epidural 17/30, spinal 3/30 *NACS (2 h):* (*P* < 0.01) < 35 (low): GA: 9/30, epidural: 6/60, spinal 0/30 *NACS (2 h):* < 35 (low): No patients in any group	Authors concluded that neurobehavioral status in the first few hours after birth better if spinal anesthesia used as compared with either GA or epidural
Yegin *et al.* 2003[21]	*Umbilical artery pH: (P = 0.38)* GA: 7.25 ± 0.07 Epidural: 7.27 ± 0.08 *Bicarbonate: (P = 0.053)* GA: 21.3 ± 4.5 Epidural: 21.0 ± 3.2	*Apgar (1 min): (NS)* GA: 7.19 ± 0.70 Epidural: 7.38 ± 0.55 *Apgar (5 min):* (*P* < 0.05) GA: 9.54 ± 0.67 Epidural: 9.87 ± 0.42		No significant difference between groups for 1 min Apgar or umbilical arterial blood gas data. Apgar scores at 5 min were significantly different
Boyle 1993[40]		*Apgar (1 min):* (*P* < 0.001) GA: 6.3 ± 2.4 Epidural: 7.9 ± 1.3 *Apgar (5 min):* (*P* < 0.001) GA: 8.1 ± 2.0 Epidural: 9.1 ± 0.7		Worsening of Apgar at both 1 and 5 min with GA
Kangas-Saarela *et al.* 1989[26]			*NACS at 3 h:* GA: Significant reduction in habituation and orientation to auditory and visual stimuli. Epidural: significant reduction in rooting	No consistent differences between anesthetic types

CSE, combined spinal epidural; GA, general anesthesia; IV, intravenous; NACS, neuroadaptive capacity score; NS, not significant; RA, regional anesthesia.

The findings of low umbilical artery pH in neonates delivered by cesarean section under regional anesthesia may be explained in the light of recent evidence that ephedrine but not phenylephrine is associated with fetal acidemia. This issue is discussed in Chapter 10. The mechanism by which ephedrine may cause fetal acidemia may be due to an increase in fetal metabolic rate resulting from direct β-sympathomimetic activity in the fetus.[45] Furthermore, phenylephrine raises maternal blood pressure at the expense of peripheral vasoconstriction; however, the uteroplacental circulation is unresponsive to vasopressors in most pregnancies. This may cause a redistribution of cardiac output to the uteroplacental circulation.[45]

In the light of these findings, it is interesting to observe that almost all those studies that demonstrate increased fetal acidemia following regional anesthesia used ephedrine as the vasopressor of choice, and that the ephedrine dose required to maintain maternal blood pressure was invariably far higher than following GA. It will be interesting to see the impact of changing patterns of vasopressor use on the development of fetal acidemia following regional anesthesia for cesarean section.

Other outcomes

Neonatal neurobehavioral function

Scanlon et al.[46] reported that neonates born to women receiving epidural lidocaine were floppy but alert, and described the Scanlon Early Neonatal Neurobehavioral Scale and tests for orientation to objectively quantify the observation. While these clinical tests are detailed and have been quantified for the purposes of scoring, the clinical implications are frequently either unclear or conflicting. For example, in a prospective non-randomized study of cesarean section using either GA or epidural anesthesia, Kangas-Saarela et al.[26] assessed 31 neonates at 3 h, 1 day, 2 days and 4–5 days following elective cesarean section. The investigators used the Scanlon Early Neonatal Neurobehavioral Scale and tests for orientation and observed that the neonates delivered with epidural anesthesia scored significantly lower on rooting at the age of 3 h than those delivered with GA, but the latter scored significantly lower on habituation and orientation to auditory and visual stimuli. What the clinical implications are of such findings are not clear. No clear pattern emerges from the data in our systematic review. Only three other studies in our systematic review assessed neurobehavioral scores. Unfortunately, all used the Neuroadaptive Capacity Score (NACS) which has recently been shown to be unreliable.[47]

The high-risk parturient

Several of the investigations in our review studied populations at risk for poor maternal and neonatal outcome. These included prematurity, intrauterine growth restriction (IUGR), pre-eclampsia and morbid obesity. These are discussed below.

Prematurity and intrauterine growth restriction

The superimposition of neonatal respiratory depression and fetal acidemia on an already compromised fetus may present additional challenges in prematurity. Data from the American College of Obstetricians and Gynecologists (ACOG) report on Neonatal Encephalopathy and Cerebral Palsy[48] showed that the risk ratio for neonatal encephalopathy was 4 : 1 for fetuses between the third and ninth percentile and was 38 : 1 for fetuses below the third percentile. No prospective studies have examined anesthesia choices in these cases. One retrospective study of 509 preterm cesarean sections prior to 32 weeks' gestation[34] demonstrated a risk ratio of 2 : 1 for low 1-min Apgar scores for GA versus epidural anesthesia. The risk ratio increased to 3 : 1 by 5 min. No data were presented on cord blood gases or neonatal outcome. In the absence of other data, a single retrospective study is probably insufficient to dictate clinical management.

IUGR may be the primary diagnosis in parturients who present for emergency cesarean section, either because of fetal "distress," preterm uterine contractions or because of associated pre-eclampsia. In a retrospective study, using multiple logistic regression and controlling for other variables, Levy et al.[32] demonstrated that among 152 cesarean deliveries for growth-restricted fetuses, GA (when compared with regional anesthesia) was an independent predictor for neonatal intubation requirement (odds ratio 6.8, $P < 0.001$), and low Apgar scores at both 1 min (odds ratio 3.5, $P = 0.008$) and at 5 min (odds ratio 6.2, $P < 0.01$). The authors also reported that GA was an independent predictor for low umbilical artery pH. This last observation is misleading as a combined population delivered by either vaginal or cesarean delivery was assessed. In this analysis GA was, not surprisingly, a predictor for neonatal acidemia because neonates requiring cesarean delivery are more likely to have low cord pH. Unlike the other outcomes, such as endotracheal intubation or low Apgar scores, GA was not a predictor for neonatal acidemia when the cesarean data was analyzed alone.

Pre-eclampsia

There often are multiple relative contraindications to GA and regional anesthesia in the pre-eclamptic patient. Endotracheal intubation during GA may provoke severe refractory hypertension, increasing the possibility of intracranial hemorrhage. In addition, airway narrowing is more profound in severe pre-eclampsia, accentuating the difficulty of airway management in these patients. Treatment with magnesium may interact with anesthetic agents, particularly muscle relaxants. Conversely, regional anesthesia may precipitate hypotension due to the contracted intravascular space. There is an increased incidence of coagulopathy which may be relative or absolute contraindication for regional block.

Pre-eclampsia may be associated with IUGR, fetal distress or prematurity. Surgery may be emergent. Data from the ACOG report on Neonatal Encephalopathy and Cerebral Palsy[48] showed that the risk ratio for neonatal encephalopathy was 6 : 1 for severe pre-eclampsia. In the presence of IUGR this is further increased. Accordingly, a severe adverse neonatal outcome is much more common than in the general obstetric population.

Five studies in our systematic review were performed in patients with severe pre-eclampsia or associated complications (HELLP syndrome or eclampsia). Of these studies, two were randomized controlled trials.[13,19]

Wallace et al.[19] randomized 80 severely pre-eclamptic patients who presented for cesarean section to receive general, epidural or CSE. Among the exclusion criteria were fetal distress, eclampsia and thrombocytopenia. No serious adverse outcomes were recorded in any group. There was no difference in either the cord pH or the Apgar scores at either 1 or 5 min among groups. There were no differences in the highest or lowest systolic or diastolic pressures during surgery, although

this was to some degree a consequence of vasopressor use, as 30% and 22% of patients in the epidural and spinal groups, respectively, received ephedrine for hypotension, as compared with none in the GA group (Table 11.3). Patients in the GA group received less fluids than those in the other anesthesia groups (1537 mL in the GA group versus 2387 mL in the CSE group, and 2255 mL in the epidural group; $P < 0.001$). This was because patients in both regional anesthesia groups received a pre-induction bolus dose of 1000 mL of Ringer's lactate while those in the GA group did not. However, all patients in the GA group received nitroglycerin, hydralazine and lidocaine pre-induction and those in the regional anesthesia group did not.

In contrast to the above investigation, Dyer et al.[13] randomized 70 parturients who had both severe pre-eclampsia and fetal distress to receive either GA or spinal anesthesia. They found no difference in maternal hemodynamic responses but there was a significant difference in the dose requirement for ephedrine (2.7 mg GA versus 13.7 mg spinal; $P = 0.002$). Unlike the study by Wallace et al.,[19] there was a significant effect on cord arterial blood gases, with a slight reduction in cord pH (7.23 GA, 7.20 spinal; $P = 0.046$) and an increase in base deficit (4.68 GA, 7.13 spinal; $P = 0.02$). Whether or not this was caused by the type of anesthesia or was a direct effect of ephedrine administration is unknown.

Moodley et al.[30] retrospectively studied 533 patients who presented for cesarean section following eclamptic seizures. Of these, 12% (n = 66) were conscious, cooperative and normovolemic without either thrombocytopenia or other maternal–fetal complications. Of these women, 56% received epidural anesthesia for cesarean section, 41% GA and 3% spinal. Fifty-seven percent of the spinal group and only 29% of the epidural group had Apgar scores below 7 at 1 min ($P = 0.03$); this difference was diminished at 5 min (NS) and there was no difference in the requirement for neonatal intensive care (34%).

The presence of coagulopathy, particularly HELLP, in which thrombocytopenia may be combined with functional impairment, is regarded by some anesthesiologists as an absolute contraindication to regional anesthesia. Vigil-De Gracia et al.[39] describes a cohort of 119 patients diagnosed with HELLP. Of these, 71 had the diagnosis prior to anesthesia. Of these women, 87% were administered epidural or spinal anesthesia and no neurologic sequelae were described. However, for an anesthesia complication with an incidence of less than 1 per 100,000, it is doubtful if this study can provide strong evidence to testify to the safety or prudence of such a decision.

Placenta previa

One small randomized controlled trial compared epidural anesthesia (n = 12) with GA (n = 13) in patients undergoing elective cesarean section who had a diagnosis of complete placenta previa.[20] Blood loss was determined by an investigator who was blinded to the type of anesthesia provided. The incidence of hypotension associated with intraoperative bleeding was higher in the GA group, but the authors did not give the incidence of this problem. Although the authors could not demonstrate any difference between groups in intraoperative blood loss, the incidence of a hematocrit less than 30% was higher in the GA group (5/12 vs 2/13). The number of units of blood transfused was higher in the GA group (1.09 vs 0.38, $P < 0.05$). Postoperative analgesia was superior in the epidural group. Other maternal outcomes and neonatal Apgar scores were similar between groups. The authors concluded that in many cases regional anesthesia is appropriate for patients with placenta previa. Epidural analgesia may reduce blood loss and provides better postoperative analgesia.

Morbid obesity

No studies in our systematic review assessed women with morbid obesity. In a prospective cohort study of 3480 women with morbid obesity (body mass index > 40) compared with controls (body mass index of 19.8–26), Cedergren[49] demonstrated that patients with morbid obesity have risk factors for multiple obstetric problems including pre-eclampsia (risk ratio 4.8), intrauterine fetal death (2.8), cesarean delivery (2.7), macrosomia (3.8) and fetal distress (2.5). Hood and Dewan,[50] in a case–controlled study, found that 48% of all laboring morbidly obese parturients needed urgent cesarean section, compared with 9% in the control population. Six of 17 morbidly obese patients who were intubated had a difficult intubation, as compared with 0/8 patients in control. Although epidural block was more difficult, as evidenced by a higher rate of initial failure, epidural analgesia was ultimately successful in 74/79 patients.

Conclusions

Many anesthesiologists prefer regional anesthesia to GA for both elective and most emergency cesarean sections. This is because of a number of advantages to regional anesthesia such as allowing the patient to be awake and to enjoy the birth of the baby and the ability to use neuraxial opioids for prolonged postoperative analgesia.

Data that emerged from our systematic review include the following:

1 Apgar score at 1 min is improved in regional anesthesia, but this effect is usually no longer evident by 5 min.

2 Regional anesthesia is associated with a higher incidence of fetal acidemia, but that this is probably related to the choice of ephedrine as a vasopressor and limited correction of maternal blood pressure.

3 Regional anesthesia is associated with a reduction in blood loss in cesarean section including patients with placenta previa. In almost all studies, this was not clinically relevant because few patients received blood transfusions.

Based on current data, maternal mortality is higher in patients who receive GA, but this finding likely reflects the increased severity of disease in these patients. We found no evidence either from randomized trials or the various prospective and retrospective studies to suggest that the choice of anesthesia in comparable patients has an impact on mortality. When properly conducted, both GA and regional anesthesia are associated with such a low incidence of serious adverse outcome that controlled trials are unable to identify anesthetic choices as independent risk factors. The use of surrogate outcome measures has not greatly contributed to the resolution of this issue because no surrogate measure has been shown to correlate maternal or neonatal death reliably. Consequently, while many clinicians strongly prefer regional anesthesia when possible, the choice should be determined by the presence of clinical risk factors and the choice of the individual patient and practitioner.

References

1 Chadwick HS, Posner K, Caplan RA, Ward RJ, Cheney FW. A comparison of obstetric and non-obstetric anesthesia malpractice claims. *Anesthesiology* 1991;**74**:242–9.
2 Rusen ID, Liston R. Health Canada. Special report on

maternal mortality and severe maternal mobidity in Canada. *Enhanced Surveillance: The Path to Prevention.* Ottawa: Canadian Ministry of Health, 2004: 7-25-2004.

3 Eltzschig HK, Lieberman ES, Camann WR. Regional anesthesia and analgesia for labor and delivery. *N Engl J Med* 2003;**348**:319–32.

4 Hawkins JL, Koonin LM, Palmer SK, Gibbs CP. Anesthesia-related deaths during obstetric delivery in the United States, 1979–1990. *Anesthesiology* 1997;**86**:277–84.

5 Chestnut DH. Anesthesia and maternal mortality. *Anesthesiology* 1997;**86**:273–6.

6 Hawkins JL, Chang J, Callaghan W, Gibbs CP, Palmer SK. Anesthesia-related maternal mortality in the United States 1991–1996: an update. *Anesthesiology* 2002;A1046.

7 Endler GC, Mariona FG, Sokol RJ, Stevenson LB. Anesthesia-related maternal mortality in Michigan, 1972–1984. *Am J Obstet Gynecol* 1988;**159**:187–93.

8 Hawkins JL. Anesthesia-related maternal mortality. *Clin Obstet Gynecol* 2003;**46**:679–87.

9 NHS maternity statistics 2002–3. http://www.publications.doh.gov.uk/public/work_health_care.htm#cat-hosp. 2004.

10 Thomas J, Paranjothy S. Royal College of Obstetricians and Gynaecologists (RCOG) Clinical Effectiveness Support Unit. *National Sentinel Caesarean Section Audit Report.* RCOG Press, 2001.

11 Shibli KU, Russell IF. A survey of anesthetic techniques used for cesarean section in the UK in 1997. *Int J Obstet Anesth* 2000;**9**:160–7.

12 Brown G, Russell IF. A survey of anesthesia for cesarean section. *Int J Obstet Anesth* 1995;**4**:214–8.

13 Dyer RA, Els I, Farbas J, Torr GJ, Schoeman LK, James MF. Prospective, randomized trial comparing general with spinal anesthesia for cesarean delivery in pre-eclamptic patients with a non-reassuring fetal heart trace. *Anesthesiology* 2003;**99**:561–9.

14 Sener EB, Guldogus F, Karakaya D, Baris S, Kocamanoglu S, Tur A. Comparison of neonatal effects of epidural and general anesthesia for cesarean section. *Gynecol Obstet Invest* 2003;**55**:41–5.

15 Kavak ZN, Basgul A, Ceyhan N. Short-term outcome of newborn infants: spinal versus general anesthesia for elective cesarean section: a prospective randomized study. *Eur J Obstet Gynecol Reprod Biol* 2001;**100**:50–4.

16 Lertakyamanee J, Chinachoti T, Tritrakarn T, Muangkasem J, Somboonnanonda A, Kolatat T. Comparison of general and regional anesthesia for cesarean section: success rate, blood loss and satisfaction from a randomized trial. *J Med Assoc Thai* 1999;**82**:672–80.

17 Kolatat T, Somboonnanonda A, Lertakyamanee J, Chinachot T, Tritrakarn T, Muangkasem J. Effects of general and regional anesthesia on the neonate: a prospective, randomized trial. *J Med Assoc Thai* 1999;**82**:40–5.

18 Mahajan J, Mahajan RP, Singh MM, Anand NK. Anesthetic technique for elective cesarean section and neurobehavioral status of newborns. *Int J Obstet Anesth* 1992;**2**:89–93.

19 Wallace DH, Leveno KJ, Cunningham FG, Giesecke AH, Shearer VE, Sidawi JE. Randomized comparison of general and regional anesthesia for cesarean delivery in pregnancies complicated by severe pre-eclampsia. *Obstet Gynecol* 1995;**86**:193–9.

20 Hong JY, Jee YS, Yoon HJ, Kim SM. Comparison of general and epidural anesthesia in elective cesarean section for placenta previa totalis: maternal hemodynamics, blood loss and neonatal outcome. *Int J Obstet Anesth* 2003;**12**:12–6.

21 Yegin A, Ertug Z, Yilmaz M, Erhman M. The effects of epidural anesthesia and general anesthesia on newborns at cesarean section. *Turk J Med Sci* 2003;**32**:311–4.

22 Gambling DR, Sharma SK, White PF, Van Beveren T, Bala AS, Gouldson R. Use of sevoflurane during elective cesarean birth: a comparison with isoflurane and spinal anesthesia. *Anesth Analg* 1995;**81**:90–5.

23 Adams HA, Meyer P, Stoppa A, Muller-Goch A, Bayer P, Hecker H. Anaesthesia for caesarean section: comparison of two general anaesthetic regimens and spinal anaesthesia. *Anaesthesist* 2003;**52**:23–32.

24 Afolabi BB, Kaka AA, Abudu OO. Spinal and general anaesthesia for emergency caesarean section: effects on neonatal Apgar score and maternal haematocrit. *Niger Postgrad Med J* 2003;**10**:51–5.

25 Ramanathan J, Coleman P, Sibai B. Anesthetic modification of hemodynamic and neuroendocrine stress responses to cesarean delivery in women with severe pre-eclampsia. *Anesth Analg* 1991;**73**:772–9.

26 Kangas-Saarela T, Koivisto M, Jouppila R, Jouppila P, Hollmen A. Comparison of the effects of general and epidural anaesthesia for caesarean section on the neurobehavioural responses of newborn infants. *Acta Anaesthesiol Scand* 1989;**33**:313–9.

27 Hodgson CA, Wauchob TD. A comparison of spinal and general anaesthesia for elective caesarean section: effect on neonatal condition at birth. *Int J Obstet Anesth* 1994;**3**:25–30.

28 Evans CM, Murphy JF, Gray OP, Rosen M. Epidural versus general anaesthesia for elective caesarean section: effect on Apgar score and acid–base status of the newborn. *Anaesthesia* 1989;**44**:778–82.

29 Mueller MD, Brühwiler H, Schüpfer GK, Lüscher KP. Higher rate of fetal acidemia after regional anesthesia for elective cesarean delivery. *Obstet Gynecol* 1997;**90**:131–4.

30 Moodley J, Jjuuko G, Rout C. Epidural compared with general anaesthesia for caesarean delivery in conscious women with eclampsia. *Br J Obstet Gynaecol* 2001;**108**:378–82.

31 Parekh N, Husaini SW, Russell IF. Caesarean section for placenta praevia: a retrospective study of anaesthetic management. *Br J Anaesth* 2000;**84**:725–30.

32 Levy BT, Dawson JD, Toth PP, Bowdler N. Predictors of neonatal resuscitation, low Apgar scores, and umbilical artery pH among growth-restricted neonates. *Obstet Gynecol* 1998;**91**:909–16.

33 Roberts SW, Leveno KJ, Sidawi JE, Lucas MJ, Kelly MA. Fetal acidemia associated with regional anesthesia for elective cesarean delivery. *Obstet Gynecol* 1995;**85**:79–83.

34 Rolbin SH, Cohen MM, Levinton CM, Kelly EN, Farine D. The premature infant: anesthesia for cesarean delivery. *Anesth Analg* 1994;**78**:912–7.

35 Hood DD, Holubec DM. Elective repeat cesarean section: effect of anesthesia type on blood loss. *J Reprod Med* 1990;**35**:368–72.

36 Petropoulos G, Siristatidis C, Salamalekis E, Creatsas G. Spinal and epidural versus general anesthesia for elective cesarean section at term: effect on the acid–base status of the mother and newborn. *J Matern Fetal Neonatal Med* 2003;**13**:260–6.

37 Lao T, Halpern SH, Crosby ET. Anesthesia and blood loss in preterm cesarean section: comparison between general and regional anesthesia. *Int J Obstet Anesth* 1993;**2**:85–8.

38 Nikolajsen L, Sørensen HC, Jensen TS, Kehlet H. Chronic pain following caesarean section. *Acta Anaesthesiol Scand* 2004;**48**:111–6.

39 Vigil-De Gracia P, Silva S, Montufar C, Carrol I, De Los Rios S. Anaesthesia in pregnant women with HELLP syndrome. *Int J Gynaecol Obstet* 2001;**74**:23–7.

40 Boyle R. Caesarean section anaesthesia and the Apgar score. *Aust NZ J Obstet Gynaecol* 1993;**33**:282–4.

41 Andrews WW, Ramin SM, Maberry MC, Shearer V, Black S, Wallace DH. Effect of type of anesthesia on blood loss at elective repeat cesarean section. *Am J Perinatol* 1992;**9**:197–200.

42 Lie B, Juul J. Effect of epidural vs general anesthesia on breastfeeding. *Acta Obstet Gynaecol Scand* 1988;**67**:207–9.

43 ACOG Comitteee on Obstetric Practice, American Academy of Pediatrics Committee on Fetus and Newborn. Use and abuse of the Apgar score. In: *Compendium of Selected Publications*. Washington, DC: American College of Obstetricians and Gynecologists, 1996.

44 Reynolds F, Sharma SK, Seed PT. Analgesia in labour and fetal acid–base balance: a meta-analysis comparing epidural with systemic opioid analgesia. *Br J Obstet Gynaecol* 2002;**109**:1344–53.

45 Riley ET. Editorial. I. Spinal anaesthesia for caesarean delivery: keep the pressure up and don't spare the vasoconstrictors. *Br J Anaesth* 2004;**92**:459–61.

46 Scanlon JW, Brown WU Jr, Weiss JB, Alper MH. Neurobehavioral responses of newborn infants after maternal epidural anesthesia. *Anesthesiology* 1974;**40**:121–8.

47 Halpern SH, Littleford JA, Brockhurst NJ, Youngs PJ, Malik N, Owen HC. The neurologic and adaptive capacity score (NACS) is not a reliable method of newborn evaluation. *Anesthesiology* 2001;**94**:958–62.

48 ACOG Task Force on Neonatal Encephalopathy and Cerebral Palsy. In: Hankins G, ed. *Neonatal Encephalopathy and Cerebral Palsy: Defining the Pathogenesis and Pathophysiology.* Washington, DC: ACOG, 2003: 112.

49 Cedergren MI. Maternal morbid obesity and the risk of adverse pregnancy outcome. *Obstet Gynecol* 2004;**103**:219–24.

50 Hood DD, Dewan DM. Anesthetic and obstetric outcome in morbidly obese parturients. *Anesthesiology* 1993;**79**:1210–8.

CHAPTER 12

Prevention and treatment of side-effects of neuraxial opioids

Niall L. Purdie & Martin van der Vyver

Introduction

The neuraxial administration of hydrophilic opioids, such as morphine and diamorphine, is a common method of providing pain relief following cesarean section. These drugs afford high-quality long-lasting analgesia without sedation. Unfortunately, side-effects such as pruritus, nausea and vomiting are common. Pruritus occurs in up to 95% of patients who receive epidural or subarachnoid hydrophilic opioids.[1–10] The incidence of nausea and vomiting may be as high as 75%.[5,10–12] Although these symptoms are usually mild and self-limiting, the intensity and severity of symptoms for some women may be sufficient to warrant therapeutic intervention. Numerous trials involving many different pharmacologic and non-pharmacologic interventions to prevent and treat these side-effects have been published. In this chapter, we attempt to answer the following question: "How may postoperative pruritus, nausea and vomiting associated with neuraxial morphine or diamorphine administration be effectively prevented or treated in women undergoing cesarean section?"

Methods

Search strategy

An initial list of published studies was obtained by searching the following databases: MEDLINE® (January 1966 to February 2004), EMBASE® (1980 to February 2004), the Cochrane Register of Controlled Trials (third quarter 2003) and the Database of Abstracts of Reviews of Effects (third quarter 2003). The date of the final search was January 25, 2004.

The following MeSH terms and text words were employed: [pruritus], [itch], [cesarean], [caesarean section], [prevention], [postoperative complications], [obstetrics], [morphine], [diamorphine], [spinal and epidural]. The search was restricted to English language. In addition, a manual hand search of major anesthetic journals (*Anesthesiology, Anesthesia and Analgesia, British Journal of Anaesthesia, Canadian Journal of Anesthesia* and *International Journal of Obstetric Anesthesia*) and the abstract proceedings of major anesthetic meetings (ASA, SOAP, CAS and IARS) between September 1998 and January 2004 was undertaken. Additional articles were identified from the reference lists of retrieved articles, review articles and obstetric anesthesia textbooks.

The same process was applied to retrieve articles on nausea and vomiting using the following MeSH terms and key words: [nausea and vomiting], [prevention], [postoperative complications], [obstetrics], [antiemetics], [cesarean section], [intrathecal opioids], [spinal opioids], [epidural opioids] and [ondansetron], [acupressure], [droperidol], [granisetron] and [dexamethasone].

Inclusion criteria
Data from the retrieved articles were included if:
1 the study was a double-blinded, randomized controlled trial (RCT);
2 all patients received neuraxial morphine or diamorphine for postoperative analgesia;
3 pruritus or nausea and vomiting were primary or secondary outcomes;
4 a pharmacologic or non-pharmacologic intervention was used to:

(i) prevent either pruritus or nausea and vomiting after cesarean section; or

(ii) provide treatment of established pruritus or nausea and vomiting after cesarean section.

Quality scoring

The authors scored relevant articles for quality using the Jadad scale[13] (see Appendix for a full description of the scale).

Data extraction

Studies on pruritus

The primary outcome was the incidence or severity of pruritus following prophylactic or active treatment interventions during the period defined by the authors. Specific side-effects of preventive and treatment methods were noted.

Studies on postoperative nausea and vomiting

The primary outcome was the incidence of nausea and vomiting between groups (assessed separately or as a combined outcome) during the period defined by authors of the studies. The secondary outcome was the need for rescue antiemetic medication (one or more doses) at any time in the postoperative period. No differentiation between early and late vomiting was attempted. Differences in nausea scores, nausea and/or vomiting at specific time intervals, number of episodes of nausea and/or vomiting or time to first vomiting episode were not examined. These outcomes were only reported in a few trials, making comparison between trials impossible. Specific side-effects of preventive methods were noted.

Results

Pruritus

Twenty-five articles were retrieved in the initial search but three were not double blinded.[14–16] In total, 22 articles met our inclusion criteria of which 16 examined prophylaxis and six examined treatment of pruritus. None of the investigators used diamorphine.

Prophylaxis of pruritus

There were 16 articles comprised of 1210 patients. Nine studies reported the administration of 0.1–0.25 mg spinal morphine[18,21–23,25,30,32,34,36] and seven

studies the administration of 2–5 mg epidural morphine[19,20,24,26,27,29,31] for post-cesarean section analgesia. All but one of the studies were placebo controlled.[30] A total of 11 different pharmacologic agents were used in the trials. Each agent was either the primary therapy under investigation or the standard control therapy with which the primary therapy was compared. The methodologic details of these studies can be found in Table 12.1 and the results in Table 12.2.

Opioid antagonists

The etiology of the pruritus induced by neuraxial opioids is not fully understood but is thought to be the result of cephalad spread of opioid in the cerebrospinal fluid (CSF) to the trigeminal nucleus, which is located superficially in the medulla.[17] In the prophylaxis and treatment of pruritus secondary to neuraxial morphine, it is perhaps not surprising that drugs possessing complete or incomplete opioid receptor antagonism have been studied widely for prophylaxis. The concern with using these agents is the possibility of reversing neuraxial opioid analgesia.

The search strategy identified a total of six studies describing the use of three pure opioid receptor antagonists: naloxone, naltrexone and nalmefene.[18–23]

Luthman *et al.*[18] administered an intravenous infusion of 0.1 mg/h naloxone or placebo for 8 h in women who had received 0.2 mg spinal morphine. During infusion, the incidence of pruritus was less in the naloxone (28%) versus the control (91%) groups ($P < 0.001$) and there was no significant difference in analgesic requirements in the first 24 h. In contrast, Thind *et al.*[19] studied 30 women who had received 4 mg epidural morphine. There was no statistically significant difference in the incidence of pruritus in the naloxone-treated patients (93%) compared with placebo control (100%), although 2/15 women in the placebo group complained of severe pruritus requiring treatment (compared with 0/15 in the naloxone group). Although they reported the incidence of pruritus for the first 24 h, they stopped the naloxone infusion after 12 h. Unfortunately, pruritus can occur for at least 18 h after injection of neuraxial morphine but the effect of naloxone rapidly dissipates after the infusion is stopped. One would therefore expect a high incidence of pruritus between 12 and 24 h after the injection of neuraxial morphine.

Table 12.1 Prophylaxis of pruritus – description of studies.

Study and reference no.	No. of patients	Dose and route of morphine administration	Timing of prophylactic intervention	Treatment groups	Quality score	Comments
Luthman et al.[18]	39	Subarachnoid morphine 0.2 mg	At cord clamping	Naloxone, 100 µg/h IV for 8 h, n = 18 Placebo n = 21	3	Number of patients randomized not stated
Thind et al.[19]	45	Epidural morphine 4 mg (n = 30)	1 h after delivery	*Group I* Epidural morphine 4 mg + 1 mL N saline IM at delivery + 1 h later 0.4 mg naloxone IV + 1.6 mg naloxone IV for 12 h, n = 15 *Group II* Epidural morphine 4 mg + 1 mL N saline IM at delivery + 1 h later 1 mL N saline IV + 1 L Hartmann's solution IV infusion over 12 h, n = 15 *Group III* Epidural saline 20 mL + 10 mg morphine IM at delivery + 1 h later 1 mL N saline IV + 1 L Hartmann's solution IV over 12 h, n = 15	4	
Abboud et al.[20]	45	Epidural morphine 4 mg	5 min after epidural morphine	*Group I* naltrexone 6 mg po n = 15 *Group II* naltrexone 9 mg po n = 15 *Group III* placebo po n = 15	5	
Abboud et al.[21]	35	Subarachnoid morphine 0.25 mg	1 h after subarachnoid morphine	*Group I* naltrexone 6 mg po n = 12 *Group II* naltrexone 3 mg po n = 10 *Group III* placebo n = 13	4	
Pellingrini et al.[22]	62	Subarachnoid morphine 0.25 mg + fentanyl 12.5 µg	At cord clamping	I nalmefene 0.25 µg/kg IV over 20 min n = 30 II placebo n = 30	5	Two patients dropped from statistical analysis as a result of protocol violation
Connelly et al.[23]	80	Subarachnoid morphine 0.2 mg + fentanyl 10 µg	At cord clamping	I IV N saline (0.1 mL/kg) at delivery, repeated 12 h later + N saline 10 mL/h for 24 h n = 20 II IV N saline (0.1 mL/kg) at delivery, repeated 12 h later + naloxone 48 µg/h for 24 h n = 20 III nalmefene (0.25 µg/kg) at delivery, repeated 12 h later + N saline 40 mL/h for 24 h n = 20 IV nalmefene (0.5 µg/kg) at delivery, repeated 12 h later + N saline 40 mL/h for 24 h n = 20	3	

Study	n	Drug/route	Timing	Groups	Quality score	Comments
Morgan et al.[24]	60	Epidural morphine 5 mg	At end of surgery	I nalbuphine 20 mg IV + 10 mg at 6 h and 12 h postoperative, n = 28; II placebo (n = 32)	3	
Charuluxananan et al.[25]	240	Subarachnoid morphine 0.2 mg	At cord clamping	I nalbuphine 4 mg IV n = 60; II ondansetron 4 mg IV n = 60; III ondansetron 8 mg IV n = 60; IV placebo n = 60	5	
Kendrick et al.[26]	51	Epidural morphine 5 mg	On leaving PACU	I nalbuphine 2.5 mg/h + PCA 1 mg n = 17; II naloxone 50 µg/h + PCA N saline n = 16; III naloxone 50 µg/h + PCA naloxone 40 µg n = 18	3	
Gambling et al.[27]	71	Epidural morphine 3 mg	20 min following delivery	I Epidural butorphanol 1 mg n = 10; II Epidural butorphanol 2 mg n = 21; III Epidural butorphanol 3 mg n = 17; IV placebo n = 23	3	Reason for unequal group sizes reported. Patients did not have an equal chance of randomization to each treatment group
Horta et al.[29]	140	Epidural morphine 2 mg	At epidural catheter insertion	I Epidural droperidol placebo n = 35; II Epidural droperidol 1.25 mg n = 35; III Epidural droperidol 2.5 mg n = 35; IV Epidural droperidol 5 mg n = 35	3	
Horta & Vianna[30]	84	Subarachnoid morphine 0.2 mg	At cord clamping	I alizapride 50 mg IV n = 42; II metoclopramide 10 mg IV n = 42	4	
Juneja et al.[32]	40	Epidural morphine 5 mg	10 min after epidural morphine	I hydroxyzine 50 mg IM n = 20; II placebo n = 20	4	
Warwick et al.[35]	60	Subarachnoid morphine 0.2 mg	At end of surgery	I propofol 10 mg IV n = 29; II placebo n = 29	4	Two patients dropped from statistical analysis; 1 lost data sheet and 1 protocol violation
Yeh et al.[33]	60	Subarachnoid morphine 0.15 mg	At cord clamping	I ondansetron 0.1 mg/kg IV n = 20; II diphenhydramine 30 mg IV n = 20; III placebo n = 20	3	
Yazigi et al.[37]	100	Subarachnoid morphine 0.1 mg + sufentanil 12.5 µg	At cord clamping	I ondansetron 8 mg IV n = 50; II placebo n = 50	4	

IM, intramuscular; IV, intravenous; PACU, post-anesthesia care unit; PCA, patient-controlled analgesia; PO, oral.

Table 12.2 Prophylaxis of pruritus – results.

Study and reference no.	Duration of follow-up (h)	Results	Complications
Luthman et al.[18]	8	Incidence of pruritus I 28% II 91% ($P < 0.001$)	No significant differences in postoperative analgesic requirements
Thind et al.[19]	24	Incidence of pruritus I 14/15 II 15/15 III 8/15 (P value not reported)	Intravenous infusion of naloxone did not ablate analgesic effects of epidural morphine
Abboud et al.[20]	24	Incidence of pruritus I 0/15 II 1/15 III 10/15 ($P < 0.05$)	Incidence of inadequate analgesia greater in group II (33%) compared with group I (7%) ($P < 0.05$)
Abboud et al.[21]	24	Incidence of pruritus I 58% II 70% III 92% ($P < 0.05$)	Trend towards shorter duration of analgesia in groups I and II compared with placebo (NSD)
Pellingrini et al.[22]	24	Incidence of pruritus not significantly different between groups Severity of pruritus reduced at 10 ($P = 0.008$) and 11 h ($P = 0.018$) following treatment with nalmefene compared with placebo	Time to first request for supplemental analgesia greater in placebo vs nalmefene 14.1 vs 6.0 h ($P = 0.037$)
Connelly et al.[23]	24	Incidence of pruritus I 95% II 90% III 95% IV 90% (P value not given)	No significant differences in postoperative analgesic requirements. Incidence of vomiting greater in both nalmefene groups ($P < 0.03$) compared with placebo
Morgan et al.[24]	18	Incidence and severity of pruritus not significantly different between groups (P value not reported)	None
Charuluxananan et al.[25]	24	Severity of pruritus significantly reduced in group I and II compared with group IV ($P < 0.001$ and $P = 0.006$, respectively)	None
Kendrick et al.[26]	24	Severity of pruritus not significantly different between groups ($P = 0.14$)	None
Gambling et al.[27]	24	Severity of pruritus not significantly different between groups (P value not reported)	Sedation scores at 8 h were higher in groups I, II and III compared with group IV ($P < 0.001$)
Horta et al.[29]	24	Incidence of pruritus I 24/35 II 18/35 III 18/35 IV 15/35 ($P < 0.001$)	Dose-dependent increase in the incidence of sedation I 2/35 II 1/35 III 6/35 IV 9/35 (P value not reported)

Continued

Table 12.2 (*continued*)

Study and reference no.	Duration of follow-up (h)	Results	Complications
Horta & Vianna[30]	24	Incidence and severity of pruritus None mild moderate severe I 12% 79% 10% 0% II 12% 55% 26% 7% Severity of pruritus between groups ($P = 0.045$)	None
Juneja et al.[32]	24	Incidence of severe pruritus I 10% II 45% ($P < 0.05$)	None
Warwick et al.[35]	8	Incidence of moderate to severe pruritus I 62% II 66% (P value not reported)	None
Yeh et al.[33]	28	Incidence of pruritus I 25% II 80% III 85% ($P < 0.01$)	None
Yazigi et al.[37]	24	Incidence and severity of pruritus None mild/moderate severe I 12/50 16/50 22/50 II 9/50 21/50 20/50 (no P value given)	None

IV, intravenous; NSD, no significant difference.

Unlike naloxone, which requires multiple intravenous injections or continuous infusion because of its short duration of action, naltrexone is a long-acting agent, which may be administered orally. Abboud et al.[20] reported the antipruritic efficacy of oral naltrexone in 45 women receiving 4 mg epidural morphine. Women receiving 6 or 9 mg naltrexone 5 min after epidural morphine administration had a lower incidence of pruritus (0% and 7%, respectively) compared with placebo (67%, $P < 0.05$). All patients in the placebo group had adequate postoperative analgesia. The authors noted that 6 mg oral naltrexone represented the optimal prophylactic dose because 9 mg was associated with a statistically significant increase in the incidence of unsatisfactory analgesia (7% vs 33%, $P < 0.05$). In a similar study by the same authors,[21] 6 mg oral naltrexone was similarly efficacious, compared with 3 mg naltrexone or placebo, in reducing the incidence of pruritus in patients who received 0.25 mg spinal morphine. There was a 58% incidence of pruritus in patients who received 6 mg naltrexone compared with 70% in patients who received 3 mg and 92% in patients who received placebo. The incidence was significantly lower in the 6-mg group compared with the placebo control. While overall there does appear to be some benefit of using oral naltrexone as a prophylactic therapy, the variability in the estimates of treatment effect is likely to be secondary to small samples sizes in both studies. In addition, neither study reported the method of assessing pruritus. More sensitive measures of treatment effect (e.g. measuring severity of pruritus over time) require further study in patients receiving oral naltrexone.

Two trials were identified comparing nalmefene with placebo[22] or naloxone.[23] Pellingrini et al.[22] randomized patients to receive either 0.25 µg/kg nalmefene or placebo by intravenous infusion over 20 min after 0.25 mg spinal morphine and 12.5 µg fentanyl. There was no difference in the incidence of pruritus between the groups, but a statistically significant difference in severity of pruritus was noted at the tenth ($P = 0.008$) and eleventh hours following nalmefene administration ($P = 0.018$). The time to first request for supplemental analgesia was greater in the placebo group compared with the nalmefene group (14.1 vs 6.0 h, $P = 0.037$). In a study comparing bolus doses of intravenous nalmefene (0.25 µg/kg or 0.5 µg/kg 12 h apart) with 48 µg/h naloxone infusion or placebo in women receiving 0.2 mg spinal morphine, Connelly et al.[23] also failed to demonstrate a reduction in the incidence of pruritus between the groups studied. While the authors noted that side-effects when present were rated as mild, moderate or severe, differences in the severity of pruritus between groups were not reported. Although there were no significant differences between the groups with respect to pain, both nalmefene groups demonstrated a higher incidence of postoperative nausea and vomiting compared with placebo ($P < 0.03$) (Table 12.2).

Overall, the results of studies examining the role of pure opioid anatgonists would suggest that none of the treatments studied reliably reduce the incidence or severity of pruritus. Naloxone, in doses of 0.1 mg/h, is effective in reducing the incidence of pruritus for the duration of the infusion without affecting the analgesic requirements. Six milligrams of oral naltrexone was effective in reducing pruritus without reducing the effectiveness of the neuraxial opioid. Three milligrams was less effective and 9 mg adversely affected analgesia. Intravenous nalmefene, while effective, also reduced the analgesic efficacy of neuraxial morphine. It should be noted that the incidence of pruritus in the treated groups was highly variable (0–100%, Table 12.2).

Opioid agonist–antagonists

Nalbuphine is an opioid analgesic drug with agonist and antagonist activity at kappa and mu opioid receptor subtypes respectively. There were two studies that compared nalbuphine with placebo[24,25] and one study compared nalbuphine with naloxone.[26] One study described the use of prophylactic epidural butorphanol, an opioid with similar actions to that of nalbuphine.[27]

Morgan et al.[24] randomized 60 women receiving 5 mg epidural morphine to receive either intravenous nalbuphine (20 mg given at end of surgery and 10 mg repeated at 6 and 12 h) or placebo. Pruritus was assessed with a 0–5 scale (0, no pruritus; 5, unbearable pruritus), at 15, 30 and 60 min followed by hourly

measurements up to 18 h. No difference in the incidence or severity of pruritus was observed. In contrast, Charuluxananan et al.[25] randomized 240 women to receive either 4 mg intravenous nalbuphine, 4 mg ondansetron, 8 mg ondansetron or placebo following 0.2 mg spinal morphine and showed a benefit of using both nalbuphine and ondansetron prophylaxis compared with placebo ($P < 0.001$). While not statistically significant, the results also suggest that nalbuphine may reduce the severity of pruritus when compared with 4 or 8 mg ondansetron. The disparity in the findings of Morgan et al.[24] and Charuluxananan et al.[25] likely rests in the differences in sample sizes between the studies and the method of measuring pruritus. While Charuluxananan et al.[25] report both the incidence and severity of pruritus at 4 h after drug administration, Morgan et al.[24] report the highest level of pruritus found over an 18-h period. The findings of the latter study may reflect higher pruritus scores obtained near the end of the study when the effect of nalbuphine was wearing off.

Kendrick et al.[26] compared three groups of women receiving a 24-h infusion of three different regimens of opioid antagonists given via a patient-controlled analgesia (PCA) device locked out at 5 min. Group A received 2.5 mL/h nalbuphine with a PCA bolus dose of 1 mg nalbuphine. Group B received 50 µg/h naloxone with a placebo bolus dose and group C received 50 µg/h naloxone with a bolus dose of 40 µg naloxone. All patients received 5 mg epidural morphine after delivery. Pruritus and pain were measured using a 10-cm visual analog scale (VAS) scale at 0, 8, 16 and 24 h. No significant differences in the severity of itching were observed among the groups ($P = 0.14$). The small sample size used per group coupled with use of active opioid antagonists in each of the groups is the likely source of failure to demonstrate a significant difference between treatments. The median scores for pruritus and their range suggest reduced pruritus in each group with considerable variability within groups. Patients who received 50 µg/h naloxone with a placebo bolus had higher pruritus scores (median 3.2) than those who received naloxone (median 2.8) or nalbuphine (median 2.2) boluses.

Gambling et al.[27] randomized 71 patients who had received 3 mg epidural morphine to receive placebo or 1, 2 or 3 mg epidural butorphanol. Pruritus, pain and somnolence were measured prior to surgery and at 2, 8 and 24 h after delivery. Butorphanol was not effective in reducing VAS pruritus scores at 8 h but significantly increased patient somnolence ($P < 0.0001$). Epidural butorphanol is therefore not recommended to prevent pruritus.

Droperidol

Empirically, some investigators have found that droperidol may decrease the incidence of pruritus associated with neuraxial opioids.[14,15] This may be because of its ability to antagonize 5-HT$_3$ receptors.[28]

Horta et al.[29] have investigated the prophylactic antipruritic efficacy of epidural droperidol. In their study of 140 post-cesarean patients receiving 2 mg epidural morphine, the investigators added either placebo (n = 35), 1.25 (n = 35), 2.5 (n = 35) or 5 mg (n = 35) droperidol to the epidural injectate. Postoperatively, a dose-dependent reduction in the incidence of pruritus was observed ($P < 0.001$). The incidence of somnolence complicating the use of droperidol increased with the dose of drug. There was a statistically significant difference between the group receiving 5 mg droperidol (26%) and the placebo group (6%).

Horta and Vianna[30] compared intravenous 50 mg alizapride with 10 mg metoclopramide in 84 women who received 0.2 mg spinal morphine. The authors of this study noted that they chose metoclopramide on the basis of findings elsewhere that showed that metoclopramide had no benefit as a treatment for pruritus. Although the authors did not find a difference in the overall incidence of pruritus between the groups, there was a marginally significant reduction in the severity of pruritus favoring the alizapride group ($P = 0.045$).

These studies suggest that both epidural droperidol and intravenous alizapride may be effective in reducing the incidence and severity of pruritus in the cesarean section population. It should be noted that necessary neurotoxicity studies have not yet been carried out and therefore epidural or subarachnoid droperidol cannot be recommended for use.[31] Further, the severity and incidence of somnolence of epidural droperidol administration limits its usefulness.

Other drugs

While the potential of morphine to release histamine systemically is widely accepted, this is not thought to be an important mechanism in the genesis of pruritus following neuraxial administration. This is supported by the finding that opioids such as fentanyl and sufentanil, which do not release histamine, may cause pruritus following neuraxial administration. Nevertheless, Juneja et al.,[32] in a study of women receiving 5 mg epidural morphine, found that prophylactically administered intramuscular 50 mg hydroxyzine is more efficacious than placebo in reducing the incidence of severe pruritus postoperatively ($P < 0.05$). However, Yeh et al.[33] reported no difference in the incidence of pruritus in patients treated with diphenhydramine compared with control (Table 12.2).

Recent interest in the antipruritic effects of subhypnotic doses of propofol in surgical patients treated with spinal morphine[34] has led to this agent being investigated in the cesarean section population. However, Warwick et al.[35] failed to demonstrate any statistically significant reduction in the incidence or severity of pruritus in women receiving a 10-mg bolus of intravenous propofol or placebo following 0.2 mg spinal morphine (Table 12.2).

The discovery that morphine can activate 5-HT$_3$ receptors by a mechanism independent of opioid receptors,[36] has led many to believe that direct effects at the level of the spinal cord and medulla may be the cause of opioid-mediated pruritus. Three studies investigating the prophylactic antipruritic effects of ondansetron in women having elective cesarean section with 0.1–0.2 mg spinal morphine revealed interesting results.

Charuluxananan et al.[25] studied 240 patients who received spinal morphine for post-cesarean section analgesia. Patients who received 4 or 8 mg ondansetron had a significantly reduced incidence of pruritus in the first 4 h after treatment compared with placebo ($P = 0.006$). However, there was no difference after 8–24 h. Yeh et al.[33] studied 60 women and similarly found a significant reduction in the incidence of pruritus in women who received 0.1 mg/kg intravenous ondansetron (1/20) compared with either placebo (17/20) or diphenhydramine (16/20) ($P < 0.01$). In contrast, Yazigi et al.,[37] in a study of 100 patients who received a combination of spinal sufentanil and morphine, failed to demonstrate a significant antipruritic effect of 8 mg intravenous ondansetron compared with placebo. The authors of this study examined pruritus every 2 h over a 24-h period following a single dose of ondansetron. The reason for these contradictory results is not apparent from the study design. Because this study did not present the incidence of pruritus over time, it is possible that sufentanil caused a high incidence of early pruritus, not prevented by ondansetron.

In summary, the efficacy of antihistamines to prevent morphine-induced pruritus is inconsistent and does not have a strong biologic basis. While there are reports that subhypnotic bolus doses of propofol may be useful in the treatment of pruritus in other settings, its prophylactic use after neuraxial morphine for cesarean section is not of benefit. Ondansetron may be more useful, provided that doses are repeated for 24 h. Further studies are required before recommending the use of ondansetron prophylaxis.

Treatment of pruritus

The six articles under review represented a total of 465 patients. Five studies considered the administration of spinal morphine (dose range 0.15–0.25 mg)[38,40–43] and one study the administration of epidural morphine (5 mg).[39] Four studies were in women undergoing spinal anesthesia for elective cesarean section. Three of the studies were placebo controlled. A total of five different drugs were used in the trials. Each agent was either the primary therapy under investigation or the standard control therapy with which the primary therapy was being compared. The methodologic details of these studies can be found in Table 12.3 and the results in Table 12.4.

Opioid agonist antagonists

Three studies examined the use of nalbuphine in the treatment of established pruritus. Cohen et al.[39] randomized women to receive either 0.2 mg intravenous naloxone or 5 mg intravenous nalbuphine for the treatment of pruritus in the 4–6 h following 5 mg epidural morphine. These investigators found that 30 min following treatment, the median verbal rating

Table 12.3 Treatment of pruritus – description of studies.

Study and reference no.	No. of patients	Dose and route of morphine administration	Requirement for treatment	Treatment groups	Quality score
Cohen et al.[39]	40	Epidural morphine 5 mg	Patients reporting pruritus approx 4–6 h following epidural morphine	I Naloxone 0.2 mg IV n = 20 II Nalbuphine 5 mg IV n = 20	3
Charuluxananan et al.[38]	90	Subarachnoid morphine 0.15 mg	Patients reporting moderate or severe pruritus up to 24 h following subarachnoid morphine	I Nalbuphine 2 mg IV n = 30 II Nalbuphine 3 mg IV n = 30 III Nalbuphine 4 mg IV n = 30	3
Alhashemi et al.[40]	45	Subarachnoid morphine 0.2 mg	Patients requesting treatment for pruritus	I Nalbuphine 5 mg IV + 10 mg q 30 min × 2 doses n = 24 II Diphenhydramine 25 mg IV + 50 mg q 30 min × 2 doses n = 21	5
Charuluxananan et al.[41]	181	Subarachnoid morphine 0.2 mg	Patients reporting moderate or severe pruritus within 4 h of subarachnoid morphine	I Nalbuphine 3 mg IV n = 91 II Propofol 20 mg IV n = 90	4
Charuluxananan et al.[42]	80	Subarachnoid morphine 0.2 mg	Patients reporting moderate or severe pruritus within 4 h of subarachnoid morphine	I Ondansetron 4 mg IV n = 41 II Placebo n = 39	3
Beilin et al.[43]*	29	Subarachnoid morphine 0.25 mg	Patients reporting pruritus approx 3–4 h following subarachnoid morphine	I Propofol 10 mg IV n = 17 II Placebo n = 12	4

* Study prematurely terminated because of poor response to therapy in both groups.
IV, intravenous.

Table 12.4 Treatment of pruritus – results.

Study and reference no.	Duration of follow-up (h)	Results	Complications
Cohen et al.[39]	8 approx	Median VAS for pruritus (30 min post-treatment) lower in group II vs group I ($P < 0.005$)	Sedation scores increased after nalbuphine ($P < 0.05$) but not naloxone Pain scores increased after naloxone ($P < 0.01$) but not nalbuphine
Charuluxananan et al.[38]	24	Treatment success rates (15 min post-treatment) I 87% II 97% III 100% ($P = 0.12$)	VAS pain scores increased ($P = 0.004$) group III vs groups I or II
Alhashemi et al.[40]	24	Treatment success rates I 83% II 43% ($P < 0.01$)	None
Charuluxananan et al.[41]	4	Treatment success rates (10 min post-treatment) I 83% II 61% ($P < 0.001$)	10 min following study drug administration an increased sedation score was found in group I vs group II patients (41% vs 28%) (NSD)
Charuluxananan et al.[42]	4	Treatment success rate I 33/41 II 14/39 ($P < 0.01$)	None
Beilin et al.[43]	6	Treatment success rate I 2/17 II 1/12 ($P = 0.75$)	Pain on injection I 6/17 II 0/12 ($P = 0.03$) Dizziness I 3/13 II 1/12 ($P = 0.61$)

NSD, no significant difference; VAS, visual analog scale.

scale for pruritus was less in the nalbuphine group compared with the naloxone group ($P < 0.005$). The authors report that sedation scores increased after nalbuphine ($P < 0.05$) and remained unchanged after naloxone, whereas pain scores increased after naloxone ($P < 0.01$) and were unchanged after nalbuphine.

In an attempt to determine the optimal dose of intravenous nalbuphine for the treatment of intrathecal morphine-induced (0.15 mg) pruritus postoperatively, Charuluxananan et al.[38] randomized women to receive 2, 3 or 4 mg intravenous nalbuphine in response to a request for antipruritic therapy. All three

doses had high treatment success rates, as defined by patients who had recovered from moderate or severe pruritus to mild or none, 15 min following treatment (87%, 97% and 100%, respectively; $P = 0.12$). The authors concluded that 3 mg intravenous nalbuphine represented the optimal treatment dose as 4 mg was associated with increased VAS pain scores postoperatively ($P = 0.004$).

Alhashemi et al.[40] have demonstrated the superiority of intravenous 5 mg nalbuphine compared with 25 mg diphenhydramine in the treatment of post-cesarean pruritus. In their study of women receiving

0.2 mg spinal morphine, treatment success rates, as defined by the proportion of patients who achieved a VAS pruritus score of zero after treatment, were 83% and 43% for nalbuphine and diphenhydramine, respectively ($P < 0.01$).

Similarly, Charuluxananan et al.[41] have reported the superior efficacy of 3 mg intravenous nalbuphine versus 20 mg propofol in the treatment of moderate to severe pruritus in the 4 h following 0.2 mg spinal morphine. These investigators report treatment success rates (as defined by patients who had recovered from moderate or severe pruritus to mild or none following treatment) of 83% and 61% for nalbuphine and propofol, respectively ($P < 0.001$). The authors report that 10 min following study drug administration, an increased sedation score was found in women receiving nalbuphine (41%) versus propofol (28%). This difference was not statistically significant.

Other drugs

Charuluxananan et al.[42] have reported the antipruritic benefits of 4 mg intravenous ondansetron compared with placebo in women receiving 0.2 mg spinal morphine. These investigators report treatment success rates (as defined by patients who had recovered from moderate or severe pruritus to mild or none following treatment) of 80% and 36% for ondansetron and placebo, respectively ($P < 0.001$).

Beilin et al.[43] found that 20 mg intravenous propofol given to women requesting therapy for pruritus following 0.25 mg spinal morphine had a very low treatment success rate (11.8%) which did not differ from placebo (8.3%, $P = 0.75$). Treatment success rates were defined by the authors as pruritus scores of 1 or 2 (on a 5-point severity scale) following treatment. There was a statistically significant increase in the occurrence of pain upon injection in the propofol group (6/17) compared with the placebo group (0/12, $P = 0.03$).

In summary, propofol is not an effective treatment for pruritus after spinal morphine in this setting. Nalbuphine, in doses between 2 and 5 mg is effective for most patients. Four milligrams of intravenous ondansetron may be a useful agent and does not cause side-effects such as drowsiness or reduction in analgesia. The role of ondansetron for the treatment of pruritus needs more study.

Nausea and vomiting

Forty-two articles were identified from the initial search. Twelve of these articles met inclusion criteria of which 11 examined prophylaxis and one examined treatment of nausea and vomiting.

Prophylaxis of nausea and vomiting

The 11 articles under review represented a total of 1307 patients. Five studies considered the administration of spinal (dose range 0.1–0.25 mg) and six studies the administration of epidural (dose range 3–5 mg) morphine, respectively. All studies were in women undergoing elective cesarean section. Ten of the studies were placebo controlled. A total of seven different pharmacologic agents and one non-pharmacologic intervention were used in the trials. Each agent was either the primary therapy under investigation or the standard control therapy with which the primary therapy was compared. The methodologic details of these studies can be found in Table 12.5 and the results in Table 12.6.

Metoclopramide

Metoclopramide has been used for many years for the prevention and treatment of postoperative nausea and vomiting. Recently, a systematic review on the efficacy of metoclopramide concluded that it was a poor antiemetic and that there was no demonstrable increase in efficacy when higher doses were used (dose–response).[44] However, we found two trials that investigated the use of metoclopramide in the prevention of postoperative nausea and vomiting. Chestnut et al.[45] administered 0.15 mg/kg intravenous metoclopramide or placebo intraoperatively to 67 women undergoing elective cesarean section who received either 4–5 mg epidural morphine or 1–1.2 mg hydromorphone. In the 4 h following surgery, women in the metoclopramide group had a lower incidence of both nausea (15 vs 36%, $P < 0.05$) and vomiting (12 vs 36%, $P < 0.05$) compared with placebo. Using a similar study design comparing intravenous 15 mg metoclopramide with 0.5 mg droperidol in women receiving 4 mg epidural morphine, Chestnut et al.[46] reported no significant differences in the incidence of postoperative nausea or vomiting between the groups studied (Table 12.6).

Table 12.5 Prophylaxis of nausea and vomiting – description of studies.

Study and reference no.	No. of patients	Dose and route of morphine administration	Timing of prophylactic intervention	Treatment groups	Quality score
Chestnut et al.[45]	67	Epidural morphine 4–5 mg or hydromorphone 1.0–1.2 mg	At cord clamping	Metoclopramide 0.15 mg/kg IV (n = 34) Placebo (n = 33)	4
Chestnut et al.[46]	81	Epidural morphine 4 mg	At cord clamping	Metoclopramide 15 mg IV (n = 40) Droperidol 0.5 mg IV (n = 41)	4
Wang et al.[49]	175	Epidural morphine 3 mg	At end of surgery	Dexamethasone 10 mg IV (n = 43) Dexamethasone 5 mg IV (n = 43) Dexamethasone 2.5 mg IV (n = 44) Placebo (n = 44)	4
Tzeng et al.[50]	120	Epidural morphine 3 mg	At end of surgery	Dexamethasone 8 mg IV (n = 38) Droperidol 1.25 mg IV (n = 38) Placebo (n = 38)	4
Nortcliffe et al.[51]	90	Subarachnoid morphine 0.2 mg	On arrival in recovery room	Cyclizine 50 mg IV (n = 30) Dexamethasone 8 mg IV (n = 30) Placebo (n = 30)	5
Kotelko et al.[53]	203	Epidural morphine 4 mg	5 min before epidural anesthesia	Scopolamine (transdermal) (n = 102) Placebo (n = 101)	3
Connelly et al.[23]	80	Subarachnoid morphine 0.2 mg + fentanyl 10 µg	At cord clamping	IV N saline (0.1 mL/kg) at delivery, repeated 12 h later + N saline 10 mL/h for 24 h (n = 20) IV N saline (0.1 mL/kg) at delivery, repeated 12 h later + naloxone 48 µg/h for 24 h (n = 20) Nalmefene (0.25 µg/kg) at delivery, repeated 12 h later + N saline 40 mL/h for 24 h (n = 20) Nalmefene (0.5 µg/kg) at delivery, repeated 12 h later + N saline 40 mL/h for 24 h (n = 20)	4
Yazigi et al.[37]	100	Subarachnoid morphine 0.1 mg + sufentanil 2.5 µg	At cord clamping	Ondansetron 8 mg IV (n = 50) Placebo (n = 50)	5
Ho et al.[54]	60	Epidural morphine 3 mg	5 min before CSE anesthesia	Sea-Band® wrist bands (n = 30) Placebo wrist bands (n = 30)	3
Harmon et al.[55]	94	Subarachnoid morphine 0.2 mg	5 min before spinal anesthesia	Sea-Band® wrist bands (n = 47) Placebo wrist bands (n = 47)	4
Duggal et al.[56]	263	Subarachnoid morphine 0.25 mg + fentanyl 10 µg	5 min before entering operating room	Sea-Band® wrist bands (n = 122) Placebo wrist bands (n = 122)	5

CSE, combined spinal epidural; IV, intravenous.

Dexamethasone

Although the mechanism of the antiemetic effect of dexamethasone is unknown, it has been established as an effective agent in the prophylaxis of postoperative nausea and vomiting[47,48] Three studies were found examining the role of prophylactic intravenous dexamethasone for antiemesis. Upon completion of surgery, Wang et al.[49] gave either intravenous dexamethasone (10, 5 or 2.5 mg) or placebo to 180 women receiving 3 mg epidural morphine.

Table 12.6 Prophylaxis of nausea and vomiting secondary – results.

Study and reference no.	Duration of follow-up (h)	Results				Complications
		Incidence of nausea	Incidence of vomiting	Combined incidence of nausea and vomiting	Requirement for rescue antiemetic medication	
Chestnut et al.[45]	4	Metoclopramide 5/34 Placebo 12/33 ($P < 0.05$)	Metoclopramide 4/34 Placebo 12/33 ($P < 0.05$)			No side-effects attributable to metoclopramide reported
Chestnut et al.[46]	4	Metoclopramide 5/40 Droperidol 5/41 (P value not reported)	Metoclopramide 3/40 Droperidol 3/41 (P value not reported)			Transient intraoperative restlessness reported (metoclopramide 3% vs droperidol 5%)
Wang et al.[49]	24	Dexamethasone 10 mg 5/43 Dexamethasone 5 mg 5/44 Dexamethasone 2.5 mg 7/44 Placebo 12/44 (P value not reported)	Dexamethasone 10 mg 3/43 Dexamethasone 5 mg 3/44 Dexamethasone 2.5 mg 7/44 Placebo 10/44 (P value not reported)	Dexamethasone 10 mg 8/43* Dexamethasone 5 mg 8/44* Dexamethasone 2.5 mg 11/44† Placebo 22/44	Dexamethasone 10 mg 4/43 Dexamethasone 5 mg 5/44 Dexamethasone 2.5 mg 8/44 Placebo 14/44	No side-effects attributable to dexamethasone reported
Tzeng et al.[50]	24	Dexamethasone 4/38 Droperidol 5/38 Placebo 11/37 (P value not reported)	Dexamethasone 3/38 Droperidol 3/38 Placebo 3/37 (P value not reported)	Dexamethasone 7/38* Droperidol 8/38† Placebo 19/37 * $P < 0.01$ † $P < 0.05$	Dexamethasone 4/38† Droperidol 5/38† Placebo 15/37 † $P < 0.05$	Restlessness reported: Dexamethasone 0/38 Droperidol 6/38 Placebo 0/38 $P < 0.05$

Study	n				
Nortcliffe et al.[51]	24	Cyclizine 10/30 Dexamethasone 18/30 Placebo 20/30 P = 0.04 (cyclizine vs dexamethasone) P = 0.02 (cyclizine vs placebo)	Cyclizine 9/30 Dexamethasone 17/30 Placebo 18/30 P = 0.04 (cyclizine vs dexamethasone) P = 0.03 (cyclizine vs placebo)	Cyclizine 4/30 Dexamethasone 17/30 Placebo 19/30 P = 0.001 (cyclizine vs dexamethasone) P = 0.001 (cyclizine vs placebo)	None
Kotelko et al.[53]	24	Scopolamine 42% Placebo 70% P < 0.005	Scopolamine 32% Placebo 52% P < 0.005	Scopolamine 28% Placebo 44% P < 0.05	Disorientation attributable to scopolamine described in 1 patient only
Connelly et al.[23]	24	N saline only 15/20 Naloxone 14/20 Nalmefene low-dose 17/20 Nalmefene high-dose 17/20 (P value not reported)	N saline only 7/20 Naloxone 9/20 Nalmefene low-dose 16/20 Nalmefene high-dose 12/20 P < 0.03	N saline only 8/20 Naloxone 8/20 Nalmefene low-dose 12/20 Nalmefene high-dose 12/20 (P value not reported)	No reversal of analgesia observed
Yazigi et al.[37]	24		Ondansetron 9/50 Placebo 24/50 P = 0.001	Ondansetron 4/50 Placebo 15/50 P = 0.004	
Ho et al.[54]	48	Sea-Band® 1/30 Placebo 13/30 P < 0.05	Sea-Band® 0/30 Placebo 8/30 P < 0.05	Sea-Band® 0/30 Placebo 2/30 (P value not reported)	No side-effects reported
Harmon et al.[55]	24	Sea-Band® 4/47 Placebo 6/47 P = 0.5	Sea-Band® 13/47 Placebo 25/47 P = 0.01	Sea-Band® 17/47 Placebo 31/47 P = 0.003	
Duggal et al.[56]	10	Sea-Band® 69/122 Placebo 80/122 P = 0.15	Sea-Band® 50/122 Placebo 56/122 P = 0.44	Sea-Band® 33/122 Placebo 42/122 (P value not reported)	Side-effects reported in Sea-Band® groups: tightness, swollen hands, problems with infusion and itching wrists

The combined incidence of nausea and vomiting was statistically less in 10 mg dexamethasone (19%, $P < 0.01$), 5 mg (18%, $P < 0.01$) and 2.5 mg (25%, $P < 0.05$) doses compared with placebo (50%). No differences in efficacy were observed between the 5 and 10 mg dexamethasone groups. Tzeng et al.,[50] in a study of similar patients, demonstrated that 8 mg intravenous dexamethasone and 1.25 mg intravenous droperidol, given immediately at the end of surgery, were both effective agents in the prevention of postoperative nausea and vomiting. In their study, of women receiving 3 mg epidural morphine, the combined incidence of nausea and vomiting was statistically less in the groups receiving dexamethasone (18%, $P < 0.01$) and droperidol (21%, $P < 0.05$) compared with those receiving placebo (51%). However, there was a higher incidence of restlessness associated with droperidol (Table 12.6). In contrast, Nortcliffe et al.[51] studied patients who received 0.25 mg spinal morphine. The patients were randomized to receive placebo, 8 mg dexamethasone or 50 mg intravenous cyclizine. The incidence of nausea was similar in the placebo and dexamethasone groups (67% and 60%, respectively). Of interest, the incidence was lower in the cyclizine group ($P < 0.02$) compared with the placebo group. This study was different from the other two because the prophylactic drugs were given in the recovery room rather than immediately after surgery. This is in keeping with evidence from other studies in which dexamethasone was more effective when given preoperatively compared with postoperatively.[52] Alternatively, dexamethasone may not a reliable drug to prevent postoperative nausea and vomiting in this setting. Of interest, no side-effects attributable to the use of dexamethasone were described in these trials.

Other drugs

Kotelko et al.[53] investigated the prophylactic efficacy of a transdermal scopolamine patch compared with placebo in their study of 203 mothers given 4 mg epidural morphine. Application of the patch, which delivered 5 µg/h scopolamine transdermally, was associated with a lower incidence of nausea (42% vs 70%, $P < 0.005$) and vomiting (32% vs 52%, $P < 0.005$). One patient in the scopolamine group experienced short-lived disorientation, which required no treatment. The incidence of dizziness (7%) and blurred vision (3% in scopolamine group vs 1.5% in placebo) was not different between groups. Side-effects such as a dry mouth or sedation were not reported.

Opioid antagonists and agonist–antagonists

Connelly et al.[23] compared two bolus doses of intravenous nalmefene (either 0.25 or 0.5 µg/kg) 12 h apart, with naloxone infusion (48 µg/h) or placebo in women receiving 0.2 mg spinal morphine. These investigators found that the incidence of vomiting was greater in both the 0.25 µg/kg (80%, $P < 0.03$) and 0.5 µg/kg (60%, $P < 0.03$) nalmefene groups compared with placebo (35%). Naloxone infusion (48 µg/h) for 24 h was no more effective than placebo for preventing nausea and vomiting or reducing the need for rescue antiemetics. These studies imply that opioid antagonists are ineffective for the prevention of postoperative nausea and vomiting.

The 5-HT receptor antagonists are highly specific and selective for postoperative nausea and vomiting. They exert their effect by binding to the chemoreceptor trigger zone (CTZ) and vagal afferents in the gastrointestinal tract. In their study of 100 women who received 0.1 mg intrathecal morphine and 2.5 µg sufentanil, Yazigi et al.[37] demonstrated a beneficial reduction in the combined incidence of postoperative nausea and vomiting in women randomized to receive 8 mg intravenous ondansetron compared with placebo (18% vs 48%, $P = 0.001$).

Acupressure

Although this antiemetic remedy has been known in Chinese medicine for a long time, the mechanism is still unclear. Peripheral nerve stimulation probably plays an essential part. Three placebo-controlled studies were identified that investigated the antiemetic efficacy of wrist bands exerting pressure upon the P-6 acupoint. In women receiving 3 mg epidural morphine, Ho et al.[54] showed that wearing acupressure wrist bands postoperatively reduced the incidence of nausea (3% vs 43%, $P < 0.05$) and vomiting (0% vs 27%, $P < 0.05$) compared with placebo.

Harmon et al.[55] also reported a beneficial effect from wearing acupressure wrist bands. These investigators showed that the combined incidence of nausea and vomiting was statistically less in the acupressure group (36 vs 66%, $P = 0.003$) compared with placebo in the first 24 h following surgery where 0.2 mg spinal morphine was used for analgesia.

In contrast, a larger study of 263 patients by Duggal et al.[56] failed to show any difference in the incidence of postoperative nausea (57% vs 66%, $P = 0.15$) or vomiting (41% vs 46%, $P = 0.44$) when acupressure bands were compared with placebo in subjects receiving 0.25 mg spinal morphine. However, postoperative nausea and vomiting were significantly reduced in a subgroup of patients who gave a history of previous postoperative nausea and vomiting. The follow-up period was only 10 h in this study compared with 48 and 24 h for the studies by Ho et al.[54] and Harmon et al.,[55] respectively. This may explain the differences in the results between studies.

Treatment of nausea and vomiting

Our search strategy identified only one study concerned with the treatment of nausea and vomiting. Cohen et al.[39] gave either 0.2 mg intravenous naloxone or 5 mg intravenous nalbuphine for the treatment of nausea and/or vomiting in the 4–6 h following epidural morphine. These researchers found that nalbuphine decreased the incidence of vomiting ($P < 0.005$) compared with naloxone. Nalbuphine completely abolished nausea in 69% of patients with this symptom, compared with only 20% for naloxone ($P < 0.05$).

Discussion

Morphine administered spinally diffuses rostrally by means of diffusion or bulk flow of the CSF, reaching the CTZ in the area postrema. Epidural morphine reaches this area by means of diffusion first to the CSF and second through systemic absorption. Morphine concentrations after epidural administration reach significant levels in the medulla oblongata within 5–6 h, as evidenced by the onset of trigeminal analgesia.[57] This is also the time when the incidence of postoperative nausea and vomiting peaks after neuraxial morphine.

The CTZ is a highly vascularized area where the blood–brain barrier is not effective. The CTZ area can be activated by direct chemical stimulation through the CSF or blood. The central structures involved in the vomiting response are rich in dopamine, acetylcholine, serotonin, histamine and opioid receptors, and blockade of these receptors is the mechanism of action of antiemetic drugs.[58] This explains why drugs from different classes can be effective. It also gives us a good reason, at least in theory, to use a multimodal approach to prevention and/or treatment of postoperative nausea and vomiting.

In a recent meta-analysis of the adverse effects of intrathecal opioids in patients undergoing cesarean section with spinal anesthesia, Dahl et al.[10] found that the number of patients needed to treat with 0.05–0.25 mg intrathecal morphine to cause nausea in one individual was 6.3 (95% confidence interval [CI], 4.2–12.5) and vomiting was 10.1 (95% CI, 5.7–41.0). Logistic regression analysis showed that increasing the dose of morphine increased the relative risk of postoperative nausea ($P < 0.00001$) and vomiting ($P < 0.006$). In contrast, Palmer et al.[59] did not find a significant correlation between dose of epidural morphine (dose range 2.5–5 mg) and the incidence of postoperative nausea and vomiting. Interestingly, the incidence of postoperative nausea and vomiting in patients receiving epidural morphine for post-cesarean section analgesia is similar to that observed with conventional parenteral opioid analgesia.[60,61] Pain itself has also been implicated as a cause of nausea.[62]

Patients have cited nausea as the most common reason for a delay in ambulation after cesarean section.[4] This symptom may also interfere with breastfeeding and bonding with the baby.

In order to analyze critically the articles on postoperative nausea and vomiting in post-cesarean section patients who received neuraxial opioids, one must look at how well these articles control for confounding variables. No studies have been published that specifically analyze risk factors for postoperative nausea and vomiting following cesarean section under regional anesthesia. The published data relate either to intraoperative nausea or vomiting during neuaraxial anesthesia[63,64] or postoperative nausea and vomiting related to non-obstetric surgical patients who received general anesthesia.[58,65] To extrapolate the risk factors identified in these studies to a population of post-cesarean section who received neuraxial opioids is controversial.

Female gender, a history of postoperative nausea and vomiting or motion sickness and duration of surgery have been established as major predictive factors in all adult patients.[65] The influence of age is controversial, while smoking seems to protect against postoperative nausea and vomiting. In a study of patients undergoing surgery under spinal anesthesia, Carpenter et al.[64]

found the following factors correlated significantly with the presence of intraoperative nausea and vomiting: development of hypotension, block height (higher than T5 compared with lower than T5), a history of motion sickness, use of procaine and the use of phenylephrine and epinephrine (added to local anesthetic).

A few studies have established the link between intraoperative hypotension and nausea during spinal anesthesia for cesarean delivery.[66,67] In current obstetric anesthesia practice, early intraoperative nausea and vomiting are considered to be symptoms of hypotension and are treated with measures to restore blood pressure (positioning, fluid, vasopressors) before antiemetic agents are administered. The mechanism is thought to be brainstem ischemia, which activates the vomiting centers grouped around the medulla. Supplemental oxygen therapy may be beneficial in these circumstances.[63] Intraoperative nausea and vomiting could contribute to early post-operative nausea and vomiting, but are unlikely to play an important part in late postoperative nausea and vomiting.

The ideal intervention to prevent postoperative nausea and vomiting in parturients who have received neuraxial opioids during cesarean section should be safe to use during lactation, cost-effective, simple to administer and free of maternal side-effects. It is not possible to conclude from this review which antiemetic is most effective or closest to the ideal but some interventions are promising and warrant further discussion.

Acupressure, a non-invasive variation of acupuncture involving constant pressure on the P6 acupoint at the wrist, is particularly attractive. Acupressure is not clinically effective if nerve stimulation is blocked by local anesthesia.[68] There have been numerous reports about the efficacy of acupressure to prevent nausea resulting from morning sickness[69] and general anesthesia.[70] In addition, it appears to be more effective than placebo in patients who did not receive neuraxial morphine for postoperative analgesia.[71] It seems as if acupressure is most effective if applied before administration of opioids.[72] Difficulties in acupuncture research, especially surrounding optimal control, still exist.[73] In studies on effectiveness of acupressure for prevention of nausea and vomiting, it is difficult to truly blind patients as the Sea-Band® is an elastic band with a stud on the inside that if correctly applied exerts pressure on a specific point in the wrist. The placebo studies either tried to blunt the stud or apply the band to a different area on the wrist. A patient who is familiar with acupressure may see or feel the difference.

Metoclopramide has a long safety record in pregnancy and lactation. However, it is not free from side-effects.[74–76] In a meta-analysis on prevention of postoperative nausea and vomiting in the non-pregnant population, Henzi et al.[44] showed that metoclopramide had no significant antinausea effect, and only a modest effect on prevention of early vomiting (number-needed-to-treat = 5.8, 95% CI 3.9–11).

No pharmacologic agents discussed in this chapter, with the exception of scopolamine and metoclopramide, have been approved for use in lactation.[77] While cyclizine has not been implicated as having deleterious effects in the pregnant women and fetus, its use in lactating women is not recommended because of the possibility of lactation inhibition. Sedation of mother and baby is also a concern.[77]

Because of the current controversy surrounding droperidol and the fact that the manufacturer plans to discontinue its production, it is unlikely to be the agent of choice in the future for preventing postoperative nausea and vomiting. Ondansetron and dexamethasone are not currently recommended for use in lactation because of a lack of evidence concerning safety. This is unfortunate, as both these agents seem effective and relatively free of side-effects.

Directions for future research would be to identify patients at high risk to develop postoperative nausea and vomiting after receiving neuraxial opioids for post-cesarean analgesia. This would allow us to stratify patients in low-, moderate- and high-risk groups according to current practice in ambulatory settings. The use of acupressure (with optimal placebo control) or dexamethasone as a single agent or a combination of dexamethasone and ondansetron in high-risk patients should be evaluated further.

The optimal treatment of nausea and vomiting warrants further investigation.

Conclusions

Successful prophylaxis and treatment of pruritus secondary to neuraxial morphine may be achieved with a number of agents. In the prophylaxis of pruritus, 4 mg intravenous nalbuphine, 50 mg alizapride and 4 mg ondansetron, 6 mg oral naltrexone and 50 mg intramuscular hydroxyzine are all effective. Although shown to be effective in one study, naloxone is not to be recommended as it is administered by a cumbersome, continuous infusion. Agents not useful in the prophylaxis of itching include intravenous propofol and epidural butorphanol. For the treatment of pruritus, 3–5 mg intravenous nalbuphine is the most effective agent in common use, while intravenous propofol is ineffective. Recent work suggests that 4 mg intravenous ondansetron may exhibit useful antipruritic effects, in addition to its role as an antiemetic.

The published evidence concerning postoperative nausea and vomiting in cesarean section patients who received neuraxial opioids is generally of a high quality. As is the case after other surgery, no single drug is totally reliable. Lack of stratification on known risk factors for postoperative nausea and vomiting associated with the use of neuraxial opioids in the post-cesarean section population makes interpretation of current literature difficult. P6 acupressure seems particularly promising because of lack of side-effects although its usefulness has not been shown to be consistent. Metoclopramide and scopolamine are the only approved drugs at present for this indication. Comparing these agents with 5 mg dexamethasone alone or combined with 4 mg ondansetron (in high-risk patients) would provide valuable information, which could guide clinical decision-making in the future.

References

1 Fuller JG, McMorland GH, Douglas MJ, Palmer L. Epidural morphine for analgesia after caesarean section: a report of 4880 patients. *Can J Anaesth* 1990;**37**:636–40.

2 Harrison DM, Sinatra R, Morgese L, Chung JH. Epidural narcotic and patient-controlled analgesia for post-cesarean section pain relief. *Anesthesiology* 1988;**68**:454–7.

3 Eisenach JC, Grice SC, Dewan DM. Patient-controlled analgesia following cesarean section: a comparison with epidural and intramuscular narcotics. *Anesthesiology* 1988;**68**:444–8.

4 Cohen SE, Subak LL, Brose WG, Halpern J. Analgesia after cesarean delivery: patient evaluations and costs of five opioid techniques. *Reg Anesth* 1991;**16**:141–9.

5 Chadwick HS, Ready LB. Intrathecal and epidural morphine sulfate for post-cesarean analgesia: a clinical comparison. *Anesthesiology* 1988;**68**:925–9.

6 Caranza R, Jeyapalan I, Buggy DJ. Central neuraxial opioid analgesia after cesarean section: comparison of epidural diamorphine and intrathecal morphine. *Int J Obstet Anesth* 1999;**8**:90–3.

7 Bloor GK, Thompson M, Chung N. A randomised, double-blind comparison of subarachnoid and epidural diamorphine for elective cesarean section using a combined spinal–epidural technique. *Int J Obstet Anesth* 2000;**9**:233–7.

8 Kelly MC, Carabine UA, Mirakhur RK. Intrathecal diamorphine for analgesia after caesarean section: a dose finding study and assessment of side-effects. *Anaesthesia* 1998;**53**:231–7.

9 Stacey RGW, Jones R, Kar G, Poon A. High-dose intrathecal diamorphine for analgesia after caesarean section. *Anaesthesia* 2001;**56**:54–60.

10 Dahl JB, Jeppesen IS, Jorgensen H, Wetterslev J, Moiniche S. Intraoperative and postoperative analgesic efficacy and adverse effects of intrathecal opioids in patients undergoing cesarean section with spinal anesthesia: a qualitative and quantitative systematic review of randomised controlled trials. *Anesthesiology* 1999;**91**:1919–27.

11 Kotelko DM, Dailey PA, Shnider SM, Rosen MA, Hughes SC, Brizgys RV. Epidural morphine analgesia after cesarean delivery. *Obstet Gynecol* 1984;**63**:409–13.

12 Rosen MA, Hughes SC, Shnider SM, *et al.* Epidural morphine for the relief of postoperative pain after cesarean delivery. *Anesth Analg* 1983;**63**:666–72.

13 Jadad AR, Moore RA, Carroll D, Jenkinson C, Reynolds DJM. Assessing the quality of reports of randomised clinical trials: is blinding necessary? *Control Clin Trials* 1996;**17**:1–12.

14 Horta ML, Horta BL. Inhibition of epidural morphine-induced pruritus by intravenous droperidol. *Reg Anesth* 1993;**18**:118–20.

15 Horta ML, Ramos L, Goncalves Z. Inhibition of epidural morphine-induced pruritus by intravenous droperidol. *Reg Anesth* 1996;**21**:312–7.

16 Sanansilp V, Areewatana S, Tonsukchai N. Droperidol and the side-effects of epidural morphine after cesarean section *Anesth Analg* 1998;**86**:532–7.

17 Ballantyne JC, Loach AB, Carr DB. Itching after epidural and spinal opiates. *Pain* 1988;**33**:149–60.

18 Luthman JA, Kay NH, White JB. Intrathecal morphine for post-cesarean section analgesia: does naloxone reduce the incidence of pruritus? *Int J Obstet Anesth* 1992;**1**:191–4.

19 Thind GS, Wells JCD, Wilkes RG. The effects of continuous intravenous naloxone on epidural morphine analgesia. *Anaesthesia* 1986;**41**:582–5.

20 Abboud TK, Afrasiabi A, Davidson J, *et al.* Prophylactic oral naltrexone with epidural morphine: effect on adverse reactions and ventilatory responses to carbon dioxide. *Anesthesiology* 1990;**72**:233–7.

21 Abboud TK, Lee K, Zhu J, *et al.* Prophylactic oral naltrexone with intrathecal morphine for cesarean section: effects on adverse reactions and analgesia. *Anesth Analg* 1990;**71**:367–70.

22 Pellingrini JE, Bailey SL, Graves J, *et al.* The impact of nalmefene on side-effects due to intrathecal morphine at caesarean section. *AANA J* 2001;**69**:199–205.

23 Connelly NR, Radii A, Parker RK. Nalmefene or naloxone for preventing intrathecal opioid mediated side-effects in cesarean delivery patients. *Int J Obstet Anesth* 1997;**6**:231–4.

24 Morgan PJ, Mehta S, Kapala DM. Nalbuphine pre-treatment in cesarean section patients receiving epidural morphine. *Reg Anesth* 1991;**16**:84–8.

25 Charuluxananan S, Kyokong O, Somboonviboon W, Narasethakamol A, Promlok P. Nalbuphine versus ondansetron for prevention of intrathecal morphine-induced pruritus after cesarean delivery. *Anesth Analg* 2003;**96**:1789–93.

26 Kendrick WD, Woods AM, Daly MY, Birch RFH, DiFazio C. Naloxone versus nalbuphine infusion for prophylaxis of epidural morphine-induced pruritus. *Anesth Analg* 1996;**82**:641–7.

27 Gambling DR, Howell P, Huber C, Kozak S. Epidural butorphanol does not reduce side-effects from epidural morphine after cesarean birth. *Anesth Analg* 1994;**78**:1099–104.

28 Szarvas S, Harmaon D, Murphy D. Neuraxial opioid-induced pruritus: a review. *J Clin Anesth* 2003;**15**:232–9.

29 Horta ML, Ramos L, Goncalves Z. The inhibition of epidural morphine-induced pruritus by epidural droperidol. *Anesth Analg* 2000;**90**:638–41.

30 Horta ML, Vianna PTG. Effect of intravenous alizapride on spinal morphine-induced pruritus. *Br J Anaesth* 2003;**91**:287–9.

31 Eisenach JC, Yaksh TL. Safety in numbers: how do we study toxicity of spinal analgesics? *Anesthesiology* 2002;**97**:1047–9.

32 Juneja MM, Ackerman WE, Bellinger K. Epidural morphine pruritus reduction with hydroxyzine in parturients. *J Kentucky Med Assoc* 1991;**89**:319–21.

33 Yeh HM, Chen LK, Lin CJ, *et al.* Prophylactic intravenous ondansetron reduces the incidence of intrathecal morphine-induced pruritus in patients undergoing cesarean delivery. *Anesth Analg* 2000;**91**:172–5.

34 Borgeat A, Wilder-Smith OHG, Saiah M, Rifat K. Subhypnotic doses of propofol relieve pruritus induced by epidural and intrathecal morphine. *Anesthesiology* 1992;**76**:510–2.

35 Warwick JP, Kearns CF, Scott WE. The effect of subhypnotic doses of propofol on the incidence of pruritus after intrathecal morphine for caesarean section. *Anaesthesia* 1997;**52**:265–75.

36 Fan P. Nonopioid mechanism of morphine modulation of the activation of 5-hydroxytryptamine type 3 receptors. *Mol Pharmacol* 1995;**47**:491–5.

37 Yazigi A, Chalhoub V, Madi-Jebara S, Haddad F, Hayek G. Prophylactic ondansetron is effective in the treatment of nausea and vomiting but not on pruritus after cesarean delivery with intrathecal sufentanil–morphine *J Clin Anesth* 2002;**14**:183–6.

38 Charuluxananan S, Kyokong O, Uerpairokit K, Singhapreecha S, Ruangrit T. Optimal dose of nalbuphine for treatment of intrathecal morphine-induced pruritus after caesarean section. *J Obstet Gynaecol Res* 1999;**3**:209–13.

39 Cohen SE, Ratner EF, Kreitzman TR, Archer JH, Mignano LR. Nalbuphine is better than naloxone for treatment of side-effects after epidural morphine. *Anesth Analg* 1992;**75**:747–52.

40 Alhashemi JA, Crosby ET, Grodecki W, Duffy PJ, Hull KA, Gallant C. Treatment of intrathecal morphine-induced pruritus following caesarean section. *Can J Anaesth* 1997;**44**:1060–5.

41 Charuluxananan S, Kyokong O, Somboonviboon W, Lertmaharit S, Ngamprasertwong P, Nimcharoendee K. Nalbuphine versus propofol for treatment of intrathecal morphine-induced pruritus after cesarean delivery. *Anesth Analg* 2001;**93**:162–5.

42 Charuluxananan S, Somboonviboon W, Kyokong O, Nimcharoendee K. Ondansetron for treatment of intrathecal morphine-induced pruritus after cesarean delivery. *Reg Anesth Pain Med* 2000;**25**:535–9.

43 Beilin Y, Bernstein HH, Zucker-Pinchoff B, Zahn J, Zenzen W. Subhypnotic doses of propofol do not relieve pruritus induced by intrathecal morphine after cesarean section. *Anesth Analg* 1998;**86**:310–3.

44 Henzi I, Walder B, Tramer MR. Metoclopramide in the prevention of postoperative nausea and vomiting: a quantitative systematic review of randomized, placebo-controlled studies. *Br J Anaesth* 1999;**83**:761–71.

45 Chestnut DH, Vandewalker GE, Owen CL, Bates JN, Choi WW. Administration of metoclopramide for prevention of nausea and vomiting during epidural anesthesia for elective cesarean section. *Anesthesiology* 1987;**66**:563–6.

46 Chestnut DH, Owen CL, Geiger M, Bates JN, Choi WW, Ostman PL. Metoclopramide versus droperidol for prevention of nausea and vomiting during epidural anesthesia for caesarean section. *South Med J* 1989;**82**:1224–7.

47 Liu K, Hsu CC, Chia YY. The effect of dose of dexamethasone for antiemesis after major gynecological surgery. *Anesth Analg* 1999;**89**:1316–8.

48 Henzi I, Walder B, Tramer MR. Dexamethasone for the prevention of postoperative nausea and vomiting: a quantitative systematic review. *Anesth Analg* 2000;**90**:186–92.

49 Wang JJ, Ho ST, Wong CS, Tzeng JI, Liu HS, Ger LP. Dexamethasone prophylaxis of nausea and vomiting after epidural morphine for post-cesarean analgesia. *Can J Anesth* 2001;**48**:185–90.

50 Tzeng JI, Wang JJ, Ho ST, Tang CS, Liu YC, Lee SC. Dexamethasone for prophylaxis of nausea and vomiting after epidural morphine for post-caesarean section analgesia: comparison of droperidol and saline. *Br J Anaesth* 2000;**85**:865–8.

51 Nortcliffe SA, Shah J, Buggy DJ. Prevention of postoperative nausea and vomiting after spinal morphine for caesarean section: comparison of cyclizine, dexamethasone and placebo. *Br J Anaesth* 2003;**90**:665–70.

52 Wang JJ, Ho ST, Tzeng JI, Tang CS. The effect of timing of dexamethasone administration on its efficacy as a prophylactic antiemetic for postoperative nausea and vomiting. *Anesth Analg* 2000;**91**:136–9.

53 Kotelko DM, Rottman RL, Wright WC, Stone JJ, Yamashiro AY, Rosenblatt RM. Transdermal scopolamine decreases nausea and vomiting following cesarean section in patients receiving epidural morphine. *Anesthesiology* 1989;**71**:675–8.

54 Ho CM, Hseu SS, Tsai SK, Lee TY. Effect of P-6 acupressure on prevention of nausea and vomiting after epidural morphine for post-caesarean section pain relief. *Acta Anaesthesiol Scand* 1996;**40**:372–5.

55 Harmon D, Ryan M, Kelly A, Bowen M. Acupressure and prevention of nausea and vomiting during and after spinal anaesthesia for caesarean section. *Br J Anaesth* 2000;**84**: 463–7.

56 Duggal KN, Douglas MJ, Peter EA, Merrick PM. Acupressure for intrathecal narcotic-induced nausea and vomiting after caesarean section. *Int J Obstet Anesth* 1998;**7**:231–6.

57 Angst MS, Ramaswamy B, Riley ET, Stanski DR. Lumbar epidural morphine in humans and supraspinal analgesia to experimental heat pain. *Anesthesiology* 2000;**92**:312–24.

58 Watcha MF, White PF. Postoperative nausea and vomiting: its etiology, treatment, and prevention. *Anesthesiology* 1992;**77**:162–84.

59 Palmer CM, Nogami WM, Van Maren G, Alves DM. Post-cesarean epidural morphine: a dose–response study. *Anesth Analg* 2000;**90**:887–91.

60 Borgeat A, Ekatodramis G, Schenker CA. Postoperative nausea and vomiting in regional anesthesia: a review. *Anesthesiology* 2003;**98**:530–47.

61 Daley MD, Sandler AN, Turner KE, Vosu H, Slavchenko P. A comparison of epidural and intramuscular morphine in patients following cesarean section. *Anesthesiology* 1990;**72**:289–94.

62 Cousins MJ. Intrathecal and epidural administration of opioids. *Anesthesiology* 1984;**61**:276–310.

63 Ratra CK, Badola RP, Bhargava KP. A study of factors concerned in emesis during spinal anesthesia. *Br J Anaesth* 1972;**44**:1208–11.

64 Carpenter RL, Caplan RA, Brown DL. Incidence and risk factors for side-effects of spinal anesthesia. *Anesthesiology* 1992;**76**:906–16.

65 Watcha MF. Postoperative nausea and emesis. *Anesthesiol Clin North America* 2002;**20**:709–22.

66 Datta S, Alper MH, Ostheimer GW, Weiss JB. Method of

ephedrine administration and nausea and hypotension during spinal anesthesia for cesarean section. *Anesthesiology* 1982;**56**:68–70.

67 Kang YG, Abouleish E, Caritis S. Prophylactic intravenous ephedrine infusion during spinal anesthesia for cesarean section. *Anesth Analg* 1982;**63**:85–7.

68 Dundee JW, Ghaly G. Local anesthesia blocks the antiemetic action of P6 acupuncture. *Clin Pharmacol Ther* 1991;**50**:78–80.

69 Dundee JW, Sourial FB, Ghaly RG, Bell PF. P6 acupressure reduces morning sickness. *J R Soc Med* 1988;**81**:456–7.

70 Dundee JW, Ghaly RG, Bill KM, Chestnutt WN, Fitzpatrick KT, Lynas AG. Effect of stimulation of the P6 antiemetic point on postoperative nausea and vomiting. *Br J Anaesth* 1989;**63**:612–8.

71 Stein DJ, Birnbach DJ, Danzer BI, *et al.* Acupressure versus intravenous metoclopramide to prevent nausea and vomiting during spinal anesthesia for cesarean section. *Anesth Analg* 1997;**84**:342–5.

72 Al-Sadi M, Newman B, Julious S. Acupressure in the prevention of postoperative nausea and vomiting. *Anaesthesia* 1997;**52**:658–61.

73 Ernst E, White AR. A review of problems in clinical acupuncture research. *Am J Chin Med* 1997;**25**:3–11.

74 Kris MG, Tyson LE, Gralla RJ. Extrapyramidal reactions with high-dose metoclopramide. *N Engl J Med* 1983;**309**:433.

75 Caldwell C, Rains G, McKiterick K. An unusual reaction to preoperative metoclopramide. *Anesthesiology* 1987;**67**:854–5.

76 Eiseanch JC, Rose JC, Castro MI. Metoclopramide exaggerates stress-induced tachycardia. *Anesthesiology* 1988;**69**:A678.

77 Coustan DR, Mochuzuki TK. *Handbook of Prescribing Medications During Pregnancy.* Philadelphia, New York: Lippincott-Raven, 2001.

CHAPTER 13

Multimodal analgesia following cesarean section: Use of non-steroidal anti-inflammatory drugs combined with neuraxial opioids

Pamela Angle & Kamal Hussain

Introduction

Post-cesarean pain management has undergone considerable evolution in recent years, shifting away from traditional opioid-based therapy toward a more multimodal or "balanced" approach. Multimodal analgesia involves use of opioid and non-opioid analgesics in combination. From a theoretical perspective, combining different classes of analgesics should provide high-quality pain relief while limiting unwanted side-effects from each drug type.[1] A typical approach would include opioids, non-opioid analgesics such as non-steroidal anti-inflammatory drugs (NSAIDs) including acetaminophen and variable addition of local anesthetic techniques.[2]

Use of NSAIDs in non-cesarean section patients has been associated with decreased opioid consumption, improved analgesia at rest and with movement, decreased uterine pain associated with pregnancy termination[3] and reduced postoperative pain.[4,5] This systematic review examined randomized trials in which NSAIDs were studied as part of post-cesarean pain relief in patients receiving neuraxial morphine or diamorphine.

Methods

Reports were sought of randomized double-blind trials examining the effectiveness of NSAIDs in which post-cesarean pain was an outcome. Trials were included if they compared regular doses of NSAIDs with placebo in patients receiving neuraxial (intrathecal/epidural) morphine or diamorphine or if these neuraxial opioids were examined either alone or in combination with an NSAID. Trials examining pain following variable doses of neuraxial morphine or diamorphine combined with a fixed regimen of NSAIDs were also included. Pain outcomes were considered valid if measured using a visual or verbal analog scale (VAS) or a 4-point pain intensity scale (none, mild, moderate or severe) or examined pain relief using a 4- or 5-point rating scale.

The two authors used different search strategies to identify potentially relevant articles or abstracts from MEDLINE® (1981–2004), EMBASE® (1980–2004), the Cochrane Database of Systematic Reviews and Cochrane Central Register of Controlled Trials (first quarter 2004), and hand searches of major anesthesia journals and abstracts of meetings from 1999–2004. The search strategy included use of the following MeSH terms and free text terms and was not restricted by language: [morphine], [diamorphine], [anesthesia or anaesthesia], [cesarean or caesarean], [spinal], [epidural], [neuraxial], [multimodal], [obstetric], [ibuprofen], [naproxen], [diclofenac], [ketorolac], [ketoprofen] and [acetaminophen].

Additional articles were identified from the reference lists of retrieved articles, review articles, textbooks and personal files of the authors. The names of authors of identified abstracts were searched in an attempt to locate published manuscripts. No attempt was made to contact the authors.

Included reports

Retrieved references were independently examined for relevance by the authors with disagreement resolved by consensus. Articles were considered relevant if they were randomized double-blind trials conducted in obstetric patients following cesarean section and at least one arm received neuraxial morphine or diamorphine in combination with an NSAID. Studies comparing neuraxial analgesia with patient-controlled intravenous analgesia or intramuscular injections or not specifically addressing the effectiveness of adding an NSAID were excluded. Relevant articles were independently examined for quality and full manuscripts were scored using the Jadad scale[6] (see Appendix for a full description of the scale). A score of 3 or more was considered good quality.

Data extraction and analysis

From each study we extracted the number of patients treated, doses of neuraxial opioid used, NSAID regimen, study duration, analgesic outcomes and information on adverse effects.

Results

Reports of 14 trials were found which examined the effectiveness of NSAIDs in combination with neuraxial morphine for post-cesarean analgesia. The NSAIDs examined included naproxen, indomethacin, diclofenac, ketorolac, tenoxicam and ketoprofen. Eleven trials were published as full manuscripts,[7–17] three were published in abstract form only.[18–20] There were two abstracts[21,22] of subsequently published manuscripts[7,14] Overall, quality scores for these trials ranged from 2 to 5. Four trials were excluded for the following reasons: two trials (manuscripts) were found not to be double blinded,[16,17] and two abstracts had non-extractable data.[19,20]

A total of 10 studies involving 828 women were eligible for inclusion. These studies received quality scores ranging from 3 to 5. No trials specifically addressing the effectiveness of NSAIDs used in combination with neuraxial diamorphine were found. No trials were found examining the effectiveness of different NSAIDs in the setting of a single dose of neuraxial opioid. Lastly, we found no trials that compared the effectiveness of route of administration of NSAIDs (intramuscular versus oral or rectal) in women receiving neuraxial opioids following cesarean delivery.

Trials are grouped and presented in accordance with their study design.

Trials comparing the addition of an NSAID versus placebo with a fixed dose of neuraxial morphine

Five trials[7–10,18] involving 390 patients undergoing elective cesarean section compared regular administration of a single type of NSAID with placebo after a single dose of spinal morphine (Table 13.1). The NSAIDs examined were naproxen (2), indomethacin (1), tenoxicam (1) and diclofenac (1). Quality scores ranged from 3 to 5 (Table 13.1). All studies found a beneficial effect of adding an NSAID to neuraxial analgesia for post-cesarean pain relief.

One placebo-controlled trial of intravenous 40 mg tenoxicam, administered following cord clamping, examined analgesia for the first 24 h in women who had 0.15 mg spinal morphine.[9] Similarly, Dennis et al.[10] examined analgesia for 48 h in women who had received 0.2 mg spinal morphine and were randomized to receive either a single dose of 100 mg rectal diclofenac or placebo. The remaining three studies examined analgesia in patients receiving scheduled doses of a naproxen or indomethacin for 72 h following 0.15–0.3 mg spinal morphine.[7,8,18]

All five studies examined incision pain at rest over time. Four examined pain with movement[7,8,10,18] and uterine pain.[7,8,9,18] Three examined pain with both rest and movement over 72 h.[7,8,18] In one study, the primary outcome was pain on sitting at 36 h with a secondary outcome of overall pain relief over 72 h.[7] All studies examined adverse outcomes such as excessive bleeding, need for additional oxytocin, pruritus, nausea and vomiting, reduced respiratory rate and neonatal side-effects.

NSAIDs were consistently associated with reductions in opioid use over time[7,8,18] and delayed time to first analgesic request.[7,8,10,18] In the majority of studies, there was a clinically modest reduction in incision and uterine pain scores over time.[7,9,18] One study reported large reductions in incision pain and peak pain scores in the NSAID group on day 1, but not in uterine pain.[8] The same study did not find a significant difference in uterine pain. This trial assessed analgesia in 30 women randomized to receive indomethacin (100 mg rectal suppository given twice daily) following 0.25–0.30 mg spinal morphine. Pain scores in this study were

Table 13.1 Effectiveness of an NSAID versus placebo following a fixed dose of neuraxial morphine.

Reference	Drug	Study design	Drug regimen	Analgesic outcome	Remediation	Quality score and comments	Adverse effects	Authors' conclusions/comments
Angle et al. 2002[7]	Naproxen vs placebo	2 groups naproxen (40) placebo (40) Elective cesarean section Spinal morphine 0.2 mg + 10 to 20 μg spinal fentanyl Primary outcome: incision pain on sitting at 36 h Follow-up: 72 h	Naproxen 500 mg po/pr q 12 h vs identical placebo for 72 h	Naproxen group compared with placebo: lower incision pain scores (sitting) × 72 h ($P < 0.0001$) and opioid use ($P < 0.01$) over time Incision pain (sitting at 36 h was reduced [38.2 ± 26.0 vs 51.4 ± 25.7; $P = 0.05$]); Uterine pain was reduced from 12–48 h Inadequate overall pain relief was reduced on day 1 9% vs 32% ($P = 0.019$) but not on days 2 or 3. Worst pain occurred from 25–36 h	Rescue analgesia: Tylenol #3® (325 mg acetaminophen and 30 mg codeine per tablet) prn; parenteral opioids prn Median time to first analgesic request: Naproxen 22 h (1–50 h) Placebo 9 h (1–49 h)	5 2 breaches in protocol (both in naproxen group; analysis by intent to treat	No differences in vaginal blood loss or pruritus: nausea/ vomiting, additional oxytocic use, sedation, respiratory rate or neonatal side-effects	Naproxen produced a modest reduction in all types of pain measured Included breastfeeding mothers, asthmatics with previous use of aspirin or NSAIDs without problems Conclusions: scheduled doses of naproxen lead to modest reductions in pain at rest and movement. Incidence of inadequate pain relief is high days 2, 3 in both groups
Pavy et al. 1995[8]	Indomethacin vs placebo	2 groups (15) indomethacin; (15) placebo Elective cesarean section Spinal morphine (0.25–0.30 μg); spinal fentanyl (10–15 μg) Follow-up: 72 h	Study group (n = 15) Indomethacin 200 mg pr followed by 12 hourly indomethacin (100 mg) × 6 doses Control group (n = 15) placebo	Mean pain on movement was decreased on day 1 in the indomethacin group (1.4 ± 1.2 vs 5.1 ± 2.1 control; $P < 0.00001$) Mean pain was reduced over 72 h in the indomethacin group ($P < 0.0003$) Median time to first analgesia request was increased in the indomethacin group (39.6 h, range 7–82 h) vs placebo group (9 h, range 2–76 h) Fewer requests for additional analgesia in the indomethacin group	Rescue analgesia: Tylenol #3® (325 mg acetaminophen and 30 mg codeine per tablet) prn; parenteral opioids prn Median total additional analgesic requests for oral medication <72 h: Indomethacin 4 (range 0–11) Placebo: 11 (range 1–20) ($P < 0.0009$) No requests for parenteral analgesia	4	No differences in vaginal blood loss, nausea/vomiting No adverse neonatal effects were noted in breastfeeding babies Pruritus: Day 1: No pruritus placebo: 1/15 indomethacin: 0/15 Day 2: No pruritus placebo: 12/15 indomethacin: 10/15 Day 3: No pruritus placebo: 11/15 indomethacin: 13/15	Addition of indomethacin to spinal morphine leads to high-quality pain relief Asthmatics excluded Breastfeeding mothers included

Study	Comparison	Groups/Methods	Pain outcomes	Rescue analgesia	Quality/Withdrawals	Side-effects	Comments
Huang et al. 2002[9]	Tenoxicam vs placebo	2 groups tenoxicam (60) placebo (60) Elective cesarean section Spinal morphine 0.15 mg Follow-up: 24 h	Tenoxicam 40 mg IV post cord clamping vs placebo No differences in wound pain scores over time Mean uterine pain scores were consistently lower in the tenoxicam group for 24 h	Meperidine 50 mg IM q 4 h prn Rescue analgesia was used in 5/58 tenoxicam vs 24/59 patients in the placebo group over 24 h	4 Withdrawals 3 patients (2 in placebo group, 1 in study group)	No differences in pruritus, nausea/vomiting, bleeding or additional oxytocic use	Single dose if IV tenoxicam improves uterine pain scores (but not wound pain scores) on day 1 Breastfeeding women excluded Overall pain relief not measured
Dennis et al. 1995[10]	Diclofenac vs placebo	2 groups diclofenac (25) placebo (25) Elective cesarean section Spinal morphine 0.2 mg in both groups ± diclofenac vs placebo Follow-up: 48 h	Single dose of 100 mg rectal diclofenac at the end of surgery vs placebo Significant increase in mean time to first analgesia request: diclofenac: 19 h (± 8) vs placebo: 14 h (± 8, $P = 0.028$) Small differences in VAS movement scores over time with diclofenac group consistently lower than placebo	Rescue analgesia: morphine IM q 6 h prn; oral co-proxamol 2 tabs q 6 h prn No difference in the type of rescue analgesics used between groups Additional morphine requested within 12 h: placebo 2/25 diclofenac 1/25 Additional morphine required within 48 h: placebo 7/25 diclofenac 6/25	3	No significant differences in side-effects: Incidence: Pruritus: diclofenac (21/25) placebo (16/25) Excessive lochia: diclofenac (2/25) placebo (0/25) Nausea: diclofenac 4/25 placebo 5/25 Vomiting: diclofenac 7/25 placebo 7/25 Respiratory rate < 12: diclofenac 0/25 placebo 0/25	Single dose of diclofenac pr led to comparable levels of analgesia and an increased time to first analgesia request
Goheen et al. 2000[18] (abstract)	Naproxen vs placebo	3 groups (n = 110 randomized; 102 analysed) Group 1 (placebo) Group 2 (1 dose naproxen followed by placebo) Group 3 (regular dose of naproxen) Elective cesarean section Spinal morphine (0.15 mg); fentanyl (15 µg) Follow-up: 3 days	Group 1 (n = 33) received placebo in PACU + placebo on the ward Group 2 (n = 34) received naproxen 500 mg in PACU + placebo on the ward Group 3 (n = 35) received naproxen 500 mg in PACU followed by naproxen 250 mg po q 8 h × 3 days Mean VAS pain scores at rest on postoperative day 1 were higher in group 1 (placebo + placebo) than group 3 (naproxen + placebo) Group 1 VAS pain scores were also higher than group 3 scores with ambulation on day 1 (5.4 ± 2.1 vs 3.9 ± 2.2)	? Rescue analgesia More additional analgesia requested over time in the placebo group Group 1: (8.9 ± 3.5 day 1; 13.3 ± 7.5 day 2) Group 2: (7.2 ± 3.2 day 1; 14.8 ± 7.8 day 2) Group 3: (6.3 ± 3.2 day 1; 9.1 ± 7.0 day 2) respectively (2.9 ± 1.3 ± 1.3)	Not rated Withdrawals 8 randomized patients were excluded from the analysis (5 patients dropped out secondary to inadequate analgesia)	No information	Naproxen improved analgesia and decreased supplemental analgesic requests Analysis was not by "intent to treat" Reasons for exclusion of 3/8 patients randomized but not analyzed were not reported

IM, intramuscular; IV, intravenous; NSAIDs, non-steroidal anti-inflammatory drugs; PACU, post-anesthesia care unit; po, oral; pr, per rectum; prn, as needed; VAS, visual analog scale.

measured once daily (every 24 h). This method of measurement may have contributed to the relatively high levels of pain reported because these may reflect pain scores more for day 2 than day 1.

Angle et al.[7] examined pain scores in patients receiving 500 mg naproxen, either orally or rectally, at regular intervals following 0.2 mg spinal morphine. Patients were asked about wound pain, gas pain, uterine cramping pain and pain on movement at frequent intervals over 72 h. Wound pain was the worst source of pain reported by women in both groups. Pain scores peaked at 36 h in the placebo group with a significant reduction found in the naproxen group at this time. Overall, pain relief was significantly improved in most patients receiving regular doses of naproxen on day 1 ($P < 0.001$) and day 2 ($P < 0.001$). There was a significant reduction in opioid use in the naproxen group compared with placebo. The incidence of poor to fair pain relief was reduced between groups on day 1 in NSAID vs placebo groups (9% vs 32%, $P = 0.019$), but not on day 2 or 3. There was no difference in the incidence of side-effects between groups (Table 13.1).

Trials examining the effect of adding an NSAID to variable doses of neuraxial morphine

Two studies, involving 180 women, were found that examined the effectiveness of regular doses of NSAIDs in the setting of variable doses of spinal morphine (Table 13.2).[11,12] In one study, diclofenac was used,[11] and in the other indomethacin followed by naproxen[12] was studied. Both studies examined incision pain at rest and followed patients up to 24 h only.

Sun et al.[11] randomized 120 women to receive varying doses of epidural morphine with the administration of one 75-mg dose of intramuscular diclofenac. The control group received 4 mg epidural morphine and intramuscular saline. Patients receiving 3 mg epidural morphine combined with diclofenac reported better analgesia and fewer requests for additional pain therapy compared with patients receiving 4 mg epidural morphine alone. Overall, pain relief was better in patients with 3 and 4 mg of epidural morphine combined with diclofenac, with fewer side-effects in the 3-mg group. The authors concluded that 3 mg epidural morphine combined with diclofenac was the optimal therapy.

Yang et al.[12] randomized 60 women to receive either 0.1 or 0.25 mg spinal morphine. Both groups received a rectal suppository of 100 mg indomethacin immediately after surgery, followed by 500 mg oral naproxen, given twice daily. The authors noted similar levels of analgesia measured at rest between groups suggesting a synergistic effect of NSAIDs. Patients in the 0.1 mg spinal morphine group had less pruritus. The authors concluded that the analgesia provided by 0.1 mg spinal morphine combined with NSAIDs produces analgesia similar to that obtained by 0.25 mg spinal morphine combined with NSAIDs. There was less pruritus and nausea in patients who received 0.1 mg spinal morphine. VAS pain scores and full opioid (codeine) use between groups were not reported.

Multigroup trials examining NSAIDs in combination with neuraxial morphine, neuraxial morphine alone or NSAID alone

Three trials involving 258 women examined the effect of adding an NSAID to varying doses of epidural[13,14] or spinal morphine (Table 13.3).[15] Two studies examined ketorolac given either intramuscularly or intravenously.[14,15] One study also examined intramuscular diclofenac.[13] All studies followed patients for 24 h and examined incision pain only at rest. Only one study examined uterine pain.[13] Quality scores ranged from 3 to 4.

In a placebo-controlled double-blind trial, Sun et al.[13] randomized 120 parturients to one of four groups. Patients received 2 mg epidural morphine with 75 mg intramuscular diclofenac, 2 mg epidural morphine alone, intramuscular diclofenac alone or placebo given both epidural and intramuscularly. All of the study drugs were given as a single dose. The use of epidural morphine combined with diclofenac provided improved overall pain relief compared with diclofenac or 2 mg epidural morphine alone.

Tzeng & Mok[14] examined the effectiveness of a single dose of intramuscular ketorolac compared with placebo given to parturients randomized to receive either 0 or 2 mg epidural morphine. Patients receiving ketorolac used less intramuscular meperidine as rescue analgesia and had consistently lower VAS pain scores compared with those receiving 2 mg intramuscular ketorolac or 2 mg epidural morphine alone.[14] The results of this study disagree with those of a study by Cohen et al.[15]

Table 13.2 Effectiveness of an NSAID with variable doses of neuraxial morphine.

Reference	Drug	Study design	Dosing regimen	Analgesic outcome	Remediation	Quality score	Adverse effects	Judgment/comments
Sun et al. 1993[11]	Diclofenac 75 mg IM Single dose NSAID vs placebo	120 women Dose response study for epidural morphine ± diclofenac Elective cesarean section Epidural anesthesia: 2% lidocaine with epinephrine 1 : 200,000 Follow-up: 24 h	Group A (20): epidural morphine 0.5 mg + diclofenac Group B (20): epidural morphine 1.0 mg + diclofenac Group C (20): epidural morphine 2.0 mg + diclofenac Group D (20): epidural morphine 3.0 mg + diclofenac Group E (20): epidural morphine 4.0 mg + diclofenac Group F (20): epidural morphine 4.0 mg + Normal saline IM	Addition of diclofenac resulted in lower uterine pain scores for the first 12 h Incision and uterine pain were highest over time in group A followed by group F Combining epidural morphine (3 or 4 mg) with a single dose of diclofenac provided the lowest mean VAS pain scores for wound and uterine pain (pain scores ≤ 1 for both) Highest ratings of overall pain relief were found in groups C, D & E with more patients in groups D & E reporting excellent pain relief	Meperidine 50 mg IM q 4 h prn No. patients requiring additional meperidine IM (no. injections) Group A: 5/20 (8) Group B: 3/20 (3) Group C: 1/20 (1) Group D: 0/20 (0) Group E: 0/20 (0) Group F: 1/20 (1)	3	Non-significant differences in pruritus; respiratory rate, nausea/vomiting, bleeding Pruritus was worst in groups E & F. Similar scores found between groups C & D (~3–4)/10 Incidence of pruritus: Group A: 17/20 Group B: 16/20 Group C: 19/20 Group D: 18/20 Group E: 19/20 Group F: 19/20 Incidence of nausea/vomiting: Group A: 2/20 Group B: 5/20 Group C: 4/20 Group D: 8/20 Group E: 7/20 Group F: 7/20	3 mg epidural morphine + diclofenac results in the best analgesia without increased side-effects Asthmatics were excluded from the study Tests of significance done without adjusting the P value for multiple testing
Yang et al. 1999[12]	Indomethacin + naproxen in both groups Multiple scheduled doses of NSAID vs placebo	60 women Elective cesarean section Spinal morphine (0.1 vs 0.25 mg dose) Spinal hyperbaric bupivacaine 0.75% Follow-up: 24 h	Group 1 (30): spinal morphine 0.1 mg + fentanyl 20 µg Group 2 (28): spinal morphine 0.25 mg + fentanyl 20 µg	VAS pain scores between groups were not reported VAS pain scores did not differ significantly over time (P = 0.33) Oral narcotics used (mg codeine for breakthrough pain) were not reported	Available Rx: Leritine®, oxycodon/acetaminophen; morphine IM or meperidine IM, Tylenol #3® No differences in parenteral opioid requests: Group 1: 4/30 Group 2: 4/28 (P = 0.99) Time to first request for acetaminophen or codeine was not different between groups (700 min)	3 Withdrawals Results of 2 patients were not analyzed because they did not receive NSAIDs	Pruritus: lower with 0.1 mg morphine (P < 0.001). And fewer requests for treatment (4/30 vs 12/28) Differences in VAS pruritus scores ranged between 0.5 and 2.5 points on the VAS scale Maximum pruritus scores were ~4.5 vs 2.5 at 4 h in group 1 vs group 2 Nausea/vomiting: Lower nausea Scores over time in the 0.1 mg group (P < 0.001) but no differences in Rx for vomiting	Similar analgesia was achieved in 0.1 mg vs 0.25 mg spinal morphine groups receiving the same NSAID regimen and pruritus was less in the 0.1 mg group Study hypothesis and conclusions relate to analgesia but the primary outcome, sample size calculation and emphasis in reporting were placed on pruritus Incidence of pruritus not reported VAS pain scores over time not reported

IM, intramuscular; NSAID, non-steroidal anti-inflammatory drug; prn, as needed; Rx, treatment; VAS, visual analog scale.

Table 13.3 Multigroup trials examining NSAIDs in combination with neuraxial morphine, neuraxial morphine alone or NSAID alone.

Reference	Drug	Study design	Outcome measures	Dosing regimen	Analgesic outcome	Remedication	Withdrawals	Quality score	Adverse effects	Authors' conclusions/ comments
Sun et al. 1992[13]	Diclofenac Single dose of NSAID vs placebo	120 women Elective cesarean section Epidural anesthesia 4 parallel groups Follow-up: 24 h	Verbal analog (0–10) wound and uterine pain scored at 2, 4, 8, 12, 24 h Overall pain relief at 24 h (4-point scale) Incidence of: Pruritus Nausea/ vomiting Respiratory rate Oxytocin use	Group A (30): placebo epidural + placebo IM Group B (30): placebo epidural + 75 mg diclofenac IM Group C (30): epidural morphine 2 mg + NS IM Group D (30): epidural morphine 2 mg + 75 mg diclofenac IM	Overall pain relief was better in group D (96% good to excellent) than group A (51%); Group B (66%); Group C (62%) Group D rated pain relief as good (9/30) to excellent (20/30) compared with group C (18/29 good) to (9/29 excellent) Group D had better analgesia (wound and uterine pain were both < 2 for the first 18 h) Less supplemental analgesia was used by group D	Meperidine 50 mg IM every 4 h as needed	Withdrawals 3 patients (1 from each of groups A, B and C for excessive lochia post-cesarean section at 12 h and increased uterine pain from oxytocin use)	4	Incidence of nausea/vomiting group: A: 3/29 B: 6/29 C: 10/29 D: 12/30 (P < 0.05 for groups C & D compared with group A) Note: P value not adjusted for multiple testing Pruritus incidence group: A: 0/29 B: 1/29 C: 27/29 D: 30/30 Excessive bleeding see comment in "Withdrawals" A: 1/29 B: 1/29 C: 1/29 D: 0/30 Bradypnea: 0 in all groups	Authors conclude that combination epidural morphine + diclofenac therapy is superior to epidural morphine alone Diclofenac alone provides inadequate pain relief Wound pain scores implied but not specifically stated as measured at rest

Study	Drug/Intervention	Population/Design	Outcomes measured	Groups	Results	Rescue analgesia	Adverse effects	Quality	Other findings	Conclusions
Cohen et al. 1996[15]	Ketorolac IV. Multiple scheduled doses of NSAID vs placebo	48 women. Elective cesarean section. 4 groups: spinal anesthesia. Follow-up: 24 h	VAS pain; Pruritus; nausea; sedation. Measurements done: post-delivery, 15 min, 2, 8, 14 and at 20 h. Overall satisfaction at 24 h	Group 1: spinal morphine 0.2 mg + IV NS; Group 2: spinal morphine 0.1 mg + IV NS; Group 3: spinal morphine 0.1 mg + IV ketorolac 60 mg IV followed by ketorolac 30 mg IV q 6 h × 3 doses. Group 4: spinal morphine (none) + IV ketorolac (as in group 3)	No differences in mean VAS pain scores between groups over time or in maximum mean VAS pain scores, time to request for first analgesics, parenteral opioid or total opioid use	Meperidine (12.5–25 mg IV) q 30 min to a maximum of 50 mg/h. 67–75% of patients in all groups received meperidine	None reported	3	Less pruritus in group 4 (no spinal morphine) compared with the other groups	There is no advantage to combining ketorolac with spinal morphine and that ketorolac alone is adequate. Very small sample size. Spinal fentanyl was given variably between groups: Group 1 (14%); Group 2 (42%); Group 3 (28%); Group 4 (14%)
Tzeng & Mok 1994[14]	Ketorolac 30 mg IM. Single dose of NSAID vs placebo	90 women. Elective cesarean section. Epidural anesthesia. 3 groups. Follow-up: 24 h	VAS wound (? rest) pain scores (0–10). Pain relief (4-point scale); measured at ½, 1, 2, 4, 6, 8, 12 h. Bleeding	N = 30 per group. Group A: 2 mg epidural morphine + IM NS; Group B: 2 mg epidural morphine + 30 mg IM ketorolac; Group C: epidural NS + ketorolac 30 mg IM	Group B had consistently lower mean VAS pain scores over 24 h compared with the other groups. 96% of group B had good to excellent analgesia	Rescue medication: meperidine 50 mg IM prn. Rescue analgesia use: Group A: 5/30 (17%); Group B: 1/30 (3%); Group C: 16/30 (53%)	None reported	3	No respiratory depression or wound hematoma. Pruritus: Group A: 13/30 (43%); Group B: 14/30 (47%); Group C: 0/30 (0%). Nausea/vomiting: Group A: 3/30 (10%); Group B: 3/30 (10%); Group C: 0/30 (0%)	That use of epidural morphine combined with ketorolac provided superior pain relief to epidural morphine alone and ketorolac alone. Wound pain measured at rest

IM, intramuscular; IV, intravenous; NS, Normal saline; NSAID, non-steroidal anti-inflammatory drug; prn, as needed; VAS, visual analog scale.

The authors of the latter study found no difference in pain scores, time to first analgesic request and overall opioid use in patients randomized to receive 0.2, 0.1 mg or no spinal morphine combined with regular doses of intravenous ketorolac compared with placebo. The authors concluded that there was no advantage to combining ketorolac with spinal morphine and that ketorolac alone provided adequate analgesia. Inconsistency of these results with those of Tzeng & Mok[14] and similar studies using different NSAIDs are probably explained by the small sample sizes studied per group in study by Cohen et al.[15] (four groups with 11–13 patients per group) which makes it unlikely that the study could have demonstrated differences if in fact they were present.

Discussion

Overall, the results suggest that the addition of an NSAID with neuraxial morphine provides valuable additional post-cesarean analgesia and is safe provided its specific contraindications are observed. None of the studies included patients with hypersensitivity to NSAIDs, renal impairment, concomitant use of known nephrotoxins or a history of peptic ulcer disease. Some of the studies included asthmatics who had previously used NSAIDs without difficulty.[1,2,5]

The addition of regular doses of an NSAID in patients receiving equivalent doses of neuraxial morphine increased the time to first analgesic request, reduced overall opioid use, and reduced pain at rest and with movement.[7,8,18] Most studies demonstrated only clinically modest reductions in pain scores (including uterine pain) in patients receiving NSAIDs over time. An overall rating of pain relief is likely to be one of the most sensitive measures of the added benefits of NSAIDs and should be included as a measure in future trials.[23] Unfortunately, only a few of the studies reported this outcome.

The studies that compare NSAIDs with neuraxial morphine suggest that NSAIDs used alone provide inferior analgesia. However, combination therapy with NSAIDs and neuraxial morphine provide analgesia superior to that found with an equivalent dose of morphine without an NSAID. This added benefit does not increase (and may decrease) the incidence of side-effects.

Trials assessing post-cesarean analgesia in patients receiving NSAIDs in combination with varying doses of neuraxial morphine provide information needed for dosing patients in the clinical setting. Sun et al.[11] found that the optimal dose of epidural morphine combined with 75 mg intramuscular diclofenac was 3.0 mg. It should be noted that while no studies were found comparing the effectiveness of NSAIDs when given by different routes, there is evidence in the non-obstetric population to suggest that oral administration of NSAIDs is equally effective with intramuscular injections.[24] For this reason, when possible, the oral route should be the preferred method of NSAID administration.

Less convincing evidence of equivalent analgesia was found in the single study comparing reduced doses of spinal morphine (0.1 vs 0.25 mg) combined with a single NSAID regimen.[12] The short duration of the study, examination of pain only at rest and failure to report VAS pain scores and oral analgesic use makes it difficult to assess analgesic outcomes. It should be remembered that the goal of multimodal analgesia is not necessarily to reduce opioid use but to improve analgesia. The relative enthusiasm for reducing neuraxial morphine doses should be tempered by evidence suggesting that approximately 25% of women receiving 0.2 mg spinal morphine combined with 500 mg oral naproxen given twice daily, reported inadequate pain relief on the second day post-cesarean section.[7] Future studies examining analgesia in this context should explore analgesia over the first 72 h with a focus on day 2, when the effect of neuraxial morphine is wearing off and patients are dependent on less potent therapies for pain relief.

Conclusions

Overall, the results suggest that short-term use of an NSAID in combination with neuraxial morphine improves analgesia and is associated with minimal adverse effects such as bleeding, additional oxytocin use or neonatal outcomes in breastfeeding mothers (in studies examining these outcomes). While NSAIDs are clearly beneficial, most trials demonstrate only clinically modest reductions in pain scores over time (including reductions in uterine pain) coupled with reductions in additional analgesic use and delayed time to first analgesic request. We found the beneficial effects of adding an NSAID were most clearly demonstrated when overall pain relief was examined but most studies did not report this outcome. The few available studies examining pain over the first 3 days suggest that further work is warranted to improve pain relief on the second and third days after cesarean section.

References

1 Kehlet H, Dahl J. The value of "multimodal" or "balanced analgesia" in postoperative pain treatment. *Anesth Analg* 1993;**77**:1048–56.

2 Angle P, Walsh V. Pain relief after cesarean section. *Tech Reg Anesth Pain Management* 2001;**5**:36–40.

3 Pagnoni B, Ravanelli A, Degradi L, Rossi R, Tiengo. Clinical efficacy of ibuprofen arginine in the management of postoperative pain associated with suction termination of pregnancy: a double blind placebo-controlled study. *Clin Drug Invest* 1996;**17**:27–32.

4 Colbert S, O'Hanlon DM, Galvin S, Chambers F, Moriarity DC. The effect of rectal diclofenac on pruritus in patients receiving intrathecal morphine. *Anaesthesia* 1999;**54**:948–52.

5 Power I, Barrat S. Analgesic agents for the postoperative period. *Surg Clin North America* 1999;**79**:275–95.

6 Jadad AR, Moore RA, Carrol D, *et al.* Assessing the quality of reports of randomized clinical trials: is blinding necessary? *Control Clin Trials* 1996;**17**:1–2.

7 Angle PJ, Halpern SH, Leighton BL, Szalai JP, Gnanendran K, Kronberg JE. A randomized controlled trial examining the effect of naproxen on analgesia during the second day after cesarean delivery. *Anesth Analg* 2002;**95**:741–5.

8 Pavy TJG, Gambling DR, Merrick PM, Douglas MJ. Rectal indomethacin potentiates spinal morphine analgesia after caesarean delivery. *Anaesth Intensive Care* 1995;**23**:555–9.

9 Huang Y, Tsai S, Huang C, *et al.* Intravenous tenoxicam reduces uterine cramps after cesarean delivery. *Can J Anesth* 2002;**49**:384–7.

10 Dennis AR, Leeson-Payne CG, Hobbs GJ. Analgesia after caesarean section: the use of rectal diclofenac as an adjunct to spinal morphine. *Anaesthesia* 1995;**50**:297–9.

11 Sun H, Wu C, Lin M, Chang C. Effects of epidural morphine and intramuscular diclofenac combination in post-cesarean analgesia: a dose–range study. *Anesth Analg* 1993;**76**:284–8.

12 Yang T, Breen TW, Archer D, Fick G. Comparison of 0.25 mg and 0.1 mg intrathecal morphine for analgesia after cesarean section. *Can J Anesth* 1999; **46**:856–60.

13 Sun H, Wu C, Lin M, Chang C, Mok MS. Combination of low-dose epidural morphine and intramuscular diclofenac sodium in post-cesarean analgesia. *Anesth Analg* 1992;**76**:64–8.

14 Tzeng JI, Mok MS. Combination of intramuscular ketorolac and low-dose epidural morphine for the relief of post-caesarean pain. *Ann Acad Med Singapore* 1994;**23**(Suppl):10–13.

15 Cohen SE, Desai JB, Ratner EF, Riley ET, Halpern J. Ketorolac and spinal morphine for post-cesarean analgesia. *Int J Obstet Anesth* 1996;**5**:14–8.

16 Ganem EM, Modolo NSP, Ferrari F, Cordon FCO, Koguti ES, Catiglia YMM. Effects of low spinal morphine doses associated with intravenous and oral ketoprofen in patients submitted to cesarean section. *Rev Bras Anesthesiol* 2003;**53**:431–9.

17 Cardoso MMS, Carvalho JCA, Amaro AR, Prado AA, Cappelli EL. Small doses of intrathecal morphine combined with systemic diclofenac for postoperative pain control after cesarean delivery. *Anesth Analg* 1998;**86**:538–41.

18 Goheen MSLB, Ong BY, Wahba RF, Lucy SJ. Effect of oral naproxen on pain following cesarean section. *Anesthesiology* 2000;**78**(Suppl): A39.

19 Roy L, Chrochetere C, Aresenault MY, Villeneuve E, Lortie L. Combined intrathecal morphine and non-steroidal anti-inflammatory drugs for post-cesarean section analgesia. *Can J Anaesth* 1997;**44**:A15.

20 Waters J, Hullander M, Kraft A, Whitten G, Burger G. Post-cesarean pain relief with ketorolac tromethamine and epidural morphine. *Anesthesiology* 1992;**77**:A813.

21 Mok MS, Tzeng JI. Intramuscular ketorolac enhances the analgesic effect of low dose epidural morphine. *Anesth Analg* 1993;**76**:S269.

22 Angle P, Halpern C, Leighton B, Wilson D, Gnanedran K, Kronberg J. Naproxen improves post cesarean analgesia after spinal morphine. *Anesth Analg* 2000;**90**:S281.

23 McQuay H, Moore A. Pain measurement, study design and validity. In: *An Evidenced-Based Resource for Pain Relief.* New York, NY: Oxford University Press, 1998: 15.

24 McQuay H, Moore A. Comparing analgesic efficacy of non-steroidal anti-inflammatory drugs given by different routes in acute and chronic pain. In: *An Evidenced-Based Resource for Pain Relief.* New York, NY: Oxford University Press, 1998: 94–101.

PART 3

Complications of obstetric anesthesia

CHAPTER 14

The use of neuraxial anesthesia in parturients with thrombocytopenia: What is an adequate platelet count?

M. Joanne Douglas

Background

The subject of administration of neuraxial (spinal, epidural or combined spinal epidural) anesthesia in the parturient with thrombocytopenia is controversial. The concern is that the woman may develop bleeding in the epidural or subarachnoid space (neuraxial hematoma) resulting in a permanent neurologic disability. In common with all controversial subjects, the quality of evidence supporting management in these situations is lacking.

In 1972, Harker and Slichter[1] used the bleeding time (BT) to compare 100 normal subjects (mean platelet count $250 \pm 40 \times 10^9$/L) and 136 thrombocytopenic patients with various platelet disorders. The BT in patients with thrombocytopenia secondary to impaired production (marrow disorders) remained normal until the platelet count was less than 100×10^9/L. In these patients there was a direct linear relationship between a platelet count of less than 100×10^9/L and BT. When the platelet count was less than 10×10^9/L, the BT exceeded 30 min (normal 4.5 ± 1.5 min). In patients with idiopathic thrombocytopenic purpura (ITP) and a mean platelet count of $17 \pm 9.9 \times 10^9$/L the BT averaged 6.5 ± 2.6 min. This study suggested that the platelets in ITP have enhanced hemostatic capacity.

There is no evidence that BT correlates with clinical bleeding but the results of the study by Harker and Slichter probably led to the belief that a platelet count of more than 100×10^9/L was necessary for the safe administration of neuraxial anesthesia. In 1991, Letsky[2] suggested that a platelet count of 80×10^9/L would be

appropriate for insertion of an epidural, providing that the prothrombin time (PT) and partial thromboplastin time (PTT) were normal.

This chapter reviews the risk of a neuraxial hematoma in the parturient who has thrombocytopenia and receives neuraxial anesthesia. A computer search of the MEDLINE® and EMBASE® databases, covering the time period 1980–August 1, 2003, was performed using the key words [pregnancy], [obstetric], [platelet count], [thrombocytop(a)enia], [an(a)esthesia/epidural], [analgesia spinal] and [epidural h(a)ematoma].

Studies included in this review were cohort studies or surveys examining the definition of thrombocytopenia and risk of neuraxial hematoma in parturients with thrombocytopenia who received neuraxial anesthesia. Excluded were case reports other than those reporting epidural hematomas. The outcomes of interest were platelet count during normal pregnancy and risk of bleeding complications, specifically neuraxial hematoma, in parturients with a platelet count less than 100×10^9/L and in those with pre-eclampsia.

Platelets in normal pregnancy

Normal platelet count

Platelets are an integral part of hemostasis. Not only do they form the initial platelet plug after trauma to a blood vessel but they also release substances that encourage formation of the permanent clot. In the non-obstetric patient, thrombocytopenia is often defined as a platelet count less than 150×10^9/L. What constitutes a normal platelet count in pregnancy and

Table 14.1 Platelet count during normal pregnancy.

Author	Country	Study type	No.	Time/place sampled	Results	Comment
Fay et al.[3]	UK	Observational, case series	2066	Antenatal clinic	Platelet count decreased throughout pregnancy, was significant after 32 weeks	No information re. derivation normal values. Platelet count decreases throughout pregnancy
Freedman et al.[4]	Canada	Random, case control	686 control, 2204 peripartum	Blood donor clinic (controls), 1621 during labor or < 24 h postpartum	Mean platelet count in donors $236 \pm 50 \times 10^9$/L, 1.02% $< 136 \times 10^9$/L; in parturients mean platelet count $274 \pm 86 \times 10^9$/L, 6.4% had platelet count $< 136 \times 10^9$/L	No indication as to how randomized; excluded those with known cause of thrombocytopenia; thrombocytopenia defined as $< 136 \times 10^9$/L
Burrows & Kelton[5]	Canada	Prospective, case series	1547	Admission to obstetric unit	6.6% platelet count $< 150 \times 10^9$/L (95%CI 6.2–7.0%)	Analyzed separately those considered at risk of hemorrhage
Boehlen et al.[6]	USA	Prospective, cohort	287 controls, 6770 parturients	Admission to labor unit or 3rd trimester visit	11.6% had platelet count $< 150 \times 10^9$/L, mean platelet count and 2.5th percentile higher in non-pregnant women, histogram shifted to left	Consecutive sampling controls and subjects
Sainio et al.[7]	Finland	Surveillance, case series	4382	Term at delivery	7.3% had platelet count $< 150 \times 10^9$/L, 0.57% $< 100 \times 10^9$/L, 0.05% $< 50 \times 10^9$/L, histogram shifted to left	No information re. derivation normal values
Summary			**16,969**			**Approximately 7% have platelet count $< 150 \times 10^9$/L, platelet histogram shifted to left in contrast to non-pregnant**

what pregnant count is safe in terms of providing neuraxial anesthesia?

The introduction of automated blood cell counters in the 1980s allowed investigators to explore the platelet count during normal pregnancy and its changes throughout gestation. There are five large studies dating from 1983 to 2000 that examined platelet count either longitudinally during pregnancy[3] or at term,[4–7] as well as some smaller studies.[8–10] The smaller studies suggested that platelet count did not decrease during pregnancy, but because of their sample size and lack of a control group they are not included in this review.

In the five large studies, all women presenting either at an antenatal clinic or admitted to the maternity unit had blood taken for platelet count. The total number of pregnant women included in these five studies was 16,969 and all found that the mean platelet count was decreased at term compared with women in early pregnancy or non-pregnant women. In some of these studies, the women were selected randomly, some had samples taken throughout pregnancy while others were at term; some noted exclusions from their data analysis while others did not (Table 14.1).

Fay et al.[3] collected 2881 blood samples from 2114 pregnant women (mixed gestational ages) attending an antenatal clinic in Bristol, UK. The original purpose for collecting the blood was to determine hemoglobin concentration and the blood was subsequently used to obtain a platelet count. Women who developed pre-eclampsia later in pregnancy were excluded, leaving 2066 women whose platelet counts were analyzed. No information is provided as to whether consecutive subjects were used or the derivation of normal values in non-pregnant women. These investigators found that the platelet count decreased throughout pregnancy, with the decrease being statistically significant from women sampled at 32 weeks' gestation (compared with those sampled at less than 20 weeks' gestation) ($P < 0.01$). Platelet volume increased significantly from 35 weeks' gestation ($P < 0.001$).

The authors postulated that increased destruction of platelets resulted in the circulation of fewer platelets that were younger and larger. Unfortunately, they did not report the mean and range of platelet count at term. Extrapolating from their graph, the mean was approximately 262×10^9/L (approximate standard error of the mean $\pm 40 \times 10^9$/L).

Freedman et al.[4] carried out platelet counts on 686 random, healthy blood donors and 2204 random prenatal and postpartum women (1621 during labor or within 24 h postpartum). Women with a clinical diagnosis that would account for thrombocytopenia were excluded. The lower limit of normal platelet count for adults in this study, defined as two standard deviations below the mean, was 136×10^9/L. Among the blood donors, 1.02% had a platelet count of less than 136×10^9/L while 4.6% (n = 74) of pregnant women had a platelet count lower than that threshold. The lowest platelet count in parturients was 21×10^9/L. This difference was statistically significant ($P < 0.001$). No cause was found for the thrombocytopenia in any of the pregnant women.

In a well-designed prospective surveillance study, Burrows and Kelton[5] performed a platelet count as part of a complete blood count of all women admitted to their obstetric unit over a 7-year period. Women who were considered at risk of hemostatic impairment were classified into a separate group (e.g. hypertensive disorders of pregnancy, immune disorders such as ITP and systemic lupus erythematosus [SLE]). The definition of thrombocytopenia was a platelet count of 150×10^9/L or less. Not included in their analysis of 15,663 deliveries were 56 women who did not have a platelet count assessed prior to birth or 136 who had a stillbirth. Therefore, a total of 15,471 pregnancies were analyzed.

One thousand and twenty-seven women had a platelet count of 150×10^9/L or less (6.6%; 95% con-

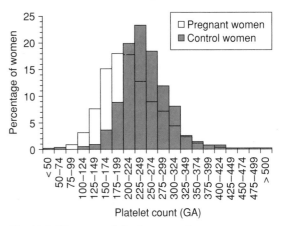

Fig. 14.1 Histogram of platelet count of pregnant women compared with non-pregnant women. From Boehlen et al.[6] with permission.

fidence interval [CI], 6.2–7%); 181 had a platelet count less than 100×10^9/L (1.2%; 95% CI, 1.0–1.4%). Seven hundred and fifty-six women were diagnosed with incidental (gestational) thrombocytopenia of pregnancy. Two previous reports from these same authors provided incremental data on the first year and first 3 years of this study.[11,12]

Boehlen et al.[6] explored the incidence of maternal and neonatal complications in women with thrombocytopenia defined as a maternal platelet count of less than 150×10^9/L. Platelet counts were performed on 6770 women consecutively admitted to the labor wards or during a prenatal visit during the last month of pregnancy. No patients were excluded. A control group consisted of 287 consecutive samples collected from all women (non-pregnant) who donated blood for the first time.

The mean platelet count of pregnant women was significantly lower than control women, as was the 25th percentile. A platelet count of 150×10^9/L was the first percentile in the control group and the 11.5th percentile in pregnant women (Fig. 14.1). Seven hundred and eighty-six pregnant women (11.6%; 95% CI, 10.8–12.4%) had a platelet count less than 150×10^9/L. In 738 women this thrombocytopenia was of unknown origin. The majority of the other cases of thrombocytopenia were related to pre-eclampsia or HELLP syndrome (**h**emolysis **e**levated **l**iver enzymes **l**ow **p**latelets). Only 21% of the thrombocytopenic women and 2.4% of all pregnant women had a platelet count below the 2.5th percentile for pregnant women (less than 116×10^9/L). No cause was found in 82% of the 136 women with a platelet count less than 116×10^9/L.

The authors reported no maternal complications, including the six women with a platelet count less than 50×10^9/L. The specific platelet count of these six is not reported. Four of these six parturients had HELLP syndrome or pre-eclampsia; one had antinuclear antibodies and one had thrombotic thrombocytopenic purpura (TTP).

As a result of this study, the authors suggest it is unnecessary to investigate more fully women who have a platelet count of more than 115×10^9/L. In women with a normal history and physical examination and a platelet count between 75 and 115×10^9/L, they suggest limited investigations such as complete blood count, blood smear, hepatic function tests as well as human immunodeficiency virus (HIV) and hepatitis C serologies. A more complete investigation is indicated if the platelet count is less than 75×10^9/L.

Sainio et al.[7] conducted a 1-year population surveillance involving 4382 women (83.8% of the population) with a term pregnancy at delivery. Blood samples were not obtained in 16.2% because of refusal or immediate delivery. The demographics of those who agreed and those who refused were comparable. The reference interval for the study population was $123-359 \times 10^9$/L (95% CI for the lower limit was $120-127 \times 10^9$/L and the 95% CI for the upper limit was $354-368 \times 10^9$/L) and showed a left shift of the distribution of platelet counts at term compared with the standard of 150×10^9/L. Their study did not include a control population. There were 317 women whose platelet counts were less than 150×10^9/L at delivery (7.3%), 25 women had a platelet count less than 100×10^9/L (0.6%), two of whom had a platelet count less than 50×10^9/L (one had ITP, one pre-eclampsia).

Eighty-one percent of the thrombocytopenic women had normal uncomplicated pregnancies or an obstetric disorder unrelated to thrombocytopenia (diabetes, cholestasis, twins without pre-eclampsia) and were diagnosed with gestational thrombocytopenia. Hemorrhage among the 317 thrombocytopenic women correlated only with known risk factors for postpartum hemorrhage, not with platelet count. There was no significant transfusion risk associated with severe or moderate thrombocytopenia. One woman with ITP (platelet count 24×10^9/L) received platelet transfusions at delivery. The diagnosis of ITP was 10 times more likely in women with a platelet count less than 70×10^9/L than in women with a platelet count less than 150×10^9/L.[7]

Shehata et al.[13] suggest that thrombocytopenia caused by increased destruction (e.g. ITP) is less likely to be associated with bleeding at a given platelet count than if it is a result of underproduction, as in marrow disorders. The rationale for this statement is that the platelets that circulate in destructive disorders are young and healthy whereas in disorders of inadequate production the circulating platelets are a mixture of young and old. This article and two other review articles discuss thrombocytopenia in pregnancy; its diagnosis, pathogenesis and management.[14,15]

In summary, maternal platelet count decreases throughout pregnancy; there is a shift to the left in the normal distribution of platelet count at term, compared with non-pregnant women.[6,7] Most authorities agree that a platelet count of more than 100×10^9/L in an otherwise healthy woman is not a cause for concern for her or for her neonate. As platelet counts of $70-100 \times 19^9$/L may occur in normal pregnancies, many authors recommend taking a "bleeding history," performing a general physical examination with careful blood pressure measurement and examining the peripheral blood film in these women to rule out more serious disorders.[15,16] As some of these women may have mild ITP, antenatal platelet counts should be reviewed.[15]

Platelet function testing

Anesthesiologists are interested in bedside testing of platelet function and for years relied on the BT to determine whether neuraxial anesthesia could be administered. The BT is influenced by many factors such as female gender, patient movement and local tissue factors. Rodgers and Levin[17] carried out a critical reappraisal of studies of BT (1083 human studies). They concluded that the BT may be useful in examining populations but not in the care of individuals and discounted BT as a test that is predictive of bleeding. Tests, such as platelet aggregometry, are not suitable for bedside testing because of the complexity and time needed to obtain results.[18–20]

Unfortunately, most studies examining platelet count and platelet function in parturients used the BT as the gold standard to evaluate platelet function or to determine the reliability of other methods of analyzing platelet function. Currently, anesthesiologists are evaluating two point of care instruments: the platelet function analyzer (PFA-100®) and the thromboelastogram (TEG). Therefore, the original MEDLINE® and EMBASE® search was expanded to include the key words [platelet function analyzer] and [thromboelastogram/thromboelastography] to answer the question: Are these tests able to predict the risk of bleeding in the epidural space following neuraxial anesthesia in a parturient with a given platelet count or a disorder such as pre-eclampsia? All of the studies are limited by small numbers.

The PFA-100® measures closure time of an aperture in response to certain agents and is thought to represent an *in vitro* BT. Two small studies have evaluated the use of this device in obstetric patients.[21,22] Over a 21-month period, Vincelot et al.[21] studied 110 full-term parturients, not in labor, at a preanesthetic visit, and other pregnant women when they presented with thrombocytopenia or gestational hypertension. They defined thrombocytopenia as a platelet count of less than 150×10^9/L and the women were divided into four groups based on the presence of complications of pregnancy (normal pregnancy, [n = 110], gestational thrombocytopenia [n = 38], pre-eclampsia without thrombocytopenia [n = 13] and pre-eclampsia with thrombocytopenia [n = 19]).

The authors concluded that platelet function was preserved in women with gestational thrombocytopenia when the platelet count was more than 70×10^9/L, unless anemia was present. In women with pre-eclampsia, PFA-100® values remained near normal until the platelet count was approximately 50×10^9/L; but it should be noted that the sample size for this group of women was very small (n = 19).

Marietta et al.[22] studied platelet aggregation using traditional platelet aggregometry and the PFA-100® in 14 normotensive and 15 hypertensive uncomplicated pregnancies. Women with proteinuria or signs of disseminated intravascular coagulation (DIC) or HELLP were excluded. There was considerable heterogeneity in both groups, with a range of gestational age from 20 to 39 weeks, even though they found that the groups were similar in this respect. Using traditional

platelet aggregometry, there was no difference in platelet aggregation between the groups even after incubation with L-arginine. The hypertensive group had a longer closure time with the PFA-100® after the samples were incubated with L-arginine. The small sample size, the heterogeneity and the failure of correlation of results with traditional aggregometry mean that further study is required before drawing any firm conclusions.

Sharma et al.[23] studied the use of TEG in a heterogeneous population of healthy non-pregnant, pregnant and postpartum women. Excluded were those with a known coagulation disorder, pre-eclampsia, hemorrhage or women on magnesium, aspirin or heparin. The pregnant women (n = 134) were at term and presenting for elective cesarean section, the postpartum women (n = 69) were 12–24 h postpartum prior to anesthesia for tubal ligation and the non-pregnant women served as controls. The study was partly designed to test new disposable plastic cups and pins for measuring TEG and the effect of celite on accelerating coagulation. The authors confirmed that normal healthy pregnancy is a hypercoagulable state and remains so for at least 24 h postpartum.

At present, there are insufficient data to indicate that the results of either the PFA-100® or thromboelastography are predictive of bleeding, especially in the epidural space.

Platelet count, platelet function and pre-eclampsia

One question frequently asked, particularly in woman with gestational hypertension (pre-eclampsia) or HELLP syndrome, is whether the platelets function normally. This concern arose from studies that used BT only to assess platelet function. BT is not considered a reliable method of determining the risk of bleeding and so the studies such as those by Ramanathan et al.[24] and McDonagh et al.[25] which only used BT are not discussed. There are four studies that used tests other than BT, often in conjunction with BT, to evaluate platelet function.

Kelton et al.[26] performed a prospective study of 26 pre-eclamptic patients and 17 healthy pregnant controls looking at platelet count, PT, activated PTT (aPTT), thrombin clotting time, stimulated thromboxane determination and platelet function using BT.

These tests were performed before delivery, on post-partum days 3 and 5, and 6 weeks postpartum. Nine of the 26 pre-eclamptic women were thrombocytopenic at presentation ($57–127 \times 10^9$/L) and six had a platelet count of less than 100×10^9/L. Five of these nine and four non-thrombocytopenic pre-eclamptic women had a prolonged BT. Collagen-induced biosynthesis of thromboxane B_2 was measured in 24 of the 26 and was reduced in 13. As a result, the authors suggested that there was a significant defect in platelet function in women with pre-eclampsia.

A prospective, observational study of 40 women with pre-eclampsia was reported by Schindler et al.[27] They measured platelet count, BT, platelet factor 3 (PF3) and thromboxane B_2 (indirect measures of assessing platelet aggregation and the release reaction). Thrombocytopenia (platelet count of less than 150×10^9/L) was present in 15%; BT was normal in all except one who had a platelet count of less than 50×10^9/L. Based on their results they concluded that neuraxial anesthesia could be performed if the platelet count was greater than 100×10^9/L and was contraindicated in women with a platelet count of less than 50×10^9/L. They also concluded that a BT should be performed if the platelet count was between 50 and 100×10^9/L and, if abnormal, neuraxial anesthesia was contraindicated. Of note, there were only two women in their study who had a platelet count between 50 and 100×10^9/L and only one with less than 50×10^9/L. Their conclusions regarding a platelet count of less than 100×10^9/L may be valid but because they are based on small numbers and the use of a BT one has to be cautious regarding their interpretation.

Others have evaluated platelet function in women with pre-eclampsia using TEG. Orlikowski et al.[28] examined platelet count, BT and TEG in 49 women with pre-eclampsia (seven mild, 33 severe, nine eclampsia). Eleven women had a platelet count between 100 and 150×10^9/L and seven had a platelet count of less than 100×10^9/L. A prolonged PT and reduced fibrinogen level occurred in two patients with a platelet count less than 100×10^9/L. The TEG was abnormal in another two women and the maximum amplitude (MA) reduced in all four (three of these had the lowest platelet counts 30, 36, 59×10^9/L). None of the women who had a platelet count of less than 100×10^9/L, a prolonged BT or an abnormal TEG received neuraxial anesthesia. They found a relationship between platelet count and abnormal TEG-derived clot formation. As the upper limit of their 95% CI was a platelet count of 75×10^9/L, they concluded that one could administer neuraxial anesthesia safely if the platelet count was above that level in women with pre-eclampsia. Women with a platelet count less than 100×10^9/L, a prolonged BT or an abnormal TEG did not receive a neuraxial anesthetic and the authors did not report how many received neuraxial anesthesia and their respective platelet counts.[28]

In a case series, Sharma et al.[29] evaluated TEG and platelet counts in 52 healthy pregnant women, 140 with mild pre-eclampsia and 114 women with severe pre-eclampsia. All were in active labor. Epidural analgesia was administered in women with a platelet count less than 100×10^9/L providing TEG parameters were normal (normal values were derived from the 52 healthy pregnant women).

Patients with severe pre-eclampsia were subdivided into those with a platelet count more than or less than 100×10^9/L. Platelet count ranges were $91–400 \times 10^9$/L in normal pregnant women, $84–409 \times 10^9$/L in those with mild pre-eclampsia and $115–351 \times 10^9$/L in those with severe pre-eclampsia and a platelet count more than 100×10^9/L. There were 34 women with severe pre-eclampsia who had a platelet count less than 100×10^9/L (mean $67 \pm 17 \times 10^9$/L). In these women the MA, as determined by TEG, was significantly hypocoagulable compared with the other three groups ($P < 0.001$). Ten women had a platelet count less than 100×10^9/L and an abnormal MA. The range of platelet counts in these 10 women was $37–66 \times 10^9$/L and they did not receive epidural analgesia. Three of these 10 also had an abnormal PT and two of those three had an abnormal aPTT, possibly indicating DIC. Otherwise, 85 mild pre-eclamptic and 63 severe pre-eclamptic patients received an uneventful epidural.[29]

DIC can occur in 21% of women with HELLP syndrome because of antecedent placental abruption, peripartum hemorrhage or subcapsular hematomas.[30] Before administering neuraxial anesthesia in the woman with HELLP syndrome or pre-eclampsia with thrombocytopenia, one should rule out a possible diagnosis of DIC. Although many suggest that TEG may be useful in predicting which patients with thrombocytopenia and pre-eclampsia could have neuraxial anesthesia, there is as yet no evidence that a normal TEG will make neuraxial anesthesia safe.[31]

Estimating the risk of epidural hematoma

Neuraxial anesthesia in healthy parturients with thrombocytopenia

Neuraxial hematomas in parturients are rare and have been published as isolated case reports. Retrospective reviews of neuraxial anesthesia in parturients with thrombocytopenia have not reported any cases. This may be because of their rarity, because of failure to report these cases or because neuraxial anesthesia is avoided in any woman considered at risk for developing a neuraxial hematoma. The rarity of neuraxial hematomas may lead an anesthesiologist to believe that administration of neuraxial anesthesia may be safe under certain circumstances. The risks and benefits of the procedure have to be assessed for each individual woman. As informed consent involves supplying a description of risks, including an approximate incidence, it is important to review the literature as to the safety of neuraxial anesthesia in parturients.

There are three studies available in which thrombocytopenic parturients received neuraxial anesthesia[32–34] (Table 14.2). All the studies were retrospective and reviewed epidural anesthesia in parturients with thrombocytopenia, recognized or unrecognized.[32–34]

Rolbin et al.[32] assessed the mean platelet count of 686 random blood donors (non-pregnant, both sexes) and 2204 randomly selected women during pregnancy and the postpartum period. Based on the results of this initial testing and the finding that there was an in-creased incidence of platelet counts of less than 150×10^9/L in obstetric patients compared with the normal blood donors (6.4% vs 2.2%), they defined peripartum thrombocytopenia as a platelet count of less than 150×10^9/L. All parturients who fell into this category were followed with serial platelet counts and their hospital charts were reviewed retrospectively to assess the type of anesthesia provided.

Sixty-one of 104 parturients with unexplained thrombocytopenia requested and received epidural anesthesia (37 continuous, 24 single shot). The platelet count was not available for most of these patients at the time of epidural anesthesia but one woman was denied epidural anesthesia based on thrombocytopenia. Seven women had platelet counts of less than 100×10^9/L and three received an epidural (two had a platelet count between 50 and 74×10^9/L and one had a count between 75 and 99×10^9/L). Seventeen patients with platelet counts of $100–125 \times 10^9$/L and 41 with platelet counts of $126–150 \times 10^9$/L also received epidural anesthesia. The lowest platelet count in this study was 21×10^9/L. No woman with a platelet count of less than 50×10^9/L received an epidural. None of the women who had epidural anesthesia had post-partum neurologic complications.[32]

Rasmus et al.[33] reviewed the charts of all women (2929) who had a vaginal or cesarean delivery over a 6-month period. All had platelet counts using the automated Coulter Counter® and the result was not available in most cases prior to administration of neuraxial anesthesia. The normal platelet count in

Table 14.2 Platelet count and type of anesthesia.

Author	Type of study, country	Population studied	No. studied	No. platelet count 50–100 $\times 10^9$/L/no. epidural	No. platelet count < 50 $\times 10^9$/L/no. epidural or spinal	Comments
Rolbin et al.[32]	Retrospective, Canada	Term parturients	686 control/ 2204 subjects	73	0	No complications
Rasmus et al.[33]	Retrospective, USA	Term parturients	2929	15/10	94	2 spinals, 2 epidurals in < 50 $\times 10^9$/L, (platelet counts of those: having neuraxial block 18, 24, 35, 38 $\times 10^9$/L)
Beilin et al.[34]	Retrospective, USA	Term parturients	15,919	80/30	?/0	No epidural placed if platelet count < 50 $\times 10^9$/L, did not state how many had platelet count < 50 $\times 10^9$/L

non-pregnant controls and males was $150–400 \times 10^9$/L ($\pm 30 \times 10^9$/L).

One hundred and eighty-three (6%) parturients had platelet counts of $100–150 \times 10^9$/L and 24 (0.8%) had platelet counts of less than 100×10^9/L. Ten of these were present on admission to hospital. Of the 10 with antepartum thrombocytopenia, one had May–Hegglin anomaly and she had a spinal for a cesarean delivery following a platelet transfusion. Another with ITP (platelet count 82×10^9/L) had an epidural. The remaining eight women had general anesthesia or no anesthesia. There were five women who had thrombocytopenia of unknown origin discovered postpartum. Four of the five had epidural anesthesia for vaginal or cesarean delivery. Ten of the 14 who had a platelet count of less than 100×10^9/L postpartum had antepartum platelet counts that were greater than 100×10^9/L. There were nine women with platelet counts of less than 50×10^9/L (range $18–42 \times 10^9$/L). Two of these women (platelet counts 18 and 32×10^9/L) had ITP. The woman with a platelet count of 18×10^9/L had an epidural for a vaginal birth. Again, no postpartum neurologic complications were reported in the women who received neuraxial anesthesia.[33]

More recently, Beilin *et al.*[34] retrospectively reviewed all charts of women who had thrombocytopenia (as defined as a platelet count of less than 100×10^9/L) during the peripartum period from March 1993 to February 1996. They sought to identify the etiology of thrombocytopenia, type of anesthesia, mode of delivery and any complications. Of 15,919 women who delivered during the period, there were 80 with platelet counts of less than 100×10^9/L. Thirty had epidural anesthesia when the platelet count was less than 100×10^9/L (range $69–98 \times 10^9$/L). Twenty-two had an epidural placed when the count was above 100×10^9/L but it subsequently decreased below 100×10^9/L ($58–99 \times 10^9$/L). Twenty-eight did not receive epidural anesthesia (platelet counts were $28–94 \times 10^9$/L). The platelet count considered by the anesthesiologist as too low to insert an epidural ranged from 34 to 90×10^9/L. Again, there were no documented neurologic complications postpartum.[34]

There is little evidence in the literature, other than that described above, to define a platelet count below which one should not perform neuraxial anesthesia in a parturient with ITP. In the studies described, several of the parturients with platelet counts below 100×10^9/L were found to have ITP. However, there are no case series specifically examining anesthetic management of parturients with ITP. In their review of management of ITP in pregnancy, Gill and Kelton[35] quoted the studies by Rolbin *et al.*[32] and Rasmus *et al.*[33] to argue that neuraxial anesthesia is safe in women with mild to moderate thrombocytopenia. A definition of mild to moderate is not given.

Guidelines for the management of ITP published by the British Society for Haematology[36] state: "In general, patients with a platelet count of more than 80×10^9/L, in the absence of pre-eclampsia are unlikely to have significantly altered platelet function." With rare exceptions, platelet function is not adversely affected in ITP and may be enhanced as it is a disorder of increased destruction. The American Society of Hematology panel recommends prophylactic platelet transfusions to prevent maternal bleeding during planned cesarean section only in women with platelet counts less than 10×10^9/L and consider platelet transfusion unnecessary in women with platelet counts more than 30×10^9/L and no bleeding symptoms.[37]

In a discussion on management of ITP in the adult in 1977, Lacey and Penner[38] presented the results of a study evaluating bleeding manifestations in ITP patients (no bleeding, minimal bleeding from trauma, spontaneous but self-limited, spontaneous, requiring special attention and massive uncontrolled or poorly controlled). These authors reported that a platelet count of more than 50×10^9/L correlated with no bleeding or minimal bleeding from trauma and they suggested that a platelet count of more than 50×10^9/L in patients with ITP did not result in an increased risk of bleeding.

In the author's own obstetric unit, spinal anesthesia is used for cesarean section in women with a stable platelet count of more than 50×10^9/L who have not previously had any evidence of bleeding or bruising at that particular count and have no additional risk factors for bleeding. We consider spinal safer than epidural anesthesia because spinal needles are smaller.

Pre-eclampsia, thrombocytopenia and neuraxial anesthesia

There are four studies that reported the results of neuraxial anesthesia in women with pre-eclampsia and a platelet count of less than 100×10^9/L[29,39–41] (Table 14.3).

Table 14.3 Neuraxial anesthesia, thrombocytopenia and pre-eclampsia.

Author	Study type, country	Population	No. of subjects	Platelet count 50–100 × 10⁹/L	Epidural with platelet count 50–100 × 10⁹/L	Comments
Hogg et al.[39]	Retrospective, USA	Severe pre-eclamptics in labor	327	18	7	No complications reported
Sharma et al.[29]	Case series, USA	Healthy pregnant controls, mild pre-eclamptics, severe pre-eclamptics in active labor	52 controls/ 140 mild/ 114 severe	34	?	10 of 34 had abnormal MA (platelet counts 37–66 × 10⁹/L, 5 of those had abnormal coagulation profile). Could have epidural if MA normal if platelet count < 100 × 10⁹/L, 63 severe pre-eclamptics received epidural. No complications
Head et al.[41]	Randomized case series, USA	Severe pre-eclamptics in labor	116: 56 epidural/ 60 PCIA	6	3	Randomized to receive epidural or intravenous PCA. Women ineligible if platelet count < 80 × 10⁹/L Outcome cesarean delivery rate, 3 of 6 with platelet count < 100 × 10⁹/L were in epidural group
Vigil-De Gracia et al.[40]	Retrospective, Panama	Parturients with HELLP	119: 71 prior to delivery	49; 40 had neuraxial anesthesia	36; 24 epidural/ 4 spinal	12 with platelet count < 50 × 10⁹/L had epidural. No reported complications

MA, maximum amplitude; PCA, patient-controlled analgesia.

Hogg et al.[39] carried out a secondary retrospective analysis of data from a multicenter trial of aspirin for women at high risk for pre-eclampsia. Their primary interest was whether epidural analgesia increased the risk of cesarean delivery, pulmonary edema and renal failure. There were 444 women with a diagnosis of severe pre-eclampsia. Among these women, 327 (74%) had labor and of those 209 (64%) had epidural anesthesia. Among the laboring women, 18 had platelet counts of less than 100 × 10⁹/L; seven had epidural anesthesia (six had platelet counts 75–99 × 10⁹/L and one 50–74 × 10⁹/L). No complications were reported.[39]

Vigil-De Gracia et al.[40] retrospectively examined the type of anesthesia and neurologic outcome in women with HELLP syndrome having cesarean section. The study covered the period July 1, 1996 to June 30, 2000. One hundred and nineteen women were diagnosed with HELLP syndrome; of the 85 who delivered by cesarean section there were 71 who were diagnosed with HELLP prior to cesarean section. The diagnosis of HELLP was based on the clinical diagnosis of pre-eclampsia and evidence of hemolysis, elevated liver enzymes and low platelet count. The PT and aPTT were normal before anesthesia was administered. Fifty-eight of the 71 women with antepartum HELLP had epidural anesthesia, four had spinal anesthesia and nine had general anesthesia for their cesarean section. Thirteen women had a platelet count less of than 50 × 10⁹/L and 12 of those had epidural anesthesia; seven had a platelet transfusion immediately before neuraxial anesthesia. There were 36 women with platelet counts of 51–100 × 10⁹/L; four had spinal anesthesia and 24 had epidural anesthesia. The remaining eight patients had general anesthesia. The other 22 women with HELLP syndrome and a platelet count of more than 100 × 10⁹/L had epidural anesthesia for their cesarean section. None of the women with HELLP syndrome who received neuraxial anesthesia had postpartum neurologic problems.[40]

In a randomized controlled trial, Head et al.[41] compared the use of intravenous patient-controlled analgesia (PCA) meperidine with patient-controlled epidural analgesia on cesarean delivery rates in women with severe pre-eclampsia. Women with a platelet count of less than 80×10^9/L were ineligible. The incidence of HELLP syndrome was similar between groups (14% epidural, 22% opioid). The mean platelet count was $186 \pm 52 \times 10^9$/L in the epidural group and $183 \pm 62 \times 10^9$/L in the opioid group. In a personal communication, Dr. John Owen stated that six of the 116 women studied had an antepartum platelet count of less than 100×10^9/L; three in the epidural group (J. Owen, personal communication via e-mail May 11, 2003). There were no maternal complications.

The rarity of epidural hematomas make it difficult to come to any firm conclusions with respect to the studies that were looking at neurologic outcome compared with platelet count. All are limited by their retrospective nature, small numbers of women with platelet counts of less than 100×10^9/L and even smaller numbers with platelet counts of less than 50×10^9/L. In a survey of American anesthesiologists (both academic and those in private practice) all would place an epidural in an "otherwise healthy parturient" with a platelet count of less than 100×10^9/L. Sixty-six percent of those in academic and 55% of those in private practice would place an epidural if the platelet count was between 80×10^9/L and 99×10^9/L. Sixteen percent of those in academic and 9% of those in private practice would place an epidural if the platelet count was between 50×10^9/L and 79×10^9/L.[42]

Reports of neuraxial hematomas following obstetric neuraxial anesthesia

In the non-obstetric population, the risk of a neuraxial hematoma in patients without known risk factors has been estimated at 0.2–3.7 in 100,000 epidural blocks.[43] In 2000, Loo et al.[43] reported that there were only seven cases of epidural hematomas after obstetric epidural anesthesia in the English literature from 1966 to November 1998. No cases were reported to that date with obstetric spinal anesthesia. Three of the epidural hematomas were managed conservatively and data on some of the seven cases were sparse. Since that time there have been three additional cases reported in the English literature following obstetric epidurals[44–46] and one following attempted spinal anesthesia.[47] In only one case was thrombocytopenia (platelet count 71×10^9/L) present prior to neuraxial block.[46]

In several of the cases included in Loo et al.'s review, the diagnosis was clinical or there was an additional risk factor at the time of neuraxial anesthesia.[43] In the recent four reports, one of the patients had unrecognized neurofibromatosis (unlikely responsible for the subsequent epidural hematoma),[44] another an ependymoma (attempted spinal)[47] and another developed DIC while the epidural was in situ.[45] In the fourth case, the woman had an eclamptic seizure in the recovery room following epidural anesthesia for cesarean section.[46] Only 4 mL of clot were removed at laminectomy. This is the only case report in the literature where the parturient had thrombocytopenia prior to neuraxial anesthesia.

It is impossible to estimate the incidence of neuraxial hematomas from case reports as many may be unreported and the denominator of women having neuraxial anesthesia in certain circumstance (e.g. preeclampsia) is unknown.

There are four large series examining complications of labor epidural analgesia.[48–50] Two were prospective and two retrospective. Two of the epidural hematomas reported in Loo et al.'s review[43] were from the retrospective studies.[48,49] Crawford[48] was the first to retrospectively review maternal complications in a consecutive series of 26,490 epidural blocks for labor analgesia and 567 patients who had an epidural for insertion of a cervical cerclage, termination of pregnancy or removal of a retained placenta. He excluded epidurals administered for elective cesarean section and eliminated minor or temporary complications. The review thus examined outcome of 27,057 epidural blocks and covered the dates October 1968 to February 1985. In this series he described a case of an epidural abscess arising in a small epidural hematoma in a woman with streptococcal bacteremia. After laminectomy the woman had complete recovery.

A report by Scott and Hibbard[49] relied on responses to a questionnaire sent to all obstetric units in the UK requesting information regarding serious adverse events following epidural anesthesia for the previous 5-year period (1982–1986). There was a 75% response rate, representing 78% of births in the UK. There were 506,000 epidurals administered for labor analgesia and cesarean section in the responding units. There was one epidural hematoma reported in this series which was treated surgically and was still improving at the time of the report.

Scott and Tunstall[50] reported on a 2-year prospective study of serious complications associated with all spinal (n = 14,856) and epidural blocks (n = 108,133) for obstetrics. Data were requested from consultant-led obstetric units and a member of the Obstetric Anaesthetists' Association was personally responsible for completing a questionnaire for each of the 2 years. Seventy-two were returned for 1990 and 79 for 1991. No epidural hematomas were reported.

Paech *et al.*[51] prospectively collected data on all epidural blocks (n = 10,995) performed for labor and delivery in a single institution for the period July 1989 to August 1994. No epidural hematomas were reported.

To date, obstetric anesthesiologists have avoided administering neuraxial blocks in patients considered at risk of developing an epidural hematoma so it is difficult to determine the specific risk related to a given platelet count or in a woman with an additional risk (e.g. pre-eclampsia). In the retrospective studies described above,[48,49] there is no indication as to the number of epidurals or spinals that were performed during the study period, making it impossible to calculate the incidence. It also is difficult to determine whether or not all cases of neuraxial hematoma that occurred were reported. In the prospective studies,[50,51] the platelet counts of the patients receiving neuraxial anesthesia were not reported. This makes it difficult to assess the risk with any particular platelet count.

To determine the 95% confidence interval around an event rate (epidural hematoma of 0%) in studies where the platelet count was reported, one can use the "rule" of zero numerators.[52] Based on that rule, using the data from Beilin's study, the upper boundary for the incidence of epidural hematomas in women with a platelet count of less than 100×10^9/L would be 10%,[34] illustrating that this type of study does not give sufficient information on which to base clinical judgment.

Conclusions

Studies of over 16,000 pregnant women have shown that the platelet count at term is lower, with the distribution shifted to the left from that of non-pregnant women. Platelet counts of $80-100 \times 10^9$/L are not uncommon in healthy women. The most common reason for mild thrombocytopenia is gestational or incidental thrombocytopenia of pregnancy and this diagnosis is not associated with any increase in morbidity for the woman or her newborn.

Studies of neuraxial anesthesia in healthy women with thrombocytopenia have shown that there is no increased risk when the platelet count is more than 100×10^9/L, but the numbers of women with a platelet count less than 100×10^9/L receiving neuraxial anesthesia are small. Current evidence, albeit based on small numbers and testing that has not been shown to be predictive of epidural space hemorrhage, suggests that a platelet count of more than 80×10^9/L is adequate for administration of neuraxial anesthesia, providing there are no additional risk factors. A recent survey confirmed that 64–78% of units were willing to administer neuraxial anesthesia if the platelet count was 80×10^9/L or above.[53]

As always, the risks and benefits for each individual patient have to be assessed before neuraxial anesthesia is administered. If the benefits of neuraxial anesthesia outweigh the risks then spinal anesthesia may be safer than epidural anesthesia.

References

1 Harker LA, Slichter SJ. The bleeding time as a screening test for evaluation of platelet function. *N Engl J Med* 1972;**287**:155–9.

2 Letsky EA. Haemostasis and epidural anaesthesia. *Int J Obstet Anesth* 1991;**1**:51–4.

3 Fay RA, Hughes AO, Farron NT. Platelets in pregnancy: hyperdestruction in pregnancy. *Obstet Gynecol* 1983;**61**:238–40.

4 Freedman J, Musclow E, Garvey B, Abbott D. Unexplained periparturient thrombocytopenia. *Am J Hematol* 1986;**21**:397–407.

5 Burrows RF, Kelton JG. Fetal thrombocytopenia and its relation to maternal thrombocytopenia. *N Engl J Med* 1993;**329**:1463–6.

6 Boehlen F, Hohfeld P, Extermann P, Perneger TV, De Moerloose P. Platelet count at term pregnancy: a reappraisal of the threshold. *Obstet Gynecol* 2000;**95**:29–33.

7 Sainio S, Kekomaki R, Riikonen S, Teramo K. Maternal thrombocytopenia at term: a population-based study. *Acta Obstet Gynaecol Scand* 2000;**79**:744–9.

8 Tygart SG, McRoyan DK, Spinnato JA, McRoyan CJ, Kitay DZ. Longitudinal study of platelet indices during normal pregnancy. *Am J Obstet Gynecol* 1986;**154**:883–7.

9 Sill PR, Lind T, Walker W. Platelet values during normal pregnancy. *Br J Obstet Gynaecol* 1985;**92**:480–3.

10 Louden KA, Broughton Pipkin F, Heptinstall S, Fox SC, Mitchell JRA, Symonds EM. A longitudinal study of platelet behaviour and thromboxane production in whole blood in normal pregnancy and the puerperium. *Br J Obstet Gynaecol* 1990;**97**:1108–14.

11 Burrows RF, Kelton JG. Incidentally detected thrombocytopenia in healthy mothers and their infants. *N Engl J Med* 1988;**319**:142–5.

12 Burrows RF, Kelton JG. Thrombocytopenia at delivery: a prospective survey of 6715 deliveries. *Am J Obstet Gynecol* 1990;**162**:731–4.

13 Shehata N, Burrows R, Kelton JG. Gestational thrombocytopenia. *Clin Obstet Gynecol* 1999;**42**:327–34.

14 Crowther MA, Burrows RF, Ginsberg J, Kelton JG. Thrombocytopenia in pregnancy: diagnosis, pathogenesis and management. *Blood Rev* 1996;**10**:8–16.

15 McCrae KR, Bussel JB, Mannucci PM, Remuzzi G, Cines DB. Platelets: an update on diagnosis and management of thrombocytopenic disorders. *Hematology* 2001;**6**:282–305.

16 ACOG Practice Bulletin. Thrombocytopenia in pregnancy. *Int J Gynaecol Obstet* 1999;**67**:117–28.

17 Rodgers RPC, Levin J. A critical reappraisal of the bleeding time. *Semin Thromb Hemost* 1990;**16**:1–20.

18 Harrison P. Progress in the assessment of platelet function. *Br J Haematol* 2000;**111**:733–44.

19 Rodgers GM. Overview of platelet physiology and laboratory evaluation of platelet function. *Clin Obstet Gynecol* 1999;**42**:349–59.

20 Kottke-Marchant K, Corcoran G. The laboratory diagnosis of platelet disorders: an algorithmic approach. *Arch Pathol Lab Med* 2002;**126**:133–46.

21 Vincelot A, Nathan N, Collet D, Mehaddi Y, Grandchamp P, Julia A. Platelet function during pregnancy: an evaluation using the PFA-100® analyser. *Br J Anaesth* 2001;**87**:890–3.

22 Marietta M, Castelli I, Piccinini F, *et al.* The PFA-100™ system for the assessment of platelet function in normotensive and hypertensive pregnancies. *Clin Lab Haematol* 2001;**23**:131–4.

23 Sharma SK, Philip J, Wiley J. Thromboelastographic changes in healthy parturients and postpartum women. *Anesth Analg* 1997;**85**:94–8.

24 Ramanathan J, Sibai BM, Vu T, Chauhan D. Correlation between bleeding times and platelet counts in women with pre-eclampsia undergoing cesarean section. *Anesthesiology* 1989;**71**:188–91.

25 McDonagh RJ, Ray JG, Burrows RF, Burrows EA, Vermeulen MJ. Platelet count may predict abnormal bleeding time among pregnant women with hypertension and pre-eclampsia. *Can J Anesth* 2001;**48**:563–9.

26 Kelton JG, Hunter DJS, Neame PB. A platelet function defect in pre-eclampsia. *Obstet Gynecol* 1985;**65**:107–9.

27 Schindler M, Gatt S, Isert P, Morgans D, Cheung A. Thrombocytopenia and platelet functional defects in pre-eclampsia: implications for regional anaesthesia. *Anaesth Intensive Care* 1990;**18**:169–74.

28 Orlikowski CEP, Rocke DA, Murray WB, *et al.* Thromboelastography changes in pre-eclampsia and eclampsia. *Br J Anaesth* 1996;**77**:157–61.

29 Sharma SK, Philip J, Whitten CW, Padakandla UB, Landers DF. Assessment of changes in coagulation in parturients with pre-eclampsia using thromboelastography. *Anesthesiology* 1999;**90**:385–90.

30 Sibai BM, Ramadan MK, Usta I, Salama M, Mercer BM, Friedman SA. Maternal morbidity and mortality in 442 pregnancies with hemolysis, elevated liver enzymes, and low

platelets (HELLP syndrome). *Am J Obstet Gynecol* 1993;**169**:1000–6.

31 Samama CM. Should a normal thromboelastogram allow us to perform a neuraxial block? A strong word of warning. *Can J Anesth* 2003;**50**:761–3.

32 Rolbin SH, Abbott D, Musclow E, Papsin F, Lie LM, Freedman J. Epidural anesthesia in pregnant patients with low platelet counts. *Obstet Gynecol* 1988;**71**:918–20.

33 Rasmus KT, Rottman RL, Kotelko DM, Wright WC, Stone JJ, Rosenblatt RM. Unrecognized thrombocytopenia and regional anesthesia in parturients: a retrospective review. *Obstet Gynecol* 1989;**73**:943–6.

34 Beilin Y, Zahn J, Comerford M. Safe epidural analgesia in thirty parturients with platelet counts between 69,000 and 98,000 mm^{-3}. *Anesth Analg* 1997;**85**:385–8.

35 Gill KK, Kelton JG. Management of idiopathic thrombocytopenic purpura in pregnancy. *Semin Hematol* 2000;**37**:275–89.

36 Guidelines for the investigation and management of idiopathic thrombocytopenic purpura in adults, children and in pregnancy. *Br J Haematol* 2003;**120**:574–96.

37 George JN, Woolf SH, Raskob GE, *et al.* Idiopathic thrombocytopenic purpura: a practice guideline developed by explicit methods for the American Society of Hematology. *Blood* 1996;**88**:3–40.

38 Lacey JV, Penner JA. Management of idiopathic thrombocytopenic purpura in the adult. *Semin Thromb Hemost* 1977;**3**:160–74.

39 Hogg B, Hauth JC, Caritis SN, *et al.* Safety of labor epidural anesthesia for women with severe hypertensive disease. *Am J Obstet Gynecol* 1999;**181**:1096–101.

40 Vigil-De Gracia P, Silva S, Montufar C, Carrol I, De Los Rios S. Anesthesia in pregnant women with HELLP syndrome. *Int J Gynaecol Obstet* 2001;**74**:23–7.

41 Head BB, Owen J, Vincent RD Jr, Shih G, Chestnut DH, Hauth JC. A randomized trial of intrapartum analgesia in women with severe pre-eclampsia. *Obstet Gynecol* 2002;**99**:452–7.

42 Beilin Y, Bodian CA, Haddad EM, Leibowitz AB. Practice patterns of anesthesiologists regarding situations in obstetric anesthesia where clinical management is controversial. *Anesth Analg* 1996;**83**:735–41.

43 Loo CC, Dahlgren G, Irestedt L. Neurological complications in obstetric regional anaesthesia. *Int J Obstet Anesth* 2000;**9**:99–124.

44 Esler MD, Durbridge J, Kirby S. Epidural haematoma after dural puncture in a parturient with neurofibromatosis. *Br J Anaesth* 2001;**87**:932–4.

45 Okuda Y, Kitajima T. Epidural hematoma in a parturient who developed disseminated intravascular coagulation after epidural anesthesia. *Reg Anesth Pain Med* 2001;**26**:383–4.

46 Yuen TST, Kua JSW, Tan IKS. Spinal haematoma following epidural anaesthesia in a patient with eclampsia. *Anaesthesia* 1999;**54**:350–4.

47 Jaeger M, Rickels E, Schmidt A, Samii M, Blomer U. Lumbar ependymoma presenting with paraplegia following attempted spinal anaesthesia. *Br J Anaesth* 2002;**88**:438–40.

48 Crawford JS. Some maternal complications of epidural analgesia for labour. *Anaesthesia* 1985;**40**:1219–25.

49 Scott DB, Hibbard BM. Serious non-fatal complications associated with extradural block in obstetric practice. *Br J Anaesth* 1990;**64**:537–41.

50 Scott DB, Tunstall ME. Serious complications associated with epidural/spinal blockade in obstetrics: a 2-year prospective study. *Int J Obstet Anesth* 1995;**4**:133–9.

51 Paech MJ, Godkin R, Webster S. Complications of obstetric epidural analgesia and anaesthesia: a prospective analysis of 10,995 cases. *Int J Obstet Anesth* 1998;**7**:5–11.

52 Hanley JA, Lippman-Hand A. If nothing goes wrong, is everything all right? Interpreting zero numerators. *JAMA* 1983;**249**:1743–5.

53 Wee L, Sinha P, Lewis M. Central nerve block and coagulation: a survey of obstetric anaesthetists. *Int J Obstet Anesth* 2002;**11**:170–5.

CHAPTER 15

A rational approach to aspiration prophylaxis

Geraldine O'Sullivan, Darren Hart & Andrew Shennan

Introduction

Mothers presenting for elective cesarean section under regional or general anesthesia, and who have received aspiration prophylaxis such as H_2 antagonists or proton pump inhibitors, do not appear to have a significant risk of aspirating gastric contents.[1] Pulmonary aspiration of gastric contents is predominantly associated with emergency cesarean section, when surgery is frequently carried out in rushed and stressed situations.

In modern obstetric practice, there is huge variation in both practice and policies regarding feeding and drinking in labor. These discrepancies have come about because of the lack of evidence to support nil-by-mouth policies and the belief by many clinicians, particularly midwives, that starving in labor is inherently wrong. Nil-by-mouth policies were introduced more than 50 years ago in an attempt to reduce pulmonary aspiration following general anesthesia. In the developed world few clinicians who care for women in labor have experience of this frightening complication. The onus has therefore shifted to the obstetric anesthesiologist to provide evidence that nil-by-mouth policies are beneficial. In the meantime, many midwives, supported by increasingly influential user groups in maternity services, support feeding and drinking in labor, because of the theoretical metabolic and psychological benefits. There is limited evidence supporting all viewpoints.

Pulmonary aspiration is now so rare it is an impossible endpoint to investigate even by large multicenter clinical trials. Even if feeding and eating in labor is related to this potentially fatal complication, its rarity may well justify the risk of allowing a more liberal approach to caloric intake in normal women in labor. Given the enormous number of women involved, this more liberal approach could be scientifically justified if an important benefit associated with intake could be proven. Whatever the practice, an informed debate is desperately needed. However, evidence that purports a benefit is lacking. Opinion leaders, whose interpretation of the available facts is based on physiologic principles and limited observational data or anecdotal reports, inevitably drive practice.

Historical perspective

In the second half of the 19th century in-hospital maternal mortality was 5–10 times higher than that seen in mothers delivered at home, with puerperal sepsis being the main cause of death. The advent of antisepsis helped to reverse this trend. However, during the period 1900–1930 the USA and UK had some of the highest rates of maternal mortality in the world. This has been attributed to excessive obstetric intervention, by hospital practitioners in the USA and in the UK by general practitioners administering general anesthesia for instrumental deliveries in the home. The decline in maternal mortality, which began in the 1930s, was dramatic and can be attributed to antibiotics, blood transfusion, ergotmetrine, improved treatment of pre-eclampsia and safer cesarean sections.[2]

The move to hospital deliveries in the early part of the 20th century in the USA and somewhat later in the UK did not *per se* influence maternal mortality but allowed the easier implementation of organized maternity care. This inevitably meant a greater number of obstetric interventions, many of which required general anesthesia. Curtis Mendelson, who died in 2002, was the obstetrician who highlighted the serious consequences of gastric aspiration in his landmark paper of 1946.[3] In this paper, he reported 66 cases of pulmonary aspiration out of a study base of 44,016 pregnancies. It is interesting that of the 45 who had the aspirated material inspected, only five aspirated solid food. It is often overlooked that only two of these women died and this was attributed to asphyxia secondary to the aspiration of solid food. In the remaining mothers, who developed aspiration pneumonitis, there were no fatalities. "Mendelson's syndrome" has since been associated with pulmonary aspiration pneumonitis. It must not be forgotten that at this time general anesthesia meant inhalational ether and was frequently administered, as Mendelson observed, by "a new and inexperienced intern." Mendelson's advice at this time became the cornerstone of anesthetic practice during subsequent decades. He advocated:

• the withholding of food during labor;
• the greater use of regional anesthesia;
• the administration of antacids;
• emptying the stomach prior to general anesthesia; and
• the competent administration of general anesthesia.

Pregnancy physiology and the risk of gastric aspiration

Gastroesophageal reflux is common in pregnancy. Studies of esophageal pH have demonstrated increased acidity, even in asymptomatic women.[4,5] This can be attributed to both an increase in intragastric pressure and a fall in lower esophageal sphincter pressure, probably as a result of the relaxing effects of progesterone.[6] Opioids and some anesthetic agents can compound these effects.[7]

Measuring gastric emptying during pregnancy and labor presents technical and ethical challenges and a variety of techniques have been used. Pregnancy does not significantly alter the rate of gastric emptying. It has been shown that gastric emptying is not delayed in healthy, non-obese, term parturients who ingest 300 mL water after an overnight fast. However, once labor begins, most studies indicate that there is a reduction in the ability of the stomach to empty physiologically[8–31] (Table 15.1). Studies using absorption of acetaminophen (paracetamol), which is not absorbed

Table 15.1 Studies of gastric emptying during pregnancy.

Method of assessment	Study period	Gastric emptying
X-ray (1938)[8]	Labor (10 subjects)	Delayed in 2 subjects
X-ray (1950)[9]	3rd trimester and labor	3rd trimester: no delay 3rd trimester + opioids: marked delay Labor: slight delay Labor + opioids: marked delay
X-ray (1956)[10]	Labor (12 subjects)	Delayed in 1 subject
Large volume test meal (1958)[11]	Serial study. Small numbers 2nd and 3rd trimester, Postpartum	No change
Double sampling test meal (1970)[12]	3rd trimester and labor	Labor: delayed, with altered pattern of emptying
Paracetamol absorption (1975)[13]	Labor with IM opioids Postpartum: 2–5 days	Labor: slight delay Labor + opioids: marked delay
Paracetamol absorption (1977)[14]	Labor	Labor: slight delay Labor + epidural analgesia (no opioid): slight delay
Epigastric impedence (1987)[15]	Non-pregnant controls, 3rd trimester, 60 min postpartum	No delay
Paracetamol absorption (1988)[16]	Non-pregnant controls, 8–11 weeks' gestation, 12–14 weeks' gestation	No delay Delayed

Continued

Table 15.1 *(continued)*

Method of assessment	Study period	Gastric emptying
Paracetamol absorption (1991)[17]	Non-pregnant controls, 1st, 2nd and 3rd trimesters	No delay in any of the three trimesters
Paracetamol absorption (1991)[18]	Post-cesarean section Epidural fentanyl 100 µg	Delayed
Paracetamol absorption (1991)[19]	Postpartum: Day 1 and day 3, 6 weeks	No delay
Real time ultrasound (1992)[20]	Non-pregnant controls 3rd trimester	No delay
Applied potential tomography (1992)[21]	Sequential study, 10 mothers: 37–40 weeks' gestation 2–3 days postpartum 6 weeks postpartum	No delay
Paracetamol absorption (1992)[22]	Labor with epidural analgesia: (i) Bupivacaine 0.375% (ii) Bupivacaine 0.375% + fentanyl 100 µg	Delayed in mothers receiving fentanyl
Paracetamol absorption (1993)[23]	Non-pregnant controls, 1st, 2nd, 3rd trimesters. Postpartum: 2 h, 18–24 h 24–48 h	Pregnancy; no change Postpartum 2 h: delayed > 24 h: no delay
Paracetamol absorption (1993)[24]	Labor: (i) Bupivacaine 0.25% (ii) Bupivacaine 0.25% + fentanyl 50 µg or 100 µg, or diamorphine 2.5 or 5 mg	Epidural opioids delayed gastric emptying
Paracetamol absorption (1994)[25]	Non-pregnant controls 8–12 weeks' gestation	Delayed
Paracetamol absorption (1995)[26]	3rd trimester and postpartum	No change
Paracetamol absorption (1996)[27]	Labor: Infusions (i) Bupivacaine 0.125% (ii) Bupivacaine 0.125% + fentanyl 2.0 µg/mL	No delay
Paracetamol absorption (1997)[28]	Labor: Infusions (i) Bupivacaine 0.125% (ii) Bupivacaine 0.125% + fentanyl 2.5 µg/mL	Up to 100 µg fentanyl: no delay > 100 µg fentanyl: delayed
Paracetamol absorption (1997)[29]	Labor: Epidural bupivacaine alone Epidural bupivacaine + fentanyl 50 µg Intrathecal bupivacaine + fentanyl 25 µg	 Delayed Delayed
Real time ultrasound (2001)[30]	Serial study in 11 women: 1st and 3rd trimester, 4–6 months postpartum	No delay
Real time ultrasound and acetaminophen absorption (2002)[31]	3rd trimester. Crossover study	No delay

IM, intramuscular.

within the stomach but rapidly so by the small intestine, have been widely used to measure gastric emptying.[32] Unfortunately, this technique is principally related to the gastric emptying of liquids and the evaluation of solids and semi-solids is more difficult. As particulate matter is more likely to be related to serious consequences, the data from these studies must be interpreted with some caution. Other techniques to investigate gastric emptying such as dye dilution,[12] epigastric impedance[15] and real time ultrasound[20,30,31] are also confounded by the same problem (i.e. they reflect liquid emptying rather than solids). Techniques using liquid test meals[11,12] require nasogastric intubation, a technique that has resulted in poor compliance amongst pregnant women.[11] In the epigastric impedance technique,[15] a constant 2-mA, 100-kHz current is applied through a pair of input electrodes while the other pair record changes in voltage, failure to accurately locate the stomach in pregnant subjects was a disadvantage with this technique. Applied potential tomography (APT)[21] generates tomographic images of the resistivity of gastric contents using electrodes placed around the epigatrium. Following ingestion of a test meal, changes in resistivity are measured. While APT can be used to assess gastric emptying of both liquid and solid meals, in pregnancy it has only been used to measure the gastric emptying of liquids. The only conclusive way to examine emptying of more particulate material is by conducting radioisotope and, to a lesser extent, X-ray studies. Although these studies are unacceptable in modern times, studies from the 1950s have demonstrated that gastric emptying of

solids is delayed in both late pregnancy and labor when parenteral opioids are administered. The delay in gastric emptying appears to be related to the duration of labor and to pain and is not reversed substantially with epidural techniques using local anesthetics.

During labor, bolus doses of epidural and intrathecal opioids further delay gastric emptying. Two studies[27,28] have evaluated the effect of epidural infusions of low-dose local anesthetics with opioids on gastric emptying during labor. In one,[27] the study began after the mother had received 90 µg fentanyl (50 µg bolus + 2 h epidural infusion at 20 µg/h) and this study showed no significant delay in gastric emptying. In the other study,[28] two groups of mothers were assessed. The study commenced in one group after 75 µg fentanyl had been infused while in the other group the study commenced after 100–125 µg had been infused. In both studies, further epidural local anesthetic with fentanyl was infused during the study period. Gastric emptying was shown to be delayed in those mothers who had received more than 100 µg fentanyl. This delay was less than that seen after the use of systemic opioids during labor, primarily in mothers who had been in labor for a significant length of time.

Decline in maternal mortality from pulmonary aspiration of gastric contents

The true reason for the decline in maternal deaths (Fig. 15.1) is difficult to ascertain but it is understandable that any new practice associated with this reduction

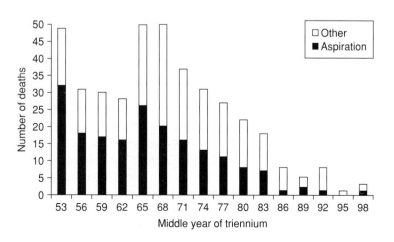

Fig. 15.1 Confidential Inquiry Triennial Reports illustrating anesthetic-related deaths.

would be eagerly accepted and rapidly introduced. In the 1940s, strategies to reduce gastric volume and increase pH were introduced because the physical properties of the stomach contents was an important cause of lethal aspiration.[3] Within obstetric anesthetic practice a number of other improvements in management were also becoming popular.

Tracheal intubation almost certainly played a significant part in reducing the incidence of pulmonary aspiration in obstetrics. However, in obstetrics its use is always in association with a rapid sequence induction of anesthesia (RSI) with cricoid pressure. The universal use of this technique in every term obstetric patient, both elective and emergency, could be questioned. A randomized controlled trial to assess the efficacy of RSI with cricoid pressure in obstetric patients has never been performed even though its use is associated with difficult or failed intubation.

Following a decline in anesthesia-related maternal mortality in the late 1950s and early 1960s, its incidence subsequently increased, at which time failed or misplaced intubation was recognized to be a significant complication of general anesthesia within the pregnant population. In these situations, extensive manipulation of the airway in the course of a difficult intubation was frequently associated with aspiration. Understandably, under these circumstances, anesthesiologists preferred a starved patient. Unfortunately, even modern obstetric practice has a significant incidence of failed intubation, reported to be as high as 1 in 250.[33] In obstetrics, anesthesia is induced with the mother lying in a tilted position so it is more likely that cricoid pressure will be incorrectly applied with consequent distortion of the larynx. Is it therefore necessary to perform a RSI with cricoid pressure in all mothers presenting for elective cesarean section under general anesthesia?

The evidence that H_2 antagonists reduce morbidity and mortality has not been conclusively demonstrated. At the time of their introduction into obstetric clinical practice, maternal mortality was already declining. Again, practice has been dictated, probably correctly, by physiologic principles. It is likely that reducing gastric volume and acidity limits damage due to aspiration pneumonitis.

Perhaps the most significant change in practice that has reduced the risk of pulmonary aspiration has been the dramatic reduction in the use of general anesthesia for cesarean section. However, the cesarean section rates have also escalated in recent decades, and therefore the decline in the overall number of general anesthetics (i.e. those most at risk of pulmonary aspiration) have not significantly reduced in absolute terms. In the UK, the National Sentinel Cesarean Section Audit (NSCSA)[34] showed that 1 in 29 mothers in England and Wales were unconscious during childbirth. This fact was not reported directly or even commented upon, but the audit found that the overall cesarean section rate in England and Wales had risen to 21.5%. As general anesthesia was used for 9.5% of the elective and 22.8% of the emergency cases (n = 10,923 and 18,534, respectively), it can be calculated that 5244 (3.5%) of the 3-month cohort of 150,139 must have delivered under general anesthesia. Therefore a reduction in the percentage use of general anesthesia cannot be the only explanation of the remarkable reduction in deaths from aspiration. Improved training in obstetric anesthesia with better understanding of the risks associated with general anesthesia may have contributed to the overall decline.

In the past 15 years the incidence of aspiration in the UK has been negligible.[1] Approximately 700,000 women deliver annually in the UK, which in a 15-year period represents approximately 10 million deliveries, during which time there have been only four fatal cases of aspiration. There has also been a reversal in the restrictive policies of nil-by-mouth and there is evidence that many more women do feed in labor.[35] Perhaps the most telling statistic will be in the forthcoming triennial reports. If, in spite of this practice, pulmonary aspiration remains low, this may be the best evidence that there is no causal relationship between feeding and mortality. However, there is still uncertainty and correct practice remains unclear.

Adverse effects of starvation

It is not surprising that labor is associated with an increased production of ketones, in particular hydroxybutyrate and acetoacetic acid.[36,37] These have been shown to occur rapidly following withdrawal of calories in pregnant women.[38] However, the increase in these acids, including non-esterified fatty acids which increase with starvation, have not been shown to be related to maternal and fetal acid–base balance.[39,40]

In the 1960s and 1970s, intravenous dextrose was given in an attempt to reduce maternal ketosis. This was soon abandoned when it became clear that this caused lactic acidosis in the babies along with jaundice and hypoglycemia.[39,41–43] The compromised fetus was particularly at risk.[42–45] Fluid overload was also a concern. It is not clear whether ketosis is as detrimental as initially thought and now it has been demonstrated that ketones can be utilized by both the mother and fetus. Indeed, this may be a normal physiologic response in labor which should not be tampered with. This understanding has also coincided with a more aggressive approach to labor management so that a long labor is far less tolerated and prolonged exposure to an intense ketotic state is rare.[46]

Whether ketosis or other effects of starvation have altered the progress and outcome of labor remain unclear. Some investigators have evaluated the effect of rehydration on labor outcome.[39,41] Infusions of normal saline have reduced maternal ketosis and possibly improved fetal well being.[47] Other investigators have demonstrated that infusing 1 L of normal saline will reduce uterine contractility.[48] A randomized controlled trial of the effect of increased intravenous hydration during labor (Ringer's lactate solution 125 vs 250 mL/h) showed that the incidence of labor lasting more than 12 h was statistically higher in the 125-mL/h group.[49] It was also suggested that the incidence of oxytocin use was less in the 250-mL/h group. This is a very large amount of fluid to give intravenously to a normal pregnant woman; perhaps it might be more physiologically acceptable to allow the mother to drink in response to thirst.

Are nil-by-mouth policies effective?

Although starving policies result in a reduced mean stomach volume over time,[50] other investigators have demonstrated that particulate matter is still present in the stomach up to 12 h after eating.[20] It is interesting that one study demonstrated that more women would choose epidural analgesia if it meant they were allowed to eat as nil-by-mouth was the policy when parenteral opioids were administered.[51] This illustrates that the desire to eat is an important factor in laboring women. In recent years there has been a significant increase in the number of units that allow food to be taken during labor.[52]

There is a large discrepancy in practices between North America and England and Wales. In 1988 less than 2% of units in the USA allowed solid intake, while this figure was almost 33% in the UK.[53] These large differences in practice have not been reflected by increased mortality from gastric aspiration in the UK. A more recent survey conducted in the USA indicates that little has changed.[54] Equally, the increased liberalization in the UK over the last decade has not resulted in an increase in maternal morbidity or mortality.

Undoubtedly, some women want to eat. In a survey of 149 women in Scotland, 30% indicated that they would liked to have eaten in the early stages of labor and a number of women had secretly eaten.[55] Many professionals argue that starvation in labor is both physiologically and psychologically detrimental for women.[56,57]

In areas where policies are less restrictive, trials have been conducted to discover the nature of oral intake during parturition. In an observational study of 5000 women conducted in US hospitals that did not have any form of restrictive policy, it was found that more than two-thirds ingested only clear fluids once in established labor.[58] Women were more likely to consume solids and non-clear fluids at home than hospital and those that labored longer consumed more. Scheepers et al.[59] conducted a retrospective survey in 2001, which monitored the influence of the caregiver on women's eating behavior during labor. Similar to the findings of Chern-Hughes,[58] they discovered that most are not advised about oral intake for labor and when left to their own devices only one-third of women will eat when in a hospital environment. It is estimated that a laboring woman may require up to 121 kcal/h once in established labor.[60] Evidence from these studies and trials confirmed that women in established labor are unable to tolerate the quantities of food and calories recommended to support them.

A key question in labor outcome is whether there are significant improvements in women who take either calories or light diet in labor. There is a scarcity of good controlled data looking specifically at delivery outcome but there are some randomized control trials that have evaluated obstetric endpoints.

We conducted a meta-analysis of all randomized controlled trials comparing effects of any form of caloric intake versus none in labor. Searches were conducted in electronic databases: MEDLINE®

Table 15.2 Randomized controlled trials included in meta-analysis.

Study	Number recruited	Randomization methods	Participants	Interventions	Outcomes
Yiannouzis & Parnell 1992[62]	297	Randomization with sealed envelopes	Multiparas and nulliparas, singleton fetus, cephalic presentation, gestation ≥ 37 weeks, cervical dilatation ≤ 3 cm	Light diet after randomization vs water only	Duration of labor, mode of delivery, Apgar scores, oxytocin requirement, vomiting – incidence
Scrutton et al. 1999[36]	88	Computer randomization with sealed envelopes	Multiparas and nulliparas, singleton fetus, cephalic presentation, gestation ≥ 37 weeks, cervical dilatation ≤ 3 cm	Light diet after randomization vs water only	Duration of labor, interventions, mode of delivery, Apgar scores, oxytocin requirement, blood gases, vomiting – incidence, volume, gastric volume Metabolic profile in early & late labor – ketones, free fatty acids, glucose, insulin, lactate
Kubli et al. 2002[37]	60	Computer randomization with sealed envelopes	Multiparas and nulliparas, singleton fetus, cephalic presentation, gestation ≥ 37 weeks, cervical dilatation ≤ 5 cm	Isotonic drinks (carbohydrate 64 g/L) after randomization vs water only	Duration of labor, interventions, mode of delivery, Apgar scores, oxytocin requirement, blood gases, vomiting – incidence, volume, gastric volume Metabolic profile in early & late labor – ketones, free fatty acids, glucose, insulin, lactate
Scheepers et al. 2002[61]	201	Double blinding randomization with sealed envelopes	Nulliparas, singleton fetus, cephalic fetus, gestation ≥ 37 weeks, cervical dilatation 2–4 cm, diabetes	Carbohydrate (126 g/L) drinks after randomization vs water only	Duration of labor, mode of delivery, Apgar scores, oxytocin requirement, arterial pH, pain medication

(1966–2002), Cochrane Pregnancy and Childbirth Group and EMBASE® (1974–2002). Reference lists were scanned for published and unpublished reports. The search terms were [randomized controlled trial], [feeding], [eating], [drinking], [labo(u)r], [nutrition], [hydration], [starvation], [ketones] and [ketosis].

To date, there are four randomized controlled trials that can be analyzed to ascertain obstetric endpoints in relation to caloric intake (Table 15.2). In 1999, Scrutton et al.[36] investigated whether a light diet would affect a woman's metabolic profile and increase her residual gastric volume. Labor outcome was also evaluated. Eighty-eight women were randomized. The light diet consisted of cereal, milk, toast, bread, semi-sweet biscuits and low-fat cheese. Light diet was compared with water only. Women beyond 37 weeks' gestation who had a singleton fetus with cephalic presentation were eligible if their cervical dilation was less than 5 cm. Women who had received intramuscular meperidine were excluded from the trial, as were women with significant obstetric or medical complications. Gastric volumes were measured with real time ultrasound all by the same investigator. Power was based on differences in metabolic endpoints, namely plasma β-hydroxybutyrate and non-esterified fatty acids and plasma glucose. Only two women withdrew from the study and four others were excluded as they had reached the second stage of labor within an hour. Women were stratified by parity, and low-dose epidural analgesia with bupivacaine and fentanyl was permitted. Glucose levels were higher in the eating group, while eating prevented the rise in hydroxybutyrate and fatty acids. There were no significant differences in other labor endpoints. Mothers in the eating group, however, did have significantly larger gastric volumes at the time of delivery and these women vomited larger volumes, which contained a considerable amount of solid residue.

A further study from the same unit randomized 60 women comparing the metabolic effects of isotonic sports drinks with water only during labor.[37] As with the previous trial, the metabolic profile was examined, along with labor outcome and residual gastric volumes. A similar protocol was followed. Those receiving sports drinks were encouraged to drink up to 0.5 L in the first hour and then a similar amount every 3–4 h. They could also take water if they wished. The water-only group had no restrictions. There were no withdrawals from the study. Despite the caloric limitation of the isotonic fluids, these drinks prevented the rise in β-hydroxybutyrate and non-esterified fatty acids seen in the starved group. Once again, there was no change in any outcome of labor but, in contrast to the light diet allowed in the original study, there was no increase in residual gastric volume in the isotonic sports drink group. While this approach may not provide the whole answer, it does at least provide a way of preventing ketosis that might be acceptable to the majority of anesthesiologists.

In Holland, Scheepers *et al.*[61] performed a randomized controlled trial in 200 women who received either carbohydrate solutions or placebo. Nulliparous women with a singleton fetus with a cervical dilation of 2–4 cm were included. Exclusion criteria included women who were scheduled for an elective cesarean section or those at "direct risk" (e.g. parturients with diabetes or multiple gestation). However, parturients with pre-eclampsia or post-term pregnancies were not excluded. Both groups were allowed to drink at will and standardized amounts of food or drink were given on demand. The main outcomes were operative deliveries, labor duration and need for analgesia. Again, envelopes were used for randomization and the trial was blinded. They found a threefold increase in cesarean section in women who received calories (21/101 vs 7/99, $P = 0.007$).

A fourth study, available only as an abstract, contains information regarding labor outcomes.[62] This trial is included in the meta-analysis of obstetric outcomes below.

Labor duration

When comparing the effect of any caloric intake versus

no caloric intake, labor was increased in duration in three trials and decreased in one. However, there was also significant heterogeneity in the trials (i.e. they disagreed with each other). The one trial in which oral intake shortened labor did not allow solid caloric intake. These data do not support the concept that caloric intake shortens the duration of labor (Fig. 15.2).

Mode of delivery

The data on outcome of labor from the four trials can be combined in a meta-analysis. When comparing any caloric intake versus no caloric intake, there were no significant differences, either in spontaneous delivery or need for cesarean section (Figs 15.3 & 15.4). There was significant heterogeneity. While three of the trials showed a slight decrease in the cesarean section rate[36,37,62] in patients who were fed, Scheepers *et al.*[61] reported a statistically significant result in the opposite direction. However, in this trial, the cesarean section rate in the placebo group was only 7% compared with the historical rate of 19% for that institution. Further, one would expect that the nulliparous high-risk population recruited for this study should have had a much higher cesarean section rate. The threefold increase in cesarean section rate (7% vs 21%) is therefore likely to be because of a type 1 statistical error (false-positive, when no difference exists). Taken together, these studies do not support the claim that oral intake decreases the cesarean section rate.

Incidence of vomiting

Three of the trials gave data on the incidence of vomiting.[36,37,62] Overall, feeding patients in labor causes a significant increase in vomiting with an odds ratio (OR) of 1.8 (Fig. 15.5). When the two trials that allowed solid oral intake are analyzed,[36,62] the odds of vomiting were greater (OR 2.423; 95% confidence interval [CI], 1.33–4.44) than in the control group. The difference in the incidence of vomiting when only clear fluid oral intake was allowed, compared with control was approximately 10% (37% vs 47%, $P = 0.46$). The difference in the volume of material vomited between patients who were fed (309 mL) and controls (104 mL) was statistically greater in the fed group when solids were allowed (difference = 205 mL; 95% CI, 99–301 mL; $P = 0.001$).[36] This was accompanied by

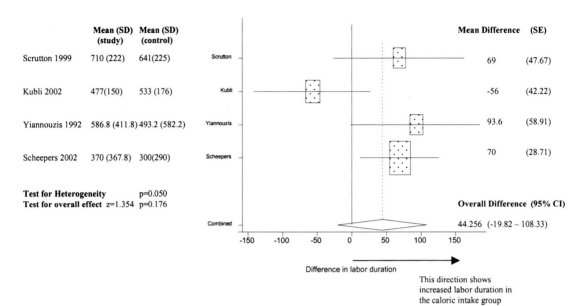

Fig. 15.2 Combined effects of caloric intake during labor versus non-caloric intake outcome: difference in labor duration. CI, confidence interval; SD, standard deviation; SE, standard error.

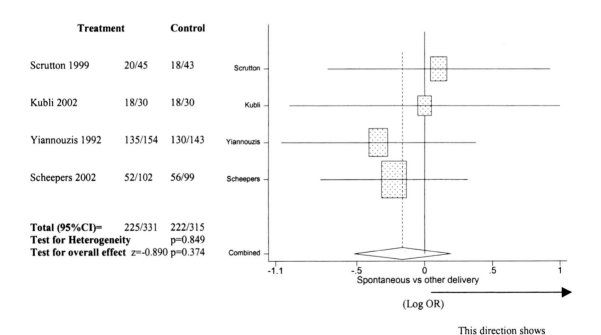

Fig. 15.3 Combined effects of caloric intake during labor versus non-caloric intake outcome: spontaneous delivery versus all other delivery types. CI, confidence interval; OR, odds ratio.

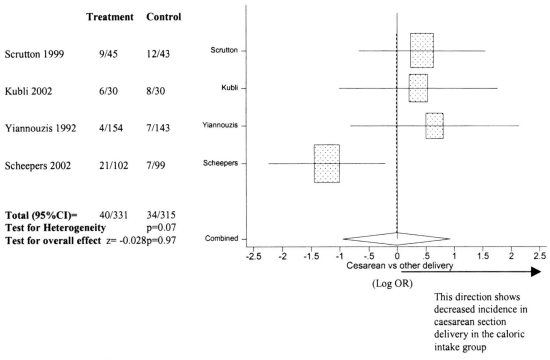

	Treatment	Control
Scrutton 1999	9/45	12/43
Kubli 2002	6/30	8/30
Yiannouzis 1992	4/154	7/143
Scheepers 2002	21/102	7/99
Total (95%CI)=	40/331	34/315
Test for Heterogeneity		p=0.07
Test for overall effect	z= -0.028p=0.97	

This direction shows decreased incidence in caesarean section delivery in the caloric intake group

Fig. 15.4 Combined effects of caloric intake during labor versus non-caloric intake outcome: cesarean delivery versus all other delivery types. CI, confidence interval; OR, odds ratio.

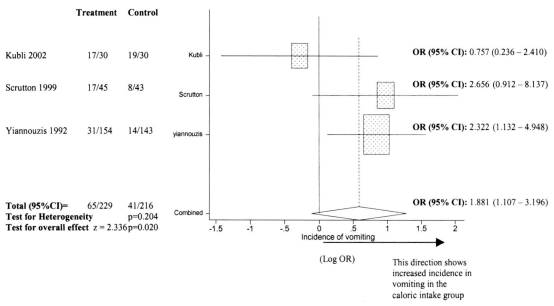

	Treatment	Control	
Kubli 2002	17/30	19/30	OR (95% CI): 0.757 (0.236 – 2.410)
Scrutton 1999	17/45	8/43	OR (95% CI): 2.656 (0.912 – 8.137)
Yiannouzis 1992	31/154	14/143	OR (95% CI): 2.322 (1.132 – 4.948)
Total (95%CI)=	65/229	41/216	OR (95% CI): 1.881 (1.107 – 3.196)
Test for Heterogeneity		p=0.204	
Test for overall effect	z = 2.336p=0.020		

This direction shows increased incidence in vomiting in the caloric intake group

Fig. 15.5 Combined effects of caloric intake during labor versus non-caloric intake outcome: incidence of vomiting versus none. CI, confidence interval; OR, odds ratio.

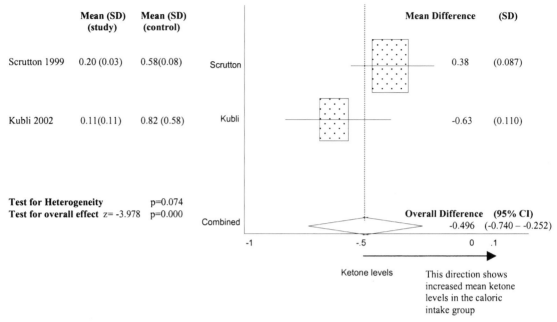

Fig. 15.6 Combined effects of caloric intake during labor versus non-caloric intake outcome: difference in plasma β-hydroxybutyrate levels (mmol/L). CI, confidence interval; SD, standard deviation.

a statistically significant increase in gastric cross-sectional area ($P < 0.001$). The volume of material vomited was not statistically different in the clinical trial that allowed a clear fluid sports drink only (difference = 66 mL; 95% CI, 115–246 mL; $P = 0.4$). In this trial, there was no significant increase in gastric cross-sectional area.[37] From the point of view of vomiting, feeding patients solid food may increase patient discomfort during labor. However, there are no data to suggest that parturients should be routinely denied clear fluids.

Plasma metabolites

In the two trials that evaluated metabolic effects,[36,37] caloric intake significantly reduced ketone levels by a mean of 0.496 mmol/L (95% CI, −0.740 to −0.252; $P = 0.0001$) (Fig. 15.6). There was a similar reduction in non-esterified fatty acids (Table 15.3). Increases in plasma glucose were also demonstrated in the meta-analysis of two of the trials, showing a significant increase of 0.6 m/L, the highest difference appearing in the trial by Kubli et al.[37] which used caloric intake with fluid.

Other outcomes

Caloric intake did not appear to affect the incidence of a low Apgar score (less than 7) at 1 min or mean umbilical artery pH. Further, there was no change in the use of intrapartum oxytocin (Table 15.3). The odds of having an Apgar score of less than 7 at 1 min was also not affected by caloric intake in the meta-analysis of the three trials, which allowed analysis of this endpoint. Mean arterial pH and use of oxytocin remained the same regardless of oral intake. Again, feeding does not seem to be an advantage, although it is difficult to draw firm conclusions from these limited numbers (Table 15.3).

Conclusions

The incidence of fatal aspiration pneumonitis in the parturient, related to general anesthesia, is extremely low. Because aspiration is a rare occurrence, there are no data on this outcome from randomized controlled trials. It is unlikely that the low incidence is directly related to a policy of restriction of oral intake during labor although it may be a factor. While a policy of

Table 15.3 Meta-analysis of other endpoints: caloric versus non-caloric intake.

Endpoint measured	Numbers analyzed	Odds ratio/ difference	Confidence intervals (95%)	Test for overall effect (P)	Test for heterogeneity (P)
Requirement for oxytocin versus none[36,37,61,62]	646	1.353	0.932–1.964	< 0.112	< 0.699
Incidence of Apgar scores < 7 at 1 min versus > 7 at 1 min[36,37,62]	445	1.150	0.455–2.910	< 0.768	< 0.486
Volume vomited during labor[36,37]	148	15.26 mL	−97.26–127.78	< 0.790	< 0.076
Mean difference in plasma non-esterified fatty acids[36,37]	148	−0.356 mmol/L	−0.438 to −0.274	< 0.001	< 0.907
Mean difference in plasma glucose levels[36,37]	148	0.669 m/L	0.350–0.988	< 0.001	< 0.682

nil-by-mouth may be responsible for unnecessary discomfort, there is very little evidence that it causes other harm. Currently available studies suggest there is no change in the length of labor, the obstetric outcome or neonatal outcome when parturients are fasted intrapartum compared with those who are fed.

Ingestion of solid foods during labor causes an increase in vomiting, but calorie-containing clear fluids do not. Clear fluids reverse the biochemical markers associated with fasting and provide some maternal comfort. Until further evidence is available, it is rational to restrict solid foods, but allow clear fluids in order to promote maternal comfort in labor. Women who wish to eat solid foods during labor should be informed of the known risks and benefits.

Acknowledgment

We would like to thank Suboshini Kugaprasad for assistance in analyzing the randomized controlled trials presented in the meta-analysis.

References

1 Department of Health and Others. *Reports on Confidential Enquiries Into Maternal Deaths in England and Wales/United Kingdom 1952–1999.* London: HMSO, 1957–2001 (Series of 16 Triennial Reports).

2 Loudon I. The transformation of maternal mortality. *BMJ* 1992;**305**:1557–60.

3 Mendelson CL. The aspiration of stomach contents into the lungs during obstetric anesthesia. *Am J Obstet Gynecol* 1946;**52**:191–206.

4 Hey VMF, Cowley DJ, Ganguli PC, *et al.* Gastro-oesophageal reflux in late pregnancy. *Anaesthesia* 1977;**32**:372–7.

5 Van Thiel DH, Gavaler JS, Shobha AB, *et al.* Heartburn of pregnancy. *Gastroenterology* 1977;**72**:666–8.

6 Van Thiel DH, Gavaler JS, Stremple J. Lower esophageal sphincter pressure in women using sequential oral contraceptives. *Gastroenterology* 1976;**71**:232–4.

7 Holdsworth JD. Relationship between stomach contents and analgesia in labour. *Br J Anaesth* 1978;**50**:1145–8.

8 Hirsheimer A, January DA, Daversa JJ. An X-ray study of gastric function during labor. *Am J Obstet Gynecol* 1938; **36**:671–3.

9 La Salvia LA, Steffen EA. Delayed gastric emptying time in labor. *Am J Obstet Gynecol* 1950;**59**:1075–81.

10 Crawford JS. Some aspects of obstetric anaesthesia. *Br J Anaesth* 1956;**28**:201–8.

11 Hunt JN, Murray FA. Gastric function in pregnancy. *Br J Obstet Gynaecol* 1958;**65**:78–83.

12 Davison JS, Davison MC, Hay DM. Gastric emptying time in late pregnancy and labour. *Br J Obstet Gynaecol* 1970;**77**: 37–41.

13 Nimmo WS, Wilson J, Prescott LF. Narcotic analgesics and delayed gastric emptying during labour. *Lancet* 1975;**1**:890–3.

14 Nimmo WS, Wilson J, Prescott LF. Further studies of gastric emptying during labour. *Anaesthesia* 1977;**32**:890–3.

15 O'Sullivan GM, Sutton AJ, Thompson SA, *et al.* Non-invasive measurement of gastric emptying in obstetric patients. *Anesth Analg* 1987;**66**:505–9.

16 Simpson KH, Stakes AF, Miller M. Pregnancy delays paracetamol absorption and gastric emptying in patients undergoing surgery. *Br J Anaesth* 1988;**60**:24–7.

17 Macfie AG, Magides AD, Richmond MN, Reilly CS. Gastric emptying in pregnancy. *Br J Anaesth* 1991;**67**:54–7.

18 Geddes SM, Thorburn J, Logan RW. Gastric emptying following caesarean section and the effect of epidural fentanyl. *Anaesthesia* 1991;**46**:1016–8.

19 Gin T, Cho AMW, Lew JKL, *et al.* Gastric emptying in the postpartum period. *Anaesth Intens Care* 1991;**19**:521–4.

20 Carp H, Jayaram A, Stoll M. Ultrasound examination of the stomach contents of parturients. *Anesth Analg* 1992;**74**: 683–7.

21 Sandar BK, Elliott RH, Windram I, Rowbotham DJ. Peripartum changes in gastric emptying. *Anaesthesia* 1992;**47**:196–8.

22 Wright PMC, Allen RW, Moore J, Donnelly JP. Gastric emptying during lumbar epidural extradural analgesia in labour: effect of fentanyl supplementation. *Br J Anaesth* 1992;**68**:248–51.

23 Whitehead E, Smith M, Dean Y, O'Sullivan G. An evaluation of gastric emptying times in pregnancy and the puerperium. *Anaesthesia* 1993;**48**:53–7.

24 Ewah B, Yau K, King M, *et al*. Effect of epidural opioids on gastric emptying in labour. *Int J Obstet Anesth* 1993;**2**:125–8.

25 Levy DM, Williams OA, Magides AD, Reilly CS. Gastric emptying is delayed at 8–12 weeks' gestation. *Br J Anaesth* 1994;**73**:237–8.

26 Stanley K, Magides A, Arnot M, *et al*. Delayed gastric emptying as a factor in delayed postprandial glycaemic response in pregnancy. *Br J Obstet Gynaecol* 1995;**102**:288–91.

27 Zimmerman DL, Breen TW, Fick G. Adding fentanyl 0.0002% to epidural bupivacaine 0.125% does not delay gastric emptying in laboring parturients. *Anesth Analg* 1996;**82**:612–6.

28 Porter JS, Bonello E, Reynolds F. The influence of epidural administration of fentanyl infusion on gastric emptying in labour. *Anaesthesia* 1997;**52**:1151–6.

29 Kelly MC, Carabine UA, Hill DA Mirakhur RK. A comparison of the effect of intrathecal and extradural fentanyl on gastric emptying in laboring women. *Anesth Analg* 1997;**85**:834–8.

30 Chiloiro M, Darconza G, Piccioli E, *et al*. Gastric emptying and orocecal transit time in pregnancy. *J Gastroenterol* 2001;**36**:538–43.

31 Wong CA, Loffredi M, Ganchiff JN, *et al*. Gastric emptying of water in term pregnancy. *Anesthesiology* 2002;**96**:1395–400.

32 Heading RC, Nimmo J, Prescott LF, *et al*. The dependence of paracetamol absorption on the rate of gastric emptying. *Br J Pharmacol* 1973;**47**:415–21.

33 Hawthorne L, Wilson R, Lyons G, *et al*. Failed intubation revisited: 17 year experience in a teaching maternity unit. *Br J Anaesth* 1996;**76**:680–4.

34 Thomas J, Paranjothy S. Royal College of Obstetricians and Gynaecologists Clinical Effectiveness Support Unit. *National Sentinel Caesarean Section Audit Report*. London: RCOG Press, 2001.

35 Hart D, Shennan AH, O'Sullivan G. To eat or not to eat? A national survey of maternity unit policies regarding oral intake during labour. Abstract. Research in Midwifery & Perinatal Health Conference; Birmingham, 2003.

36 Scrutton MJL, Metcalfe GA, Lowy C, *et al*. Eating in labour. *Anaesthesia* 1999;**54**:329–34.

37 Kubli M, Scrutton MJ, Seed PT, *et al*. An evaluation of isotonic "sport drinks" during labor. *Anesth Analg* 2002;**94**:404–8.

38 Metzger BE, Vileisis RA, Ramikar V, *et al*. "Accelerated starvation" and the skipped breakfast in late normal pregnancy. *Lancet* 1982;**1**:588–92.

39 Dumoulin JG, Foulkes JEB. Ketonuria during labour. *Br J Obstet Gynaecol* 1984;**91**:97–8.

40 Bencini FX, Symonds EM. Ketone bodies in fetal and maternal blood during parturition. *Aust NZ J Obstet Gynaecol* 1972;**12**:176–8.

41 Romney SL, Gabel PV. Maternal glucose loading in the management of fetal distress. *Am J Obstet Gynecol* 1966;**96**:698–708.

42 Kenepp NB, Shelley WC, Gabbe SG, *et al*. Fetal and neonatal hazards of maternal hydration with 5% dextrose before caesarean section. *Lancet* 1982;**1**:1150–2.

43 Lawrence GF, Brown VA, Parsons RJ, *et al*. Feto-maternal consequences of high-dose glucose infusion during labour. *Br J Obstet Gynaecol* 1982;**89**:27–32.

44 Feeney JG. Water intoxication and oxytocin. *BMJ* 1982;**284**:243.

45 Tarno-Mordi WO, Shaw JCL, Lin D, *et al*. Iatrogenic hyponatraemia of the newborn due to maternal fluid overload: a prospective study. *BMJ* 1981;**283**:639–42.

46 O'Driscoll K, Jackson JA, Gallagher JT. Prevention of prolonged labour. *BMJ* 1969;**2**:447–80.

47 Morton KE, Jackson MC, Gillmer MDG. A comparison of the effects of four intravenous solutions for the treatment of ketonuria during labour. *Br J Obstet Gynaecol* 1985;**92**:473–9.

48 Cheek TG, Samuels P, Miller F, *et al*. Normal saline IV fluid load decreases uterine activity in active labor. *Br J Anaesth* 1996;**77**:632–5.

49 Garite TJ, Weeks J, Peters-Phair K, *et al*. A randomized controlled trial of the effect of increased intravenous hydration on the course of labor in nulliparous women. *Am J Obstet Gynecol* 2000;**183**:1544–8.

50 Roberts RB, Shirley MA. The obstetrician's role in reducing the risk of aspiration pneumonitis with particular reference to the use of oral antacids. *Am J Obstet Gynecol* 1976;**124**:611–7.

51 Armstrong T, Johnston I. Epidural service implications of feeding policy in labour. *Anaesthesia* 1997;**52**:798–9.

52 Berry H. Feast or famine? Oral intake during labour: current evidence and practice. *Br J Midwifery* 1997;**5**:413–7.

53 Michael S, Reilly CS, Caunt M. Policies for oral intake during labour: a survey of maternity units in England and Wales. *Anaesthesia* 1991;**46**:1071–3.

54 Hawkins J, Gibbs C, Martin-Salvaj G, *et al*. Oral intake policies on labor and delivery: a national survey. *J Clin Anesthesia* 1998;**10**:449–51.

55 Armstrong TSH, Johnston IG. Which women want food during labour? Results of an audit in a Scottish DGH. *Health Bull* 2000;**58**:141–4.

56 Lewis P. Food for thought: should women fast or feed in labour? *Modern Midwife* 1991;**Jul**:14–7.

57 Champion P, McCormick C. *Eating and Drinking in Labour*. Oxford: Miriad, Books for Midwives, 2001.

58 Chern-Hughes B. Oral intake in labor: trends in midwifery practice. *J Nurs Midwifery* 1999;**44**:135–8.

59 Scheepers HCJ, Thans MCJ, de Jong PA, *et al*. Eating and

drinking in labor: the influence of practitioner's advice on womens' behaviour. *Birth* 2001;**28**:119–23.

60 British Nutrition Foundation. Nutrition requirements [online]. 2003. Available from: http://www.nutrition.org.uk

61 Scheepers HCJ, Thans MCJ, de Jong PA, *et al.* A double-blind randomised, placebo controlled study on the influence of carbohydrate solution intake during labor. *Br J Obstet Gynaecol* 2002;**109**:178–81.

62 Yiannouzis C, Parnell C. A randomised controlled trial measuring the effects on labour of offering a light, low fat diet. Abstract. London: Miriad, Books for Midwives, 1992.

CHAPTER 16

Postdural puncture headache

Peter T-L. Choi & Stefan Lucas

Introduction

In 1898, August Bier and his assistant, Dr. Hildebrandt, performed the first successful spinal anesthetic with cocaine. Coincidentally, Bier also described the first account of postdural puncture headache (PDPH) and hypothesized that the symptoms could be a result of escape of a considerable amount of cerebrospinal fluid (CSF).[1] Since the publication of his seminal paper, over 100 years of observational and experimental data have been published. To date, no consensus exists on the management of this complication. This chapter reviews the current definition and epidemiology of PDPH and summarizes the evidence for its prevention and treatment. Where possible, the evidence from studies of obstetric patients is emphasized.

Identification of postdural puncture headache literature

To identify relevant observational and experimental studies of PDPH for this chapter, the McMaster Obstetrical PDPH Evidence Database (MOPED) was initially searched. This bibliographic database references literature published from 1949 to February 2002. Citations were identified by computerized searches (MEDLINE® 1966–February 2002, CINAHL® 1982–February 2002, HealthSTAR 1975–February 2002, Cochrane Library 2002 Issue 1), citation review and hand searches of abstracts and conference proceedings.[2] In addition to MOPED, additional studies of PDPH in obstetric and surgical patients were sought using search strategies similar to those described for the development of MOPED.[3] These searches were conducted in MEDLINE® (July 2003), EMBASE® (July 2003) and the Cochrane Library (2003 Issue 3).

Definition and clinical features

To date, no single definition of PDPH has been used consistently in the clinical or research settings. The International Headache Society provided diagnostic criteria for PDPH in 1988 (Table 16.1).[4] However, researchers continue to vary in their definitions. Choi *et al.*[5] reviewed studies of PDPH in obstetric patients published from 1949 to 2002 and found wide variation in the definition of PDPH. In general, most authors have defined PDPH as a headache that occurred following dural puncture, either accidentally with an epidural needle or intentionally with a spinal needle, worsened with sitting or standing and improved with lying down. The headache could be frontal, occipital or nuchal, with or without cervical or shoulder involvement. Some authors have included additional signs and symptoms, such as ocular (diplopia), vestibular (dizziness, vertigo, nausea) or cochlear (tinnitus, hyperacusis, transient hearing loss) findings to distinguish PDPH from other headaches.

Severity of PDPH is also inconsistently defined. The definition proposed by Lybecker *et al.*[6] has been used most often (Table 16.1). Another grading system that combines visual analog scores and the patient's functional ability (Table 16.1), described by Corbey *et al.*,[7,8] has been used in some clinical studies. The reliability of the various measures of severity of PDPH has not yet been determined.

Onset and duration

The onset and duration of PDPH in obstetric patients have been reported infrequently. Of 51 studies from 1949 to 2002, only 20 (39.2%) reported the onset of PDPH and 10 (19.6%) reported the duration of

Table 16.1 Diagnostic criteria for PDPH and classification of severity.

International Headache Society diagnostic criteria[4]
A Bilateral headache developed less than 7 days after lumbar puncture

B Headache occurs or worsens less than 15 min after assuming the upright position, and disappears or improves less than 30 min after resuming the recumbent position

C Headache disappears within 14 days after lumbar puncture

Lybecker classification of severity for PDPH[6]
Score 1 Mild PDPH
    Postural headache with slight restriction of daily activities
    Not bedridden
    No associated symptoms

Score 2 Moderate PDPH
    Postural headache with significant restriction of daily activities
    Bedridden part of the day
    Associated symptoms may or may not be present

Score 3 Severe PDPH
    Postural headache with complete restriction of daily activities
    Bedridden all day
    Associated symptoms present

Corbey classification of severity of PDPH[7,8]
Grade I   Headache does not interfere with normal daily activity
    VAS pain score 1–3 out of 10

Grade II   Headache relieved by periodical bed rest
    VAS pain score 4–7 out of 10

Grade III Headache prevents patient from sitting up to eat
    VAS pain score 8–10 out of 10

PDPH, postdural puncture headache; VAS, visual analog score.

PDPH.[5] Determining the onset and duration of PDPH from the literature is further confounded by varying co-interventions for prevention and treatment of PDPH and the lack of details regarding the length of follow-up. Only eight studies have reported lengths of follow-up; their median length was 6 days, which may be insufficient. Thus, our current knowledge is limited, especially of the duration of PDPH.

The onset of PDPH has ranged from less than 1–6 days after accidental dural puncture with epidural needles and from 1–7 days after dural puncture with spinal needles.[5] The variation in the presentation of the data amongst the various studies precludes any pooling of the data to determine median or mean onset in the obstetric population.

There have been few reports concerning the duration of PDPH after accidental dural puncture with epidural needles. Holdcroft and Morgan[9] followed a cohort of 1000 consecutive obstetric patients who had received epidural analgesia and reported that PDPH may last as long as 6 days. The duration of PDPH following dural puncture with spinal needles ranged 1–7 days in obstetric patients.[5] In one large prospective case series of 9277 non-obstetric surgical patients undergoing spinal anesthesia, the investigators found that 18.3% (185/1011) of individuals with PDPH had symptoms for more than 7 days; however, over 96% (974/1011) of PDPHs arose from dural punctures with needles larger than 24 gauge.[10]

Risk factors

Patient-related risk factors
Risk factors for PDPH have been systematically reviewed by a number of researchers.[11,12] In 1964, Tourtellotte *et al.*[12] exhaustively examined the world

Needle	Total patients with PDPH/ total patients studied	Frequency of PDPH (%; 95% CI)*
Epidural needles		
Tuohy 16 G	13/18	34.7 (18.1–51.3)
Tuohy 18 G	3/15	20.1 (14.6–25.6)
Hustead 18 G	65/148	41.3 (39.1–43.5)
All epidural needles	239/385	52.1 (51.4–52.8)
Cutting spinal needles		
Quincke 24 G	15/238	11.2 (10.2–12.2)
Quincke 25 G	90/1624	6.3 (6.3–6.4)
Quincke 26 G	139/2467	5.6 (5.6–5.7)
Quincke 27 G	28/1007	2.9 (2.8–3.0)
Polymedic 25 G	22/292	6.6 (5.9–7.4)
Becton–Dickinson 26 G	205/2560	5.8 (5.6–5.9)
Atraumatic spinal needles		
Sprotte 24 G	57/1767	3.5 (3.5–3.5)
Whitacre 25 G	103/6366	2.2 (2.2–2.2)
Whitacre 27 G	10/668	1.7 (1.6–1.8)

Table 16.2 Pooled estimates of the frequency of PDPH based on needle shape and diameter.

CI, confidence interval; G, gauge; PDPH, postdural puncture headache.
* Pooled frequency calculated using single-proportion meta-analysis using a random effects model. All data from Choi *et al*.[5]

literature on PDPH. Based on the existing evidence, they concluded that female gender and younger age were risk factors for PDPH. Subsequent large prospective follow-up studies using multivariate analyses have confirmed the inverse relationship between age and the risk of PDPH.[13,14]

A number of case series, published as abstracts, have suggested a decreased risk of PDPH in morbidly obese parturients. One retrospective study of 99 parturients with accidental dural puncture from 17 or 18 gauge epidural needles reported a significantly lower incidence of PDPH in patients with a body mass index of more than 30 kg/m^2 (8/33, 24%) compared with patients with a body mass index of less than 30 kg/m^2 (50/67, 45%; $P < 0.05$).[15] An earlier retrospective study, published as an abstract, also found a lower incidence of PDPH in patients with a body mass index of 30 kg/m^2 or more (6/11) compared with patients with lower body mass indices (18/20; $P = 0.0239$).[16] To date, these observations have not been confirmed with prospective data.

Procedure-related risk factors

Characteristics of the epidural or spinal needle have been suggested as risk factors for PDPH. Tourtellotte *et al.*[12] noted an association between increasing needle

diameter and increased risk, an observation that had been made as early as 1914.[17] Subsequently, Halpern and Preston[18] systematically reviewed the influence of spinal needle design on the frequency of PDPH based on data from randomized controlled trials (RCTs) in surgical populations. They demonstrated an increased risk of PDPH with the use of cutting needles compared with atraumatic needles (odds ratio [OR] 0.26; 95% confidence interval [CI], 0.11–0.62; $P < 0.05$). Similarly, there was an increased risk of PDPH with the use of larger diameter needles compared with smaller diameter needles (OR 0.18; 95% CI, 0.09–0.36; $P < 0.05$).[18]

As age and gender could influence the incidence of PDPH, Choi *et al.*[5] estimated the frequency of PDPH in obstetric patients in a third systematic review. Estimates were based on the shape and diameter of the needle (Table 16.2). Both epidural and spinal needles were evaluated. Their meta-analysis, which pooled data from clinical trials and observational studies, confirmed the findings of Halpern and Preston:[18] cutting needles and needles of larger diameters increased the risk of PDPH. The authors also noted that PDPH was a common complication following neuraxial block using small diameter atraumatic needles. They found that the incidence in parturients was 1 in 59

Table 16.3 Randomized controlled trials evaluating the effect of needle bevel direction relative to the dural fibers on the risk of PDPH.

| Reference | Population | Proportion of PDPH | | RR (95% CI)* | NNP (95% CI)[†] |
		Parallel	Perpendicular		
Norris et al. 1989[20]	Parturients with ADP from Hustead 17 or 18 G needle	11/21	16/20	0.66 (0.41–1.04)	
Huffnagle et al. 1998[21]	Parturients with ADP from Hustead 18 G needle	0/4	0/4	1.00 (0.02–41.2)	
Richardson & Wissler 1999[22]	Parturients with ADP from Tuohy 17 G needle	1/9	2/6	0.33 (0.04–2.91)	
Mihic 1985[23]	Patients undergoing spinal anesthesia with 22 or 25 G spinal needles	1/140 (22 G) 0/280 (25 G)	5/29 (22 G) 5/33 (25 G)	0.05 (0.01–0.40)[‡] 0.01 (0.001–0.20)[‡]	7.1 (4–50) 6.3 (4–28)
Casagrán et al. 1992[24]	Patients undergoing spinal anesthesia with Quincke 26 G needle	1/150	6/120	0.13 (0.02–1.09)	
Friedrich & Kainz 1988[25]	Patients undergoing lumbar puncture with 20 or 21 G needles	2/20	14/20	0.14 (0.04–0.55)[‡]	1.7 (1–3)

ADP, accidental dural puncture; CI, confidence interval; G, gauge; NNP, number-needed-to-prevent; PDPH, postdural puncture headache; RR, relative risk.

* Relative risk < 1 indicates a lower risk in the parallel orientation group. Relative risk = 1 indicates no difference between groups. Relative risk > 1 indicates a higher risk in the parallel orientation group. A 95% confidence interval that includes the value of 1 is indicative of a difference that is not statistically significant ($P \geq 0.05$).

[†] Number-needed-to-prevent are calculated for results with statistically significant differences between the two groups.

[‡] $P < 0.0001$.

when a Whitacre 27 gauge needle was used for dural puncture.[5]

The relationship between the number of dural punctures and the risk of PDPH remains unclear. Intuitively, based on the pathophysiology of PDPH, the risk of PDPH should increase with the number of dural punctures. Data from prospective observational studies have produced conflicting results. Lybecker et al.[13] did not find a relationship between the number of perforations and the risk of PDPH in 1021 spinal anesthetics. In contrast, Seeberger et al.[14] noted a statistically significant increase in the frequency of PDPH after repeated dural puncture (7/165) compared with a single dural puncture (123/7869, $P < 0.02$).

The direction of the needle bevel of epidural and spinal cutting needles, in relation to the fibers of the dura mater, could affect the size, shape and duration of the hole resulting from dural puncture. Hypothetically, a needle with its bevel oriented parallel to the dural fibers would split the fibers, result in a smaller

hole and lead to less CSF leakage compared with a needle with its bevel oriented perpendicular to the dural fibers.[19] Six RCTs have tested this hypothesis (Table 16.3).[20–25] Three RCTs examined accidental dural punctures with epidural needles and the development of PDPH in obstetric patients.[20–22] Pooled dural puncture rates did not differ between groups. The pooled frequency of PDPH showed a trend in favor of the group with the needle bevel oriented parallel to the dural fibers but the difference was not statistically significant. Although the results are promising, they must be considered as "hypothesis-generating" based on the small number of patients reported to date in peer-reviewed publications. One RCT of 515 patients allocated patients undergoing spinal anesthesia to four groups based on patient position (sitting or lateral decubitus) and needle bevel direction (parallel or perpendicular). No significant differences were seen in the frequencies of PDPH but both groups with parallel orientation of the needle bevel had trends toward fewer PDPHs.[26] Unfortunately, the study has not been published as a full manuscript.

The anatomic rationale for the influence of bevel orientation on the risk of PDPH may need to be revisited. A study using electron microscopy of cross-sections of dura mater from human cadavers has shown that the dural fibers run longitudinally on the epidural surface but criss-cross each other on the intrathecal surface.[27] In human cadaveric dura, Angle et al.[28] found that the rate of CSF leakage was influenced by the epidural needle diameter rather than the bevel orientation of the needle.

Another possible risk factor is the approach used to enter the intrathecal space. Hypothetically, the paramedian approach would result in a dural puncture with a "flap valve" that would seal the hole and prevent CSF leakage compared with the median approach.[19,29] The published data are scarce. Janik and Dick[30] randomized 250 patients undergoing transurethral prostate surgery with spinal anesthesia to either a paramedian or a median approach. Frequencies of PDPH were similar between the two groups (paramedian 15/125 vs median 11/125). Two other studies, published as abstracts, have also failed to find any differences between the two approaches.[31,32] Interestingly, all three studies reported higher frequencies of PDPH in the paramedian groups, yet the paramedian approach is still suggested as a potential technique to reduce the risk of PDPH.[29] The current data do not suggest a difference between the two approaches.

For spinal anesthesia, the intrathecal injectate may affect the risk of PDPH. One large prospective study found statistically significant differences in the frequency of PDPH following spinal anesthesia with tetracaine–procaine (47/804) compared with spinal anesthesia with bupivacaine–glucose (84/842) or lidocaine–glucose (73/765).[33] It is unclear whether the difference was caused by the type of local anesthetic (ester vs amide) or because of the absence or presence of glucose.[33]

Three RCTs have studied the effect of the intrathecal injectate on the risk of PDPH in obstetric patients.[34–36] Runza et al.[34] randomized patients undergoing elective cesarean section with spinal anesthesia to either 11.25 mg bupivacaine 0.75% (25 patients) or 11.25 mg bupivacaine 1% (25 patients). There was no statistically significant difference in the frequencies of PDPH (0/25 bupivacaine 0.75% vs 4/25 bupivacaine 1%).

Two RCTs studied the effect of intrathecal opioids.[35,36] Abboud et al.[35] randomized patients undergoing cesarean section with spinal anesthesia to hyperbaric bupivacaine 0.75% with intrathecal morphine (40 patients) or without intrathecal morphine (42 patients). There were no statistically significant differences in the frequencies of PDPH (9/40 with morphine vs 8/42 without morphine). In a similar population, Meininger et al.[36] randomized 100 patients (20 patients per group) to hyperbaric mepivacaine 2% with placebo, fentanyl 5 μg, fentanyl 10 μg, sufentanil 2.5 μg or sufentanil 5 μg. Again, no differences were seen in the incidence of PDPH. At this time, based on the scant data, the concentration of local anesthetic, the presence or absence of opioids and the type of opioid do not appear to affect the incidence of PDPH.

Management

Symptoms of PDPH are believed to result from loss of CSF and the cranial fluid cushion, dural traction and compression of cranial contents, and cerebral vasodilation with an increased arteriovenous pressure gradient. Interventions to prevent or treat PDPH can be divided into conservative management, pharmacologic interventions and invasive procedures. In general, pharmacologic interventions aim to reduce the arteriovenous pressure gradient by vasoconstriction; invasive procedures aim to reduce the rate and volume of CSF lost by occluding, sealing or reducing the size of the puncture site.

Tourtellotte et al.,[12] writing in 1964, identified nearly 50 interventions for prevention or treatment of PDPH. This chapter reviews the small number of interventions that are commonly used or are under investigation. For interventions that have been evaluated in RCTs, in the absence of clinical and statistical heterogeneity, the data have been pooled using meta-analysis to provide a summary estimate (odds ratio or relative risk) and a number-needed-to-prevent (NNP), number-needed-to-treat (NNT), or number-needed-to-harm (NNH) along with their 95% CIs. The NNP and NNT are the numbers of patients that must be administered the intervention to successfully prevent or treat one PDPH, respectively. The NNH is the number of patients that must be administered the intervention to cause harm to one patient.

Conservative measures to prevent postdural puncture headache

Some authors suggest that bed rest after dural puncture prevents PDPH, presumably by altering the rate of CSF loss. This intervention was studied in 16 RCTs in patients undergoing neuraxial anesthesia, diagnostic lumbar puncture or myelography. Two systematic reviews summarized the data.[37,38] Both meta-analyses concluded that bed rest did not reduce the frequency of PDPH compared with immediate or early mobilization.[37,38] In the subgroup of RCTs involving neuraxial anesthesia, bed rest *increased* the frequency of PDPH (OR 2.03; 95% CI, 1.20–3.43) with an NNH of 9.2 (95% CI, 5.2–37.6).[38]

Some suggest that aggressive fluid administration reduces the risk of PDPH. The mechanism is unclear as CSF production is autoregulated and appears unaffected by intravascular volume status. Two RCTs have evaluated the efficacy of this intervention.[39,40] The incidence of PDPH did not differ between patients who received 1 L 0.9% saline and 1 L 5% glucose intravenously (19/41) and patients who did not receive any intravenous fluids (22/51) prior to lumbar myelography.[39] The incidence and duration of PDPH were identical (36%) in the 50 patients who received 1.5 L/day oral fluids and the 50 patients who received 3 L/day oral fluids for 5 days after diagnostic lumbar puncture.[40]

Some investigators have suggested that the maneuver of avoidance of second-stage pushing in parturients with accidental dural puncture from epidural needles may reduce the risk of PDPH. The data have been conflicting: retrospective studies suggest a decreased risk of PDPH with avoidance of pushing[41] while prospective observational studies do not.[42] One RCT randomly allocated parturients receiving spinal analgesia using 22 gauge spinal needles to second-stage pushing and spontaneous vaginal delivery (100 patients) or avoidance of second-stage pushing and forceps delivery (100 patients).[43] The difference in the number of PDPHs was not statistically significant (9/100 active pushing vs 10/100 no pushing); however, the results may be confounded by the high frequency of forceps delivery (30%) in the active pushing group because patients were not permitted to push more than 10 times. Further investigation is required before recommending that second-stage pushing should be limited.

Drug interventions

Caffeine

Caffeine was first suggested as an intervention for the management of PDPH by Holder in 1944.[44] The presumed mechanism of action of caffeine, a vasoconstrictor, is cerebral vasoconstriction and decrease in the cerebral arteriovenous pressure gradient.[45–47] Caffeine is currently the only drug used commonly to prevent PDPH. Three RCTs have evaluated its prophylactic efficacy, but only one has been published as a peer-reviewed publication.[48] Yücel *et al.*[48] randomized patients undergoing lower abdominal or lower extremity surgery with spinal anesthesia to receive 1 L intravenous 0.9% saline either with 500 mg caffeine sodium benzoate or without caffeine during the first 90 min after dural puncture. Caffeine reduced the frequency of moderate or severe headache (3/30 caffeine vs 11/30 no caffeine; $P = 0.03$). The severity of the headache was rated by the patient on a 5-point scale (0 = no headache, 4 = severe headache), which was not tested for reliability. Furthermore, the statistically significant difference between the two groups disappeared (11/30 caffeine vs 16/30 no caffeine; $P = 0.30$) when all PDPHs were included. The other two RCTs, which were published as abstracts,[49,50] evaluated prophylactic intramuscular caffeine benzoate and oral anhydrous caffeine and found non-significant trends toward more frequent PDPH with the use of caffeine. Thus, prophylactic caffeine requires further investigation before its use can be recommended.

Several studies have evaluated the therapeutic efficacy of caffeine.[51–57] Three studies were RCTs.[51–53] Sechzer and Abel[51] randomized patients with PDPH after spinal anesthesia for obstetric or non-obstetric surgery to receive 500 mg intravenous caffeine sodium benzoate (20 patients) or placebo (21 patients). A single dose of caffeine relieved PDPH in 15 of 20 subjects; placebo relieved PDPH in three of the 21 subjects but all three experienced relapse. These results suggest an NNT of 1.6 (95% CI, 1–3) for therapeutic intravenous caffeine. In addition, all 18 patients who did not obtain relief after the single dose of study medication (caffeine or placebo) were given a rescue dose of intravenous caffeine; 10 of the 18 subjects achieved relief with this dose.[51]

Camann *et al.*[52] randomized postpartum patients with PDPH to receive either 300 mg oral anhydrous caffeine (20 patients) or placebo (20 patients). Four hours after ingestion, 18 patients in the caffeine group had improved based on visual analog scores compared with 12 patients in the placebo group and the magnitude of decrease in the severity of the PDPH was significantly greater with caffeine (36.1 ± 5.5 mm) than with placebo (10.9 ± 6.7 mm; $P = 0.014$). However, differences in visual analog scores disappeared 24 h after ingestion. The authors did not report the number of patients who obtained complete relief in each group.

In contrast to the two previous RCTs, Lang and Yip[53] did not find any benefit with 500 mg intravenous caffeine sodium benzoate compared with epidural blood patch for the treatment of PDPH. Only two of eight patients achieved relief after two doses of caffeine. Seven of eight patients obtained relief after one epidural blood patch and the eighth patient had relief after a second blood patch.

For any pharmacologic intervention in the postpartum patient, potential harm to the mother and the nursing infant must be considered. In lactating women, caffeine, in doses up to 336 mg, did not diffuse freely into breast milk with only 0.06–3.2% of the maternal dose being available for absorption by the nursing infant.[58,59] Caffeine ingestion, as a single dose up to 336 mg, appears to be safe for nursing.[58,59] Information on higher doses, which may be used for prevention or treatment of PDPH, is currently unavailable. With regards to maternal safety, there are three case reports of grand mal seizures following intravenous caffeine infusions.[60–62] Although the data are insufficient to draw conclusions regarding association or causation, in patients who are predisposed to seizures, caffeine, at the doses suggested for management of PDPH, should be used with caution.

In summary, current evidence suggests that caffeine may be a promising drug for the management of PDPH but the evidence, based on the small number of patients studied to date in well-designed RCTs, is insufficient to establish clinical practice guidelines regarding its use. Caffeine appears safe for nursing but should be used with caution if the risk for seizures exists.

Theophylline

Like caffeine, theophylline is a methylxanthine and acts via similar vasoconstrictive mechanisms.[46,47] Its role in the prevention of PDPH has not been reported in peer-reviewed publications. In one abstract, Holmes et al.[63] randomized patients with accidental dural puncture from Tuohy 17 gauge needles to receive either 300 mg/day oral theophylline for 2 days (four patients) or prophylactic epidural blood patch (six patients). Visual analog scores were lower in the epidural blood patch (EBP) group; however, the sample size was extremely small. At least two studies have evaluated its therapeutic efficacy but only one study was published as a full manuscript.[64,65] Fuerstein and Zeides[64] randomized 11 patients with severe PDPH following diagnostic lumbar puncture to receive either 281.7 mg oral theophylline (six patients) or placebo (five patients). Subjects graded the severity of their PDPH on a 3-point score (1 = mild PDPH, 3 = severe PDPH) thrice daily until resolution of their headache. The sum of all pain scores was used as the outcome variable for each patient. The total pain score was lower in the theophylline group (mean $\pm$ standard error 16 ± 3.9) than in the placebo group (28 ± 4.7; $P = 0.04$). The authors indicated that their "results should be considered preliminary. Nevertheless... additional trials on the benefits of methylxanthines in the treatment of post-puncture headache are called for."[64] Until further trials clarify the risks and benefits of theophylline, it should not be used for prevention of PDPH.

Sumatriptan

Sumatriptan is a 5-hydroxytryptamine type 1 receptor agonist with potent vasoconstricting properties. Used for the treatment of migraine headaches, sumatriptan has been suggested as a potential treatment for PDPH. To date, the published literature consists of case reports and case series,[66–71] which report variable success. One small RCT, published as an abstract, did not demonstrate any benefit with sumatriptan compared with placebo, but the study only involved 10 patients.[72] Currently, although there is biologic rationale to support its use, there are insufficient data to draw conclusions on the efficacy of this drug in the management of PDPH.

With regards to harm, a single dose of 6 mg subcutaneous sumatriptan does not pose a significant risk to the nursing infant. Only 0.24% of the administered maternal dose is available in the breast milk. This amount equates to a mean infant weight-adjusted exposure of 3.5% (95% CI, 0.3–6.7%) of the maternal exposure.[73] As sumatriptan is a vasoconstrictor, like the methylxanthines, its use should probably be avoided in patients at risk for seizures.[74,75]

Adrenocorticotropic hormone

Adrenocorticotropic hormone (ACTH) has been suggested as a possible treatment for PDPH. The therapeutic mechanism is unknown but it may work by increasing sodium retention and intravascular volume.[75] Over 22 patients have been treated successfully with 20 IU intramuscular ACTH or 1.5 IU/kg intravenous ACTH infusion.[76–78] Current evidence is entirely anecdotal; thus, the use of ACTH for the treatment of PDPH is still experimental.

Invasive interventions

Invasive interventions include epidural patching and insertion of an intrathecal catheter. Autologous blood, saline, dextran 40, gelatin and fibrin glue have been suggested as injectates for epidural patches. Few of these interventions have been studied in rigorous clinical trials.

Epidural blood patch

The EBP was suggested originally by Gormley[79] as a treatment for PDPH. The technique in current use was described over 30 years ago by DiGiovanni and Dunbar.[80] The efficacy of prophylactic and therapeutic EBP was evaluated in a recent systematic review but meta-analysis was not performed because of the clinical and methodologic heterogeneity observed between studies.[81]

Cohort studies have shown discrepant results regarding the efficacy of prophylactic EBP with reduction in the incidence of PDPH after diagnostic lumbar puncture[82] and myelography,[83] but not in parturients undergoing epidural analgesia or anesthesia.[84] Prophylactic EBP after anesthesia has been studied in six controlled clinical trials.[63,85–89] Four trials studied parturients with accidental dural puncture from large-diameter Tuohy needles during epidural catheter insertion;[85–88] one RCT studied surgical patients with accidental dural puncture from Tuohy 17 gauge needles,[63] and one RCT studied patients undergoing spinal anesthesia for extracorporeal shock wave lithotripsy.[89] In the five studies that reported incidences of PDPH, all reported lower incidences with prophylactic

EBP compared with conservative management (Table 16.4). The differences in four of these studies were statistically significant; however, all of the studies had small sample sizes.

In contrast, comparison of therapeutic EBP with conservative management has been reported in only one RCT (Table 16.5).[90] Seebacher et al.[90] randomized patients with PDPH after spinal or epidural anesthesia, lumbar puncture or myelography to receive either therapeutic EBP with 10–20 mL autologous blood or sham EBP (with epidural needle insertion, venipuncture and withdrawal of autologous blood, but no epidural injection). A neurologist, blinded to the treatment allocation, evaluated each patient prior to the treatment and 2 and 24 h after the intervention. Five of the six patients in the EBP group had complete relief of symptoms; no patient in the sham EBP group had complete relief. Although impressive, the sample size of this study was small.

Bart and Wheeler[91] compared EBP with epidural saline patch in a pseudorandomized trial, with allocation based on hospital registry number, of patients with dural puncture from 25 gauge needles for spinal anesthesia or accidental dural puncture from 17 gauge needles for epidural anesthesia. For both types of dural puncture, the frequency of PDPH was significantly lower in the EBP group compared with the epidural saline group (Table 16.5).

Various aspects relating to the EBP procedure remain unclear. The timing and volume of the EBP and the duration of bed rest after an EBP have been investigated in RCTs. Loeser et al.[92] randomized 50 patients with PDPH after dural puncture with 18 or 20 gauge needles to receive an EBP with 10 mL autologous blood either less than 24 h after dural puncture (immediate group, 17 patients) or more than 24 h after dural puncture (delayed group, 31 patients). Only five patients obtained relief with an EBP in the immediate group compared with 30 patients in the delayed group ($P < 0.001$). The authors did not report the actual duration of time from dural puncture to performance of the EBP, the onset of PDPH after dural puncture, the severity of PDPH or the duration of follow-up; therefore, one cannot determine whether differences in onset or severity or insufficient duration of follow-up may have influenced their results. No other RCTs have examined the timing of EBP administration.

Table 16.4 Randomized controlled trials of EBP for the prevention of PDPH.

Reference	Population	Intervention	Control	Proportion of PDPH		RR (95% CI)*
				EBP	Control	
Colonna-Romano & Shapiro 1989[85]	Parturients with ADP from Tuohy 17 G needles	15 mL autologous blood via *in situ* epidural catheter postpartum	Oral fluids and avoidance of ambulation	4/19	16/20	0.26 (0.11–0.65)[†]
Ackerman *et al.* 1990[86]	Parturients with ADP from epidural needles	18–20 mL autologous blood via *in situ* epidural catheter postpartum	Conservative management	1/7	4/7	0.25 (0.04–1.71)
Trivedi *et al.* 1993[87]	Parturients with ADP from Tuohy 18 G needles	15 mL autologous blood via *in situ* epidural catheter postpartum	Oral fluids ± analgesics	1/20	21/24	0.06 (0.01–0.39)[‡]
Trivedi *et al.* 1993[87]	Parturients with ADP from Tuohy 18 G needles	15 mL autologous blood via *in situ* epidural catheter postpartum	40–60 mL saline bolus via *in situ* epidural catheter postpartum	1/20	20/30	0.08 (0.01–0.52)[§]
Lowenwirt *et al.* 1998[88]	Parturients with ADP from Tuohy 16 or 17 G needles	15–20 mL autologous blood via *in situ* epidural catheter ≥ 5 h after last local anesthetic dose	IV fluids, bedrest, theophylline or caffeine	4/25	24/24	0.18 (0.08–0.41)[‡]
Sengupta *et al.* 1989[89]	Surgical patients aged 18–60 undergoing ESWL with spinal anesthesia using 25 G needles	10 mL autologous blood injected at same level as dural puncture via Tuohy 16 G needle	10 mL epidural 0.9% saline injected at same level as dural puncture via Tuohy 16 G needle	2/24	11/24	0.18 (0.04–0.74)[**]
Holmes *et al.* 1994[63]	Surgical patients with ADP from Tuohy 17 G needles	Blood injected via *in situ* epidural catheter after resolution of epidural block	Oral theophylline 300 mg	NR	NR	

ADP, accidental dural puncture; CI, confidence interval; EBP, epidural blood patch; ESWL, extracorporeal shock wave lithotripsy; G, gauge; IV, intravenous; NNP, number-needed-to-prevent; NR, not reported; PDPH, postdural puncture headache; RR, relative risk.

* Relative risk < 1 indicates a lower risk in the epidural blood patch group. Relative risk = 1 indicates no difference between groups. Relative risk > 1 indicates a higher risk in the control group. A 95% confidence interval that includes the value of 1 is indicative of a difference that is not statistically significant ($P \geq 0.05$).

[†] $P = 0.001$; NNP 1.7 (95% CI, 1–3).

[‡] $P < 0.0001$; NNP 1.2 (95% CI, 1–2).

[§] $P < 0.0001$; NNP 1.6 (95% CI, 1–2).

[**] $P = 0.009$; NNP 2.7 (95% CI, 2–7).

Table 16.5 Randomized controlled trials of EBP for the treatment of PDPH.

Reference	Population	Intervention	Control	Proportion of PDPH		RR (95% CI)*
				EBP	Control	
Seebacher et al. 1989[90]	Patients aged 18–70 with PDPH > 4 days duration after neuraxial anesthesia, LP or myelography	10–20 mL autologous blood 1 interspace below level of DP	Sham EBP – needle inserted into epidural space without injection of blood	1/6	6/6	0.23 (0.06–0.97)[†]
Bart & Wheeler 1978[91]	Postpartum patients with PDPH after DP with 17 or 25 G needles	10 mL autologous blood at level of DP	30 mL epidural 0.9% saline at level of DP	3/11 (17 G) 0/11 (25 G)	6/6 (17 G) 6/15 (25 G)	0.31 (0.13–0.78)[‡] 0.10 (0.01–1.65)
Loeser et al. 1978[92]	Patients with PDPH after DP after epidural anesthesia or LP with 18 or 20 G needles	10 mL autologous blood administered < 24 h after DP	10 mL autologous blood administered > 24 h after DP	12/17	1/31	21.9 (3.11–154)[§]
Taivainen et al. 1993[93]	Patients with PDPH after spinal anesthesia or myelography	10 mL autologous blood at same level or 1 level below DP	10–15 mL autologous blood, depending on patient height, at same level or 1 level below DP	8/25	8/24	0.96 (0.43–2.14)

CI, confidence interval; DP, dural puncture; EBP, epidural blood patch; G, gauge; LP, lumbar puncture; NNT, number-needed-to-treat; PDPH, postdural puncture headache; RR, relative risk.

* Relative risk < 1 indicates a lower risk in the intervention group. Relative risk = 1 indicates no difference between groups. Relative risk > 1 indicates a higher risk in the control group. A 95% confidence interval that includes the value of 1 is indicative of a difference that is not statistically significant ($P \geq 0.05$).

[†] $P = 0.03$; NNT 1.4 (95% CI, 1–3).

[‡] $P = 0.03$; NNT 1.6 (95% CI, 1–3).

[§] $P < 0.0001$; NNT 1.0 (95% CI, 1–2).

Table 16.6 Frequency of back pain after epidural blood patching.

Reference	Study design	Volume of blood (mL)	Back pain (%)
Sengupta et al. 1989[89]	Randomized trial	10	12/24 (50)
Seebacher et al. 1989[90]	Randomized trial	10–20	6/6 (100)
Abouleish et al. 1975[95]	Prospective cohort	7–10	20/81 (25)
Cheek et al. 1988[96]	Prospective cohort	17–20	3/10 (30)
Taivainen et al. 1993[93]	Prospective cohort	10–15	20/81 (25)
Tarkkila et al. 1989[97]	Retrospective	5–20	49/133 (25)
Pooled frequency (95% CI)*			42.1% (40.9–43.5%)

CI, confidence interval.
* Pooled frequency calculated using single-proportion meta-analysis using a random effects model.

Taivainen et al.[93] studied the effect of the volume of blood on the success of therapeutic EBP. Patients with PDPH after spinal anesthesia or myelography were randomized to receive an EBP with a volume of either 10 mL (low-volume group) or 10–15 mL autologous blood (high-volume group), depending on the patient's height. There were no statistically significant differences between the two groups in the proportion of patients with complete relief 2 h after the EBP (26/27 low-volume group vs 23/26 high-volume group) or 4 weeks later (17/25 low-volume group vs 16/24 high-volume group). More importantly, the study suggested that the success rate of therapeutic blood patching was actually lower than previous estimates. Although 88–96% of patients had complete relief of symptoms within 2 h of the intervention, 16–36% of patients experienced recurrence of symptoms after discharge with duration of PDPH lasting as long as 14 days.[93]

The duration of bed rest after epidural blood patching may be a potential determinant of the success or failure of an EBP. Martin et al.[94] randomized 30 patients with PDPH to receive an EBP followed by 30, 60 or 120 min of bed rest (10 patients per group). Twenty-four hours after the EBP, although all patients noted an improvement in the severity of their headaches, symptoms of PDPH were still present in four patients of the 30-min group, two of the 60-min group and none of the 120-min group. The authors concluded that longer durations of bed rest increased the success of an EBP. Information on the number of patients with recurrence of symptoms after 24 h is unavailable as the duration of follow-up did not extend beyond the first 24 h after the EBP.

Harm from epidural blood patching has not been rigorously evaluated. The most frequently reported adverse effect from EBP is back pain, which usually resolved without treatment. The frequency of back pain has varied from 25% to 100% with a pooled frequency of 42.1% (95% CI, 40.9–43.5%; Table 16.6).[89,90,93,95–97] Other symptoms such as neckache,[95] paresthesia,[95] sensory disturbances,[97] auditory disturbances,[97] visual disturbances[97] and abdominal discomfort[96] have been described but the numbers are too few to provide accurate estimates of frequency. Rarely reported complications include neurologic complications (cerebral ischemia,[98] aseptic meningeal irritation,[99] radiculopathy,[100–102] and lumbovertebral syndrome[103]) and transient bradycardia.[104] A number of case reports have described seizures after EBP;[60,62,105–107] however, the seizures were usually attributed to other causes such as eclampsia[60,62,106] and subdural hematoma.[107] Injection of air into the intrathecal space during the EBP procedure could result in pneumocephalus and result in seizures.[108] Infection, adhesive arachnoiditis and epidural hematoma are potential rare complications but the frequencies of these events are unknown. To date, there has been one case report of an epidural hematoma that required surgical evacuation. The patient had received six EBPs.[109]

Epidural saline

Epidural saline has been studied in five controlled clinical trials (Tables 16.4, 16.5 and 16.7).[87,89,91,110,111] One compared epidural saline boluses with conservative management,[110] two compared epidural saline boluses

Table 16.7 Randomized controlled trials of epidural saline for management of PDPH.

| Reference* | Population | Intervention | Control | Proportion of PDPH | | RR (95% CI)† |
				Intervention	Control	
Santos et al. 1986[110]	Parturients with ADP from epidural in situ needles	2 doses of saline via epidural catheter postpartum	No intervention	3/13	9/16	0.41 (0.14–1.21)
Thomas et al. 1992[111]	Parturients with ADP from 17 G epidural needles	30 mL saline bolus via in situ epidural catheter every 6 h for 3 doses postpartum	Saline infusion via in situ epidural catheter postpartum	5/15	5/15	1.00 (0.36–2.75)
Trivedi et al. 1993[87]	Parturients with ADP from Tuohy 18 G needles	40–60 mL saline bolus via in situ epidural catheter postpartum	Oral fluids ± analgesics	20/30	21/24	0.76 (0.57–1.02)

ADP, unintentional dural puncture; CI, confidence interval; G, gauge; PDPH, postdural puncture headache; RR, relative risk.
* See Tables 16.4 and 16.5 for comparison between epidural saline and epidural blood patch.
† Relative risk < 1 indicates a lower risk in the intervention group. Relative risk = 1 indicates no difference between groups. Relative risk > 1 indicates a higher risk in the control group. A 95% confidence interval that includes the value of 1 is indicative of a difference that is not statistically significant ($P \geq 0.05$).

with EBP,[89,91] one compared epidural saline boluses with epidural saline infusions[111] and one compared epidural saline boluses with conservative management and with EBP.[87] Prophylactic epidural saline showed a trend towards lower frequencies of PDPH compared with conservative management but the differences were not statistically significant (Table 16.7).[87,110] Epidural saline was inferior to EBP for prevention or treatment of PDPH (Tables 16.4 and 16.5).[87,89,91] There was no difference between epidural saline boluses and epidural saline infusion for the prevention of PDPH (Table 16.7).[111] Given the small sample sizes, wide dispersion of the estimates of effect and the variation in the interventions, larger RCTs are still needed to elucidate the role of epidural saline in the management of PDPH.

Other epidural patches

Dextran 40, gelatin and fibrin glue have been suggested as substitute injectates for epidural patching. The data are anecdotal. Epidural dextran 40, at doses of 20–30 mL, have been used successfully in the prevention and treatment of PDPH.[112–116] One case report of two patients described the successful use of epidural gelatin (Gelfoam®) 600–700 mg in 10 mL plasma as an epidural patch.[117] Epidural fibrin glue has been used to treat chronic CSF leak and PDPH in three patients.[118–120]

Conclusions regarding the efficacy of these interventions await further data, preferably from large RCTs.

Intrathecal catheter after accidental dural puncture

Insertion of an intrathecal catheter upon discovery of an accidental dural puncture from an epidural needle may reduce PDPH. The hypothesis arose from the observation, based on retrospective data, that women receiving continuous spinal anesthesia had frequencies of PDPH that were lower than expected for the size of needles used. The mechanism of action is unknown; however, authors have speculated that an intrathecal catheter causes an inflammatory response with subsequent fibrin sealing of the dural hole when the catheter is removed.[121] Restoration of CSF volume may also contribute.[122] A cohort study by Norris and Leighton[123] has compared the efficacy of intrathecal catheter insertion with conservative therapy for the prevention of PDPH following accidental dural puncture with Hustead 17 or 18 gauge needles. No difference was seen in the frequency of PDPH between the two groups (15/35 intrathecal catheters vs 9/21 conservative therapy). Liu et al.[124] randomized 87 orthopedic patients with continuous spinal anesthesia, administered via a 20-gauge intrathecal catheter, to withdrawal of the catheter either immediately or 12–24 h after the procedure.

The difference in the frequency of PDPH was not statistically significant between the two groups (5/47 immediate vs 3/40 delayed). There were no differences in the frequency or the severity of PDPH, as measured by a 10-cm visual analog scale, between the two groups.

Conclusions

PDPH is an iatrogenic complication arising from dural puncture. Strict definitions of PDPH have been recommended but they have been used inconsistently in PDPH research. Risk factors for PDPH include female gender, younger age, cutting needles and large-diameter needles. In parturients, the risk for PDPH remains significant even with small-diameter atraumatic spinal needles. The approach of the needle (median or paramedian), the bevel orientation and the intrathecal injectate do not appear to modify the risk of PDPH. The efficacy of bed rest remains uncertain although the data from RCTs involving neuraxial anesthesia suggest harm. Aggressive fluid administration does not appear to be beneficial. The role of caffeine in the prevention or treatment of PDPH is unclear based on current discrepant evidence; however, further investigation is needed before recommending its use. Theophylline, sumatriptan and ACTH also require further study. The evidence for prophylactic and therapeutic blood patch suggests that they are efficacious, but larger RCTs are still needed for definitive answers concerning their timing and volume. The efficacy of other epidural patches and intrathecal catheter insertion await further trials. For all interventions, inadequate data exist regarding adverse effects and harm.

References

1 Bier A. Verusche über cocainisirung des rückenmarkes. *Deutsch Ztschr Chir* 1899;**51**:361–9.

2 Choi PT, Galinski SE, Lucas S, Takeuchi L, Jadad AR. Examining the evidence in anesthesia literature: a survey and evaluation of obstetrical postdural puncture headache reports. *Can J Anesth* 2002;**49**:49–56.

3 Choi PT. Best evidence in anesthesia: an evaluation of information of PDPH. MSc thesis. Hamilton: McMaster University, 2001.

4 Headache Classification Committee of the International Headache Society. Classification and diagnostic criteria for headache disorders, cranial neuralgias, and facial pain.

Diagnostic criteria 7.2.1. Post-lumbar puncture headache. *Cephalalgia* 1988;**8**(Suppl 7):1–96.

5 Choi PT, Galinski SE, Takeuchi L, Lucas S, Tamayo C, Jadad AR. PDPH is a common complication of neuraxial blockade in parturients: a meta-analysis of obstetrical studies. *Can J Anesth* 2003;**50**:460–9.

6 Lybecker H, Djernes M, Schmidt JF. Postdural puncture headache (PDPH): onset, duration, severity, and associated symptoms. An analysis of 75 consecutive patients with PDPH. *Acta Anaesthesiol Scand* 1995;**39**:605–12.

7 Corbey MP, Berg P, Quayhor H. Classification and severity of postdural puncture headache: comparison of 26-gauge and 27-gauge Quincke needle for spinal anaesthesia in day-care surgery patients under 45 years. *Anaesthesia* 1993;**48**:776–81.

8 Corbey MP, Bach AB, Lech K, Frørup AM. Grading of severity of postdural puncture headache after 27-gauge Quincke and Whitacre needles. *Acta Anaesthesiol Scand* 1997;**41**:779–84.

9 Holdcroft A, Morgan M. Maternal complications of obstetric epidural analgesia. *Anaesth Intens Care* 1976;**4**:108–12.

10 Vandam LD, Dripps RD. Long-term follow-up of patients who received 10,998 spinal anesthetics. *JAMA* 1956;**161**:586–91.

11 Thorsén G. Neurological complications after spinal anaesthesia and results from 2493 follow-up cases. *Acta Chir Scand Suppl* 1947;**121**:1–272.

12 Tourtellotte WW, Haerer AF, Heller GF. *Post-Lumbar Puncture Headache.* Springfield, IL: Charles C Thomas, 1964.

13 Lybecker H, Møller JT, May O, Nielsen HK. Incidence and prediction of postdural puncture headache: a prospective study of 1021 spinal anesthesias. *Anesth Analg* 1990;**70**:389–94.

14 Seeberger MD, Kaufmann M, Staender S, Schneider M, Scheidegger D. Repeated dural punctures increase the incidence of postdural puncture headache. *Anesth Analg* 1996;**82**:302–5.

15 Faure E, Moreno R, Thisted R. Incidence of postdural puncture headache in morbidly obese parturients. *Reg Anesth* 1994;**19**:361–3.

16 Heyman HJ, Salem MR, Joseph NJ. Maternal obesity and headache following unexpected dural puncture. *Anesthesiology* 1990;**73**:A971.

17 Huston JW, Lebherz TB. Spinal anesthesia for vaginal delivery with special reference to prevention of postpartum headache. *Am J Obstet Gynecol* 1952;**63**:139–45.

18 Halpern S, Preston R. Postdural puncture headache and spinal needle design: meta-analyses. *Anesthesiology* 1994;**81**:1376–83.

19 Kempen PM, Mocek CK. Bevel direction, dura geometry, and hole size in membrane puncture laboratory report. *Reg Anesth* 1997;**22**:267–72.

20 Norris MC, Leighton BL, DeSimone CA. Needle bevel direction and headache after inadvertent dural puncture. *Anesthesiology* 1989;**70**:729–31.

21 Huffnagle SL, Norris MC, Arkoosh VA, *et al.* The influence of epidural needle bevel orientation on spread of sensory

blockade in the laboring parturient. *Anesth Analg* 1998;**87**: 326–30.

22 Richardson MG, Wissler RN. The effects of needle bevel orientation during epidural catheter insertion in laboring parturients. *Anesth Analg* 1999;**88**:352–6.

23 Mihic DN. Postspinal headache and relationship of needle bevel to longitudinal dural fibers. *Reg Anesth* 1985;**10**:76–81.

24 Casagrán B, Busquets A, Brull J. Incidencia de cefaleas tras anestesia intradural con agujas del número 26 según que la punción sea con el bisel perpendicular o paraleo a las fibras de la duramadre. *Rev Esp Anestesiol Reanim* 1992;**39**:227–9.

25 Friedrich G, Kainz J. Die prophylaxe postpunktioneller beschwerden durch das drehen der punktionskanüle um 90 grad. *Wein Klin Wochenschr* 1988;**100**:23–5.

26 Culling RD, Rubin A, Culclasure J, Hansen T, Epps J. Spinal headache: bevel orientation not an important factor. *Reg Anesth* 1990;**15**(1S):32.

27 Runza M, Pietrabissa R, Mantero S, Albani A, Quaghini V, Contro R. Lumbar dura mater biomechanics: experimental characterization and scanning microscopy observations. *Anesth Analg* 1999;**88**:1317–21.

28 Angle PJM, Kronberg JEM, Thompson DEM, *et al.* Dural tissue trauma and cerebrospinal leak after epidural needle puncture: effect of needle design, angle, and bevel orientation. *Anesthesiology* 2003;**99**:1376–82.

29 Hatfalvi BI. Postulated mechanisms for postdural puncture headache and review of laboratory models: clinical experience. *Reg Anesth* 1995;**20**:329–36.

30 Janik R, Dick W. Der postspinale kopfschmerz: häufigkeit nach medianer und paramedianer technik. *Anaesthesist* 1992;**41**:137–41.

31 Stasiuk RBP, Jenkins LC. Post spinal headache: a comparison of midline and laminar approaches. *Can J Anaesth* 1990;**37**:S58.

32 Jorgensen NH. Postdural puncture is more common with the paramedian approach. *Anesth Analg* 1991;**72**:S131.

33 Naulty JS, Hertwig L, Hunt CO, Datta S, Ostheimer GW, Weiss JB. Influence of local anesthetic solution on postdural puncture headache. *Anesthesiology* 1990;**72**:450–4.

34 Runza M, Albani A, Tagliabue M, Haiek M, LoPresti S, Birnbach DJ. Spinal anesthesia using hyperbaric 0.75% versus hyperbaric 1% bupivacaine for cesarean section. *Anesth Analg* 1998;**87**:1099–104.

35 Abboud TK, Zhu J, Reyes A, *et al.* Effect of subarachnoid morphine on the incidence of spinal headache. *Reg Anesth* 1992;**17**:34–6.

36 Meininger D, Byhahn C, Kessler P, *et al.* Intrathecal fentanyl, sufentanil, or placebo combined with hyperbaric mepivacaine 2% for parturients undergoing elective cesarean delivery. *Anesth Analg* 2003;**96**:852–8.

37 Thoennissen J, Herkner H, Lang W, Domanovits H, Laggner AN, Müllner M. Does bed rest after cervical or lumbar puncture prevent headache? A systematic review and meta-analysis. *CMAJ* 2001;**165**:1311–6.

38 Sudlow C, Warlow C. Posture and fluids for preventing post-dural puncture headache (Cochrane review). *Cochrane Database Syst Rev* 2003;**3**:CD001790.

39 Eldevik OP, Nakken KO, Haughton VM. The effect of dehydration on the side-effects of metrizamide myelography. *Radiology* 1978;**129**:715–6.

40 Dieterich M, Brandt T. Incidence of post-lumbar puncture headache is independent of daily fluid intake. *Eur Arch Psychiatr Neurol Sci* 1988;**237**:194–6.

41 Angle P, Thompson D, Halpern S, Wilson DB. Second stage pushing correlates with headache after unintentional dural puncture in parturients. *Can J Anesth* 1999;**46**:861–6.

42 Stride PC, Cooper GM. Dural taps revisited: a 20-year survey from Birmingham Maternity Hospital. *Anaesthesia* 1993;**48**:247–55.

43 Ravindran RS, Viegas OJ, Tasch MD, Cline PJ, Deaton RL, Brown TR. Bearing down at the time of delivery and the incidence of spinal headache in parturients. *Anesth Analg* 1981;**60**:524–6.

44 Holder HG. Reactions after spinal anesthesia. *JAMA* 1944;**124**:56–7.

45 Denker PG. The effect of caffeine on the cerebrospinal fluid pressure. *Am J Med Sci* 1931;**181**:675–81.

46 Loman J, Myerson A. The action of certain drugs on the cerebrospinal fluid and on the internal jugular venous and systemic arterial pressures of man. *Arch Neurol Psychiatr* 1932;**27**:1226–44.

47 Moyer JH, Tashnek AB, Miller SI, Snyder H, Bowman RO, Smith CP. The effect of theophylline with ethylenediamine (aminophylline) and caffeine on cerebral hemodynamics and cerebrospinal fluid pressure in patients with hypertensive headaches. *Am J Med Sci* 1952;**224**:377–85.

48 Yücel A, Özyalçin S, Talu GK, Yücel EC, Erdine S. Intravenous administration of caffeine sodium benzoate for postdural puncture headache. *Reg Anesth Pain Med* 1999;**24**:51–4.

49 Ilioff G, Strelec SR, Rothfus W. Does prophylactic intramuscular caffeine sodium benzoate decrease the incidence of postdural puncture headache? *Reg Anesth* 1990;**15**(1S):65.

50 Strelec S, Prylinski J, Sakert T. The efficacy of multi-dose oral caffeine in prevention of post-dural puncture headache. *Reg Anesth* 1994;**19**(2S):79.

51 Sechzer P, Abel L. Post-spinal anesthesia headache treated with caffeine: evaluation with demand method. Part I. *Curr Ther Res* 1978;**24**:307–12.

52 Camann WR, Murray RS, Mushlin PS, *et al.* Effects of oral caffeine on postdural puncture headache: a double-blind, placebo-controlled trial. *Anesth Analg* 1990;**70**:181–4.

53 Lang SA, Yip RW. Intravenous caffeine as a treatment for postdural puncture headaches: will it replace the epidural blood patch? *Anesth Analg* 1993;**76**:S207.

54 Jarvis AP, Grenawalt JW, Pagraeus L. Intravenous caffeine for post-dural puncture headache. *Anesth Analg* 1986;**65**: 316–7.

55 Aguilera L, Rodríguez-Sasiain JM, Castrillo J, *et al.* Cafeína intravenosa en el tratamiento de la cefalea pospunción dural. *Rev Esp Anest Reanim* 1988;**35**:78–9.

56 Abboud TK, Zhu J, Reyes A, Steffens Z, Afrasiabi A, Gendein D. Efficacy of intravenous caffeine for post dural puncture headache. *Anesthesiology* 1990;**73**:A936.

57 Yang S-F, Tsai M-H. Cafergot in the treatment of post-dural puncture headache: a 21 cases report. *Anesthesiology* 1994;**81**:A1012.

58 Tyrala EE, Dodson WE. Caffeine secretion into breast milk. *Arch Dis Child* 1979;**54**:787–800.

59 Berlin CM, Denson HM, Daniel CH, Ward RM. Disposition of dietary caffeine in milk, saliva, and plasma of lactating women. *Pediatrics* 1984;**73**:59–63.

60 Bolton VE, Leicht CH, Scanlon TS. Postpartum seizure after epidural blood patch and intravenous caffeine sodium benzoate. *Anesthesiology* 1989;**70**:146–9.

61 Cohen SM, Laurito CE, Curran MJ. Grand mal seizure in a postpartum patient following intravenous infusion of caffeine sodium benzoate to treat persistent headache. *J Clin Anesth* 1992;**4**:48–51.

62 de Van V, Corneillie M, Vanacker B, *et al.* Treatment for postdural puncture headache associated with late postpartum eclampsia. *Acta Anaesthesiol Belgica* 1999;**50**:99–102.

63 Holmes M, Waters J, Leivers D, Burger G. Prophylactic epidural blood patch versus prophylactic theophylline following accidental dural puncture. *Anesthesiology* 1994;**81**:A1177.

64 Fuerstein TJ, Zeides A. Theophylline relieves headache following lumbar puncture: placebo-controlled, double-blind pilot study. *Klin Wochenschr* 1986;**64**:216–8.

65 Schwalbe SS, Schiffmiller MW, Marx GF. Theophylline for post-dural puncture headache. *Anesthesiology* 1991;**75**:A1082.

66 Carp H, Singh PJ, Vadhera R, Jayaram A. Effects of the serotonin-receptor agonist sumatriptan on postdural puncture headache: report of six cases. *Anesth Analg* 1994;**79**:180–2.

67 Rohmer C, Le Bourlot G. Céphalées après rachianesthésie traitées par le sumatriptan. *Ann Fr Anesth Réanim* 1995;**14**:237.

68 von Hornstein WF, Reich A. Limites du sumatriptan dan le traitement des céphalées après ponction de la dure-mère. *Ann Fr Anesth Réanim* 1996;**15**:229–30.

69 Lhussier G, Mercier FJ, Dounas M. Sumatriptan: an alternative to the blood patch? *Anaesthesia* 1996;**51**:1078.

70 Hodgson C, Roitberg-Henry A. The use of sumatriptan in the treatment of postdural puncture headache. *Anaesthesia* 1997;**52**:808.

71 Sprigge JS. The use of sumatriptan in the treatment of postdural puncture headache after accidental lumbar puncture complicated a blood patch procedure. *Anaesthesia* 1999;**54**:95–6.

72 Connelly NR, Parker RK, Rahimi A, Gibson C. Sumatriptan in patients with postdural puncture headache. *Anesthesiology* 1999;**90**:A31.

73 Wojnar-Horton RE, Hackett LP, Yapp P, Dusci LJ, Paech M, Ilett KF. Distribution and excretion of sumatriptan in human milk. *Br J Clin Pharmacol* 1996;**41**:217–21.

74 Oliver CD, White SA. Unexplained fitting in three parturients suffering from postdural puncture headache. *Br J Anaesth* 2002;**89**:782–5.

75 Rice I, Radhakrishnan D, Nelson-Piercey C. Cerebral vasoconstrictors and postdural puncture headache: the big squeeze. *Br J Anaesth* 2003;**90**:527–8.

76 Kshatri A, Foster PA. Adrenocorticotropic hormone infusion as a novel treatment for postdural puncture headache. *Reg Anesth* 1997;**22**:432–4.

77 Collier BB. Treatment for postdural puncture headache. *Br J Anaesth* 1994;**72**:366–7.

78 Foster P. ACTH treatment for post-lumbar puncture headache. *Br J Anaesth* 1994;**72**:429.

79 Gormley JB. Treatment of postspinal headache. *Anesthesiology* 1960;**21**:565–6.

80 DiGiovanni AJ, Dunbar BS. Epidural injection of autologous blood for postlumbar puncture headache. *Anesth Analg* 1970;**49**:268–71.

81 Sudlow C, Warlow C. Epidural blood patching for preventing and treating post-dural puncture headache (Cochrane review). *Cochrane Database Syst Rev* 2003;**3**:CD001791.

82 Heide W, Diener H-C. Epidural blood patch reduces the incidence of postlumbar puncture headache. *Headache* 1990;**30**:280–1.

83 Gutterman P, Bezier HS. Prophylaxis of postmyelogram headaches. *J Neurosurg* 1978;**49**:869–71.

84 Palahniuk RJ, Cumming M. Prophylactic blood patch does not prevent post lumbar puncture headache. *Can Anaesth Soc J* 1979;**26**:132–3.

85 Colonna-Romano P, Shapiro BE. Unintentional dural puncture and prophylactic epidural blood patch in obstetrics. *Anesth Analg* 1989;**69**:522–3.

86 Ackerman WE, Juneja MM, Kaczorowski DM. Prophylactic epidural blood patch for prevention of postdural headache in the parturient. *Anesthesiology* 1990;**17**:45–9.

87 Trivedi ND, Eddi D, Shevde K. Headache prevention following accidental dural puncture in obstetric patients. *J Clin Anesth* 1993;**5**:42–5.

88 Lowenwirt I, Cohen S, Zephyr J, Hamer R, Hronkova B, Rovner JS. Treatment of accidental dural puncture in obstetric patients: prophylactic vs therapeutic blood patch. *Anesthesiology* 1998;**88**:A38.

89 Sengupta P, Bagley G, Lim M. Prevention of postdural puncture headache after spinal anaesthesia for extracorporeal shockwave lithotripsy: an assessment of prophylactic epidural blood patching. *Anaesthesia* 1989;**44**:54–6.

90 Seebacher J, Ribeiro V, LeGuillou JL, *et al.* Epidural blood patch in the treatment of post dural puncture headache: a double blind study. *Headache* 1989;**29**:630–2.

91 Bart AJ, Wheeler AS. Comparison of epidural saline placement and epidural blood placement in the treatment of post-lumbar puncture headache. *Anesthesiology* 1978;**48**:221–3.

92 Loeser EA, Hill GE, Bennet GM, Sederberg JH. Time vs success rate for epidural blood patch. *Anesthesiology* 1978;**49**:147–8.

93 Taivainen T, Pitkänen M, Tuominen M, Rosenberg PH. Efficacy of epidural blood patch for postdural puncture headache. *Acta Anaesthesiol Scand* 1993;**37**:702–5.

94 Martin R, Jourdain S, Clairoux M, Tétrault JP. Duration of decubitus position after epidural blood patch. *Can J Anaesth* 1994;**41**:23–5.

95 Abouleish E, de la Vega S, Blendinger I, Tio T-O. Long-term

follow-up of epidural blood patch. *Anesth Analg* 1975; **54**:459–63.

96 Cheek TG, Banner R, Sauter J, Gutsche BB. Prophylactic extradural blood patch is effective: a preliminary communication. *Br J Anaesth* 1988;**61**:340–2.

97 Tarkkila PJ, Miralles JA, Palomaki EA. The subjective complications and efficiency of the epidural blood patch in the treatment of postdural puncture headache. *Reg Anesth* 1989;**14**:247–50.

98 Mercieri M, Mercieri A, Paolini S, *et al.* Postpartum cerebral ischaemia after accidental dural puncture and epidural blood patch. *Br J Anaesth* 2003;**90**:98–100.

99 Oh J, Camann W. Severe, acute meningeal irritative reaction after epidural blood patch. *Anesth Analg* 1998;**87**:1139–40.

100 Cornwall RD, Dolan W. Radicular back pain following lumbar epidural blood patch. *Anesthesiology* 1975;**43**:692–3.

101 Rainbird A, Pfitzner A. Restricted spread of analgesia following epidural blood patch: case report with a review of possible complications. *Anaesthesia* 1983;**38**:481–4.

102 Tekkök IH, Carter DA, Brinker R. Spinal subdural haematoma as a complication of immediate epidural blood patch. *Can J Anaesth* 1996;**43**:306–9.

103 Seeberger MD, Urwyler A. Lumbovertebral syndrome after extradural blood patch. *Br J Anaesth* 1992;**69**:414–6.

104 Andrews PJD, Ackerman WE, Juneja M, Cases-Cristobal V, Rigor BM. Transient bradycardia associated with extradural blood patch after inadvertent dural puncture in parturients. *Br J Anaesth* 1992;**69**:401–3.

105 Christensen K. A generalized seizure in connection with epidural blood-patch. *Ugeskr Laeger* 1989;**151**:3405–6.

106 Marfurt D, Lyrer P, Rüttimann U, Strebel S, Schneider MC. Recurrent post-partum seizures after epidural blood patch. *Br J Anaesth* 2002;**90**:247–50.

107 Kardash K, Morrow F, Beique F. Seizures after epidural blood patch with undiagnosed subdural hematoma. *Reg Anesth Pain Med* 2002;**27**:433–6.

108 Srinivasa V, Eappen S, Schlossmacher MG, Gerner P. Seizures after epidural blood patch. *Reg Anesth Pain Med* 2003;**28**:71.

109 Reynolds AF, Hameroff SR, Blitt CD, Roberts WL. Spinal subdural epiarachnoid hematoma: a complication of a novel epidural blood patch technique. *Anesth Analg* 1980;**59**:702–3.

110 Santos DJ, Barrett T, Lachica R, Coyle D. Efficacy of epidural saline patch in preventing post-dural puncture headache. *Reg Anesth* 1986;**11**:42–3.

111 Thomas DI, Suresh MS, Stride PC, Wilkey AD. Prophylaxis of dural headache: epidural saline bolus versus infusion. *Anesth Analg* 1992;**74**:S319.

112 Salvador L, Carrero E, Castillo J, Villalonga A, Nalda MA. Prevention of post dural puncture headache with epidural-administered dextran 40. *Reg Anesth* 1992;**17**:357–8.

113 Barrios-Alarcon J, Aldrete JA, Paragas-Tapia D. Relief of post-lumbar puncture headache with epidural dextran 40: a preliminary report. *Reg Anesth* 1989;**14**:78–80.

114 Stevens DS, Peeter-Asdourian C. Treatment of postdural puncture headache with "epidural dextran patch." *Reg Anesth* 1993;**18**:324–5.

115 Aldrete JA. Persistent post-dural puncture headache treated with epidural infusion of dextran. *Headache* 1994;**34**:265–7.

116 Reynvoet MEJ, Cosaert PAJM, Desmet FR, Plasschaert SM. Epidural dextran 40 for postdural puncture headache. *Anaesthesia* 1997;**52**:886–8.

117 Epidural gelatin (Gelfoam®) patch treatment for post dural puncture headache. *Anaesth Intens Care* 1991;**19**:444–53.

118 Gerritse BM, van Dongen RT, Crul BJ. Epidural fibrin glue injection stops persistent cerebrospinal leak during long-term intrathecal catheterization. *Anesth Analg* 1997;**84**:1140–1.

119 Crul BJ, Gerritse BM, van Dongen RT, Schoonderwaldt HC. Epidural fibrin glue injection stops persistent postdural puncture headache. *Anesthesiology* 1999;**91**:576–7.

120 Gentili ME. Epidural fibrin glue injection stops postdural puncture headache in patient with long-term intrathecal catheterization. *Reg Anesth Pain Med* 2003;**28**:70.

121 Dennehy KC, Rosaeg OP. Intrathecal catheter insertion during labour reduces the risk of postdural puncture headache. *Can J Anaesth* 1998;**45**:42–5.

122 Kuczkowski KM, Benumof JL. Decrease in the incidence of post-dural puncture headache: maintaining CSF volume. *Acta Anaesthesiol Scand* 2003;**47**:98–100.

123 Norris MC, Leighton BL. Continuous spinal anesthesia after unintentional dural puncture in parturients. *Reg Anesth* 1990;**15**:285–7.

124 Liu N, Montefiore A, Kermarec N, Rauss A, Bonnet F. Prolonged placement of spinal catheters does not prevent postdural puncture headache. *Reg Anesth* 1993;**18**:110–3.

CHAPTER 17

Epidural analgesia and back pain

Terrance W. Breen

Background

In 1990, MacArthur *et al.*[1] reported that epidural anesthesia for labor and delivery was associated with long-term backache; furthermore, they contended that the association was "probably causal."[1] Around the same time, other researchers questioned the impact of labor analgesia on obstetric and neonatal outcomes.[2,3] A recurring message in these studies was to advocate for "full disclosure" of known and unknown risks of labor epidural analgesia so parturients could make informed choices. The international obstetric anesthesia community acknowledged these issues and rose to the challenge of addressing them, performing more and better studies until the controversies were addressed. Patients can now be given "full disclosure" about back pain after labor and delivery. This chapter reviews the literature on back pain after pregnancy, how labor epidural analgesia came to be associated with back pain after delivery and current beliefs about back pain after labor and delivery.

Epidemiology terminology[4]

Most back pain studies describe back pain in terms of rate and/or proportion, and use the terms incidence and prevalence extensively. *Incidence* refers to the rate of occurrence of an event in a defined population over a specified period of time. For example, MacArthur *et al.*[1] compared the incidence of *new-onset* backache after delivery in women who received epidural anesthesia with those who did not, where postpartum backache was defined as backache beginning within 3 months of delivery and lasting at least 6 weeks. Many back pain studies examine the *lifetime cumulative incidence* of back pain, reporting the proportion of the population that has experienced back pain at some

point in their lives. The lifetime cumulative incidence begins at zero and rises until equilibrium, where the rate of new cases equals the death rate in the population. *Prevalence* refers to the number of affected persons in the population at a specific time. *Point prevalence* reflects a snapshot of a problem at a particular moment in time, such as the proportion of individuals who report back pain on the 90th day after delivery (at the time of answering a questionnaire or survey 3 months after delivery). *Period prevalence* refers to the proportion of affected individuals who report a problem over a defined period of time, such as those who experience any low back pain in the 3 months after childbirth, whether or not they have low back pain at the time of the questionnaire or survey.

Low back pain

Low back pain may be defined as pain, muscle tension or stiffness localized below the costal margin and above the gluteal folds, with or without leg pain (sciatica).[5] A simpler definition of low back pain is pain felt in the lumbosacral spinal and paraspinal regions.[6] Low back pain is common, affecting more than 50% of the population over the course of their lives.[5,6] The duration of pain is used to categorize different populations of low back pain: *acute* low back pain lasts 0–6 weeks; *subacute* low back pain lasts 5–13 weeks; and *chronic* low back pain lasts longer than 3 months. The majority of low back pain improves within 1 month, but symptoms persist or recur in 25–50% of individuals over the ensuing year.

When patients present with low back pain, a specific treatable cause is found in fewer than 10% of patients. Specific causes of low back pain include herniation of the nucleus pulposus, infection, inflammation, arthritis, osteoporosis, fractures, tumors and visceral disorders such as pancreatitis and renal calculi. Rare but serious causes of back pain after anesthesia include epidural abscess, epidural hematoma, meningitis and direct spinal cord or nerve damage. More than 90% of patients with low back pain have non-specific low back pain.

The important hallmarks of non-specific low back pain are pain and disability. Low back pain is a significant burden to all healthcare systems and is the second most common symptomatic reason to see a physician in the USA and the most common reason to seek care from an alternative medicine practitioner such as a chiropractor or massage therapist.[6] Low back pain accounts for approximately one-third of workers' compensation costs and is the most costly common workers' compensation complaint. Against this background, any association between labor epidural analgesia and low back pain would be a cause for great concern.

Age and back pain

Low back pain is common and is experienced by most people at some point in their lives. A large postal questionnaire study of 29,424 individuals (52% female) reported information about the prevalence, lifetime cumulative incidence and severity of low back pain across the ages 12–41 years.[7] The lifetime cumulative incidence of any low back pain rises rapidly from < 10% for 12-year-olds to > 50% for 20-year-olds. The rate of rise of lifetime low back pain then slows reaching approximately 70% by age 41 (Table 17.1). The point prevalence for back pain on any given day is 8–14% for 20–40-year-olds. These investigators also graded the severity of low back pain by duration but did not report the impact of the low back pain. Information about pregnancy and anesthesia is not included in this study or many other studies of back pain in women of reproductive age.

Table 17.1 One-year period prevalence of back pain in men and women.[7]

Duration of LBP	Age 20	Age 25	Age 30	Age 35
0–7 days (%)	13	16	16	17
8–30 days (%)	20	25	24	22
> 30 days (%)	8	1	11	10

LBP, low back pain.

Studies of back pain and pregnancy

Ostgaard and Andersson[8] studied 429 pregnant women with a history of back pain before pregnancy and 375 women with no previous back pain. The risk of experiencing back pain in pregnancy was 58% for women with a previous history of back pain compared with 28% in women without a previous history of back pain. The point prevalence of back pain during pregnancy was approximately 35% in women with previous back pain and did not change over gestation. In contrast, women without a history of back pain had a steady increase in back pain over pregnancy from 3% to 12%. The average intensity of back pain was 4–5 on a scale of 0–10 and was not different between multiparous and nulliparous women or through gestation. Regression analysis showed that the main predictor of back pain in pregnancy was pre-existing back pain. Younger age was also a risk factor for back pain in pregnancy and multiparity was predictive for longer periods of back pain.

Ostgaard and Andersson[9] mailed questionnaires to the above women approximately 1 year after delivery; the mean time from delivery to response was 18 months. Women were retrospectively asked about sick-leave because of back pain during pregnancy, current back pain and the time interval between delivery and the disappearance of back pain during the index pregnancy. Twenty-one percent of parturients took time off work because of low back pain during pregnancy and the average duration of leave was 7.5 weeks. Back pain at the time of delivery was reported by 67% of women. At follow-up, 63% had no back pain, leaving 37% with some back pain. Of these, 26% with back pain were "much improved," 4% "somewhat improved" and 7% reported "serious back pain" 18 months after delivery. Women who reported serious back pain were more likely to have experienced back pain before delivery and had more frequent back pain after delivery. This was more common in women who performed monotonous and heavy work antenatally. In addition, these women took more sick-leave because of back pain. Of the women with postpartum back pain who recovered, 50% were back pain free by 17 weeks. Women without a history of back pain before pregnancy were less likely to have back pain after delivery. The prevalence of low back pain after delivery is shown in Fig. 17.1.

Ostgaard et al.[10] have also studied "posterior pelvic

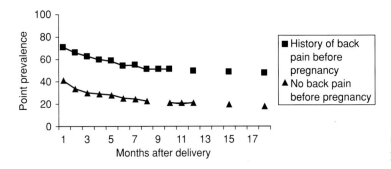

Fig. 17.1 Point prevalence of postpartum back pain.[8]

Table 17.2 The difference between back pain and posterior pelvic pain.[10]

Back pain	Posterior pelvic pain
A pain drawing with markings *above* the sacrum	A pain drawing with well-defined markings of stabbing pain in the buttocks distal and lateral to the L5–S1 area, with or without radiation to the posterior thigh or knee, but not into the foot
Back pain experienced when the patient was in forward flexion	A history of pain related to time and weight-bearing in the posterior pelvis, deep in the gluteal area
Decreased range of motion in the lumbar spine	Pain-free intervals
Pain from palpation of the erector spina muscle	Free range of motion in the hips and spine and no nerve root syndrome
Negative posterior pelvic pain provocation test results	Positive posterior pain provocation test results

pain" in addition to back pain during and after pregnancy (Table 17.2). Forty-two percent of women complained of pain at 25 weeks' gestation (similar to previous studies), 35% of posterior pelvic pain and 7% of back pain. By 11 weeks postpartum, 20% of women complained of pain: 15% back pain and 5% posterior pelvic pain. By 23 weeks, 12% of women complained of pain: 8% back pain and 4% posterior pelvic pain. Posterior pelvic pain was more problematic during pregnancy and back pain more so after delivery. Ostgaard *et al.* emphasize the importance of differentiating between posterior pelvic and back pain as the therapies during pregnancy and the natural history after delivery are different.[11,12]

Low back pain after epidural analgesia and anesthesia

In January 1987, MacArthur *et al.*[1] mailed out postal questionnaires to 30,096 women who had delivered at Birmingham Maternity Hospital between 1978 and 1985. Women were asked questions concerning a broad range of obstetric, anesthetic and maternal issues in the postpartum period (ranging 1–9 years from delivery to completion of the questionnaire). The overall findings of the study were published in a book.[13] Questionnaires were returned by 11,701 women (38.9%). Long-term backache, defined as backache occurring within 3 months of delivery and lasting at least 6 weeks, was reported by 23.3% of women. Backache on a previous occasion was reported by 40% of these women. They were excluded from the analysis, leaving a study population of 1634 women (14.0% of the study population) with new-onset backache after delivery. Backache lasted more than 1 year for 69% of these women and was still present at the time of the questionnaire in 65% (9.1% of the total sample reporting chronic back pain beginning after childbirth). Women who received epidural anesthesia were much more likely to report back pain (18.9%)

than those who did not receive epidural anesthesia (10.5%). As the researchers had detailed information about patients including demographics and obstetric information, they performed logistic regression analysis to determine which factors were most associated with backache after delivery. Epidural anesthesia was the factor most strongly associated with postpartum backache, followed by nulliparity, Asian race, younger age, no episiotomy, spinal anesthesia, a longer second stage of labor, spontaneous onset of labor and social class III, IV or V. Epidural anesthesia was associated with postpartum backache for both "normal" deliveries and "abnormal" deliveries, where "normal" was defined as singleton pregnancy, with occiput anterior presentation at delivery, spontaneous onset of labor, no forceps, no cesarean section, active phase of labor < 12 h and a second stage of labor < 2 h. The investigators examined women who received epidural anesthesia and underwent labor and vaginal delivery, labor and emergency cesarean section or elective cesarean section. Backache was associated with labor and delivery (vaginal or emergency cesarean) but not with elective cesarean section. The authors proposed that labor epidural analgesia allowed women to adopt a "stressed posture" and to remain in a position that they would not otherwise tolerate because of the anesthesia. This hypothesis seemed possible and amenable to further study.

Why might the investigators have found an association between labor epidural analgesia and backache at all? Less than 40% of patients responded to the survey so the results may not reflect the population. As the survey asked about health issues after delivery, perhaps patients who experienced health issues were more likely to respond. The authors did not collect information about back pain before or during pregnancy, so those potential confounding factors were not controlled for.

This study created significant controversy, in part because the finding of backache after epidural analgesia was unexpected, and in part because of the authors' assertion that the relationship between labor epidural analgesia and postpartum backache was "probably causal" and not just association. The stated primary purpose of the overall study was "to ascertain the nature and prevalence of morbidity after childbirth and, secondly, to examine its relationship with a wide range of obstetric, anesthetic, and maternal factors."

The investigators collected a large amount of information, entered it into a database and then began querying the database, looking for expected and unexpected associations. The investigators should have published their descriptive findings, listed any associated or predictive factors, acknowledged the limitations of their data, and possibly speculated on avenues for future research.

In addition to the other deficiencies in this study, retrospective studies yield unreliable results when parturients are asked whether or not they experienced back pain in the past. Macarthur et al.[14] documented the frequency of back pain after childbirth in a cohort of 244 patients. Approximately half of these received epidural analgesia and half did not. At day 1, day 7 and week 6 after delivery, the patients reported the incidence of back pain. One year after delivery, the investigators again requested information on back pain but also asked the women to recall whether or not they had had back pain during the previous time intervals. They measured the correlation (kappa) between the information gathered prospectively and the recalled information. Of note, a kappa of less than 0.4 is considered poor correlation. They found that the information recorded at 1 year after delivery was poorly correlated with the results obtained at all three time points in women who received epidural analgesia and those who did not. The range of kappa for the epidural group was 0.11–0.25, compared with −0.09 to 0.18 in the non-epidural group. This study did not demonstrate "recall bias" because there was no statistical difference in kappas between groups. However, it showed that retrospective data were extremely unreliable.

In order to determine whether or not epidural analgesia causes an increased incidence in long-term (more than 6 weeks) back pain, MEDLINE®, EMBASE® and Science Citation Index® were reviewed from 1980 until March 2004 using the following key words and text terms: [analgesia], [obstetrical], [anesthesia obstetrical], [analgesia epidural], [back pain], [back ache] and [pregnancy]. Studies comparing parturients who received epidural analgesia with those who did not were included if they were prospective cohort or randomized controlled trials (RCTs). Retrospective studies,[15,16] studies without a control group[17] and those that reported short-term effects[18–20] were excluded. In all there were nine studies. Of the three RCTs, two were available as full manuscripts[21,22] and one as an

Table 17.3 Epidural analgesia and long-term back pain. Characteristics of studies.

Study	Design	Response rate (%)	Epidural (N)	Non-epidural (N)	Duration of follow-up	Incidence of back pain: epidural vs non-epidural
Breen et al.[24]	Prospective cohort	72	589	453	1–2 months	44% vs 45%
Patel et al.[27]	Prospective cohort	?	242	53	6 months	32% vs 34%
Russell et al.[28]	Prospective cohort	75	319	131	3 months	34% vs 31%
Macarthur et al.[25]	Prospective cohort	100	164	165	6 weeks	14% vs 7%
Macarthur et al.[26]	Prospective cohort	74	121	123	1 year	10% vs 14%
To & Wong[30]	Prospective cohort	58	40	149	21–24 months	25% vs 12.5%
Thompson et al.[29]	Prospective cohort	92	433	850	24 weeks	OR = 1.15 (95% CI, 0.9–1.46)
Breen et al.[23]	Randomized controlled trial (by treatment received)	71	120	52	6–8 weeks	48% vs 53%
Howell et al.[21,31]	Randomized controlled trial	80	162 166	151 158	3 months 1 year	39% vs 34% 35% vs 27%
Loughnan et al.[22]	Randomized controlled trial	83	249	259	6 months	48% vs 50%

CI, confidence interval; OR, odds ratio.

abstract[23] with additional information from the primary investigator (T.W. Breen, personal communication). There were six prospective cohort studies,[24–30] but one study reported two follow-up time periods of the same patients in different manuscripts.[25,26] One study is available only as an abstract.[27] In all, data on approximately 2400 women with and 2400 women without epidural analgesia are available. A summary of the results of the studies is shown in Table 17.3. The studies available in complete manuscript form are described in more detail below.

Prospective cohort studies

Breen et al.[24] interviewed 1185 women in a Boston hospital after delivery and recruited them to a study of back pain after delivery. Information concerning demographic variables, labor analgesia, method of delivery and history of back pain were collected. Two months later, a questionnaire was mailed to all participants. Non-responders were sent a second questionnaire and an attempt was made to contact persistent non-responders by telephone. The primary study outcome was back pain at the time of the postpartum survey. Anesthetic technique was not specified in the study but was consistent in the institution where the vast majority of patients received epidural bupivacaine 0.04–0.125% and fentanyl 1–2 µg/mL with or without epinephrine 1 : 600,000. Labor analgesia was maintained by continuous infusion and supplemented by intermittent top-ups as needed. Follow-up data were obtained from 1042 patients (88%) with 754 (72%) returning questionnaires and the other 288 contacted by telephone. Postpartum back pain was reported by 460 responders (44%) and 68 women (6.5%) rated the pain as "severe." The prevalence of postpartum back pain was equivalent in women who received epidural analgesia (45%) and those who did not (44%). Method of delivery did not affect the prevalence of back pain, which occurred in 45% of women after vaginal delivery and 42% after cesarean section. The investigators performed stepwise logistic regression analysis of the entire database and found a positive relationship between postpartum back pain and back pain before or during the pregnancy and weight, and a negative association with age. Factors not associated with back pain after deliveries were height, mode of delivery, neonatal birth weight and epidural analgesia.

The investigators applied logistic regression analysis to women with new-onset back pain and found an inverse association with height and a positive association with weight. Factors not associated with new-onset postpartum back pain included age, mode of delivery, neonatal birth weight and epidural administration. In contrast to the retrospective studies, this study found that labor epidural analgesia did not cause postpartum back pain.

Macarthur et al.[25] recruited 329 women in Montreal to a prospective cohort study: 164 women who received epidural analgesia and 165 who did not. Their anesthetic technique differed from that of Breen et al.[24] as intermittent top-ups of 0.25% bupivacaine were used rather than a continuous infusion. Back pain was assessed the day after delivery, 7 days and 6 weeks postpartum and all assessments were by a trained research nurse. Some demographic differences were noted between women who did, and did not, receive labor epidural analgesia. Specifically, women who received epidural analgesia spent longer in the lithotomy position, were more likely to be nulliparous, had more cesarean sections and were more likely to be Caucasian. Back pain during pregnancy was reported by 34% of women who received labor epidural analgesia and 35% of women who did not. Back pain after labor epidural was more common on the first postpartum day but no more frequent at 7 days or 6 weeks postpartum. There were no differences in interference with activities at 1, 7 or 42 days postpartum. Women with a history of back pain during pregnancy were removed from the dataset and the analysis repeated. Again, there were no differences in the prevalence of postpartum back pain or its functional impairment. The investigators contacted 74% of study participants 1 year after delivery and again found no difference in the prevalence or severity of back pain in women who did, and did not, receive labor epidural analgesia.[26]

Russell et al.[28] performed a prospective study in follow-up to their retrospective study.[16] The study design included women who received epidural analgesia and who were randomized to plain epidural bupivacaine 0.125% or bupivacaine 0.0625% plus fentanyl or sufentanil. One control patient who did not receive labor epidural analgesia was recruited for every two epidural patients. The study was designed to produce two different epidural groups: a traditional epidural group with local anesthetic alone, which was expected to produce more motor block, and a low-dose epidural group who received local anesthetic plus opioid and were expected to experience less motor block. Women who received epidural analgesia were asked about various symptoms after successful analgesia but before delivery. Women without epidural analgesia were asked the questions the day after delivery. Three months after delivery, a postal questionnaire was sent to study participants. If a completed questionnaire was not returned within 6 weeks, attempts were made to contact mothers by telephone. A total of 616 women were initially recruited and 17 were excluded for obstetric or anesthesia reasons. The response rate of the 599 women was 75% but varied among the groups (79% and 81% in the epidural groups, 66% in the non-epidural group). A total of 150 women (33.3%) experienced backache lasting at least 3 months and, of these, 33 represented new-onset backache. Motor blockade was more common in the epidural group receiving more bupivacaine. The prevalence of back pain before pregnancy, during pregnancy and at 3 months postpartum did not differ among the three study groups (bupivacaine alone 38.9%; bupivacaine plus opioid 30.3%; no epidural 30.5%). Similarly, the incidence of new-onset backache was 6.4%, 8.6% and 6.9%, respectively, not statistically different between groups. Logistic regression analysis of all patients showed that the only predictor for postpartum backache, either persistent or new onset, was previous backache before or during pregnancy.

To and Wong[30] surveyed 326 pregnant Chinese women and prospectively collected back pain data at 28 weeks' gestation and 21–24 months postpartum. Back pain during pregnancy was reported by 250 women (76%). The majority of back pain was mild, intermittent and did not require specific treatment. Women with back pain during pregnancy were more likely to have experienced back pain when not pregnant and/or with a previous pregnancy. The most common patterns of back pain were:

1 lower back pain (56.4%);
2 sciatic pain (26.8%); and
3 lower back plus sciatic pain (10.4%).

Labor and delivery outcomes were not different between parturients who experienced antenatal back pain and those who did not. Interestingly, 14% of women who experienced back pain in pregnancy received labor epidural analgesia compared with 18%

of women who did not experience back pain in pregnancy. At the 2-year follow-up, complete data were available for 189 patients (58%), 40 of whom were experiencing persistent back pain (21%). Ten women in the persistent back pain group (25%) had received labor epidural analgesia compared with 18 women (12%) in the group without back pain; this was not statistically different ($P = 0.07$). The investigators found that greater weight gain during pregnancy and smaller weight loss after delivery were related to persistent back pain. The investigators did not report a logistic regression analysis.

A population-based cohort study was conducted in the Australian Capital Territory involving women who gave birth from March to October 1997.[29] The aim of the study was to describe changes in the prevalence of maternal health problems in the 6 months after birth. Questionnaires were administered 4 days, and 8, 16 and 24 weeks postpartum. Of women eligible for the study, 1295 (70%) agreed to participate and 1193 (92%) completed all questionnaires. Of health issues surveyed, fatigue and backache were significantly more common than other problems. The point prevalence of backache was 53% at 8 weeks postpartum, 47% by 16 weeks and 45% by 24 weeks. One-third of women in this study received labor epidural analgesia. No statistically significant association occurred between epidural use and backache:

- *8 weeks:* odds ratio (OR) 1.04 (95% confidence interval [CI], 0.83–1.33)
- *16 weeks:* OR 1.29 (95% CI, 1.02–1.64)
- *24 weeks:* OR 1.15 (95% CI, 0.90–1.46)

Randomized controlled trials

It is difficult to find pregnant women willing to be randomized to epidural or non-epidural analgesia but two published trials have succeeded. Over 4.5 years,

Howell *et al.*[31] enrolled 369 primigravid women into a study where they were randomized to receive epidural analgesia with intermittent boluses of 0.25% bupivacaine or intramuscular injections of 50–100 mg meperidine as needed. A total of 184 women were randomized to receive labor epidural analgesia and 123 (66.8%) actually received epidural analgesia (the most common reason for not receiving epidural analgesia was rapid progress of labor). Of 185 women randomized to non-epidural analgesia, 52 (28%) eventually received epidural analgesia (failure of meperidine to provide adequate pain relief). Data analysis was by intention-to-treat, not by treatment received. There were no differences in the prevalence of lower or middle back pain during pregnancy (at 32 weeks' gestation), 3 months or 12 months postpartum (Table 17.4). The patients in this study were asked to participate in a follow-up study approximately 2 years after delivery.[21] Of the 184 women originally randomized to labor epidural analgesia, 151 were contacted in follow-up, 119 by personal interview and the other 32 by telephone interview (20) or postal questionnaire (12). In the non-epidural group, 155 of the original 185 women agreed to the follow-up study. Assessment was by personal interview for 122 women, telephone interview for 18 women and postal questionnaire for the other 15. Analysis was on the basis of intention-to-treat and the researchers found no differences between subjective measures of back pain reported by patients or objective measures of spine mobility.

The other RCT involved 611 women who were randomized to receive epidural bupivacaine or intramuscular meperidine.[22] Each woman was interviewed and asked about back pain 24 h after delivery. A follow-up questionnaire was mailed out 6 months after birth with 508 women returning completed forms: 249 in the epidural group and 259 in the meperidine group (83%). Considering all questionnaire responders, the

Table 17.4 Backache during pregnancy, and at 3 and 12 months postpartum. Values are given as N (%).[21]

	Antenatal		3 months postpartum		12 months postpartum	
	Epidural N = 176	Non-epidural N = 181	Epidural N = 162	Non-epidural N = 151	Epidural N = 166	Non-epidural N = 158
Middle backache	44 (25)	54 (30)	35 (22)	30 (20)	26 (16)	25 (16)
Lower backache	91 (52)	93 (51)	56 (35)	52 (34)	58 (35)	43 (27)

prevalence of postpartum backache was not different in the epidural and meperidine groups (48% vs 50%). Stepwise logistic regression showed the only association with postpartum backache was the duration of the first stage of labor. Women with a history of backache before delivery were removed, leaving the prevalence of backache 6 months postpartum as 29% in the epidural group and 28% in the meperidine group. Logistic regression again failed to find any associations with postpartum backache. The new-onset backache data was analyzed one final time by analgesia received rather than intention-to-treat. Women with new-onset backache were more likely to have received epidural analgesia ($P = 0.02$, Mann–Whitney U-test). However, after stepwise logistic regression analysis, the only positive associations with new-onset backache were non-Caucasian women and the duration of the first stage of labor. Type of analgesia received was not associated with new-onset backache.

Conclusions

Back pain is a common problem with an annual prevalence of 25–50% in women of reproductive age and a period prevalence during pregnancy of up to 76%. There are numerous factors that correlate with postpartum back pain that are independent of the type of analgesia received by the parturient. When determining whether or not epidural analgesia causes an increased incidence of back pain, it is important to balance these predisposing factors. Ideally, this is performed using RCTs in which women are assigned to receive epidural analgesia or non-epidural analgesia. When this is carried out, there is no difference in the incidence of back pain. However, the main methodologic problem with this approach is that some patients receive epidural analgesia even though they are assigned to the non-epidural group. The reverse may also occur. In the studies cited above, the incidence of this type of crossover was approximately 30%. When analyzing the data as "intent-to-treat," these patients "contaminate" the data and reduce the apparent difference between groups. When studying chronic back pain in this setting, prospective studies have the advantage that the exposure (epidural or non-epidural analgesia) is well documented and there is no contamination. However, it is possible that the

antecedent risk factors for postpartum low back pain may not be equally distributed.

In this case, RCTs and prospective cohort studies yield the same result – new, long-term postpartum back pain is not caused by intrapartum epidural analgesia. This statement can be made with confidence because two different types of study design give the same answer.

References

1 MacArthur C, Lewis M, Knox EG, Crawford JS. Epidural anaesthesia and long-term backache after childbirth. *BMJ* 1990;**301**:9–12.
2 Lieberman E, O'Donoghue C. Unintended effects of epidural analgesia during labor: a systematic review. *Am J Obstet Gynecol* 2002;**186**:S31–S68.
3 Thorp JA, Breedlove G. Epidural analgesia in labor: an evaluation of risks and benefits. *Birth* 1996;**23**:63–83.
4 Coggon D, Rose G, Barker DJP. *Epidemiology for the Uninitiated.* London: BMJ Publishing Group, 1997.
5 van Tulder M, Koes B, Bombardier C. Low back pain. *Best Pract Res Clin Rheumatol* 2002;**16**:761–75.
6 Atlas SJ, Nardin RA. Evaluation and treatment of low back pain: an evidence-based approach to clinical care. *Muscle Nerve* 2003;**27**:265–84.
7 Leboeuf-Yde C, Kyvik KO. At what age does low back pain become a common problem? A study of 29,424 individuals aged 12–41 years. *Spine* 1998;**23**:228–34.
8 Ostgaard HC, Andersson GB. Previous back pain and risk of developing back pain in a future pregnancy. *Spine* 1991;**16**:432–6.
9 Ostgaard HC, Andersson GB. Postpartum low-back pain. *Spine* 1992;**17**:53–5.
10 Ostgaard HC, Roos-Hansson E, Zetherstrom G. Regression of back and posterior pelvic pain after pregnancy. *Spine* 1996;**21**:2777–80.
11 Noren L, Ostgaard S, Johansson G, Ostgaard HC. Lumbar back and posterior pelvic pain during pregnancy: a 3-year follow-up. *Eur Spine J* 2002;**11**:267–71.
12 Perkins J, Hammer RL, Loubert PV. Identification and management of pregnancy-related low back pain. *J Nurs Midwifery* 1998;**43**:331–40.
13 MacArthur C, Lewis M, Knox EG. *Health after Childbirth.* London: HMSO, 1991.
14 Macarthur C, Macarthur A, Weeks S. Accuracy of recall of back pain after delivery. *BMJ* 1996;**313**:467.
15 Macintyre C, McClure JH, Whitfield A. Backache and epidural analgesia: a retrospective survey of mothers 1 year after childbirth. *Int J Obstet Anesth* 1995;**4**:21–5.
16 Russell R, Groves P, Taub N, O'Dowd J. Assessing long-term backache after childbirth. *BMJ* 1993;**306**:1299–303.
17 Butler R, Fuller J. Back pain following epidural anaesthesia in labour. *Can J Anaesth* 1998;**45**:724–8.

18 Crawford JS. Lumbar epidural block in labour: clinical analysis. *Br J Anaesth* 1972;**44**:66–74.

19 Dawkins CJM. An analysis of complications of extradural and caudal block. *Anaesthesia* 1969;**24**:554–63.

20 Ong B, Cohen MM, Cumming M, Palahniuk RJ. Obstetrical anaesthesia at Winnipeg Women's Hospital 1975–83: anaesthetic techniques and complications. *Can J Anaesth* 1987;**34**:294–9.

21 Howell CJ, Dean T, Lucking L, Dziedzic K, Jones PW, Johanson RB. Randomised study of long-term outcome after epidural versus non-epidural analgesia during labour. *BMJ* 2002;**325**:357–9.

22 Loughnan BA, Carli F, Romney M, Dore CJ, Gordon H. Epidural analgesia and backache: a randomized controlled comparison with intramuscular meperidine for analgesia during labour. *Br J Anaesth* 2002;**89**:466–72.

23 Breen TW, Campbell DC, Halpern SH, Muir HA, Blanchard W. Epidural analgesia and back pain following delivery: a prospective randomized study. *Anesthesiology* 1999;**90**:A7.

24 Breen TW, Ransil BJ, Groves PA, Oriol NE. Factors associated with back pain after childbirth. *Anesthesiology* 1994;**81**:29–34.

25 Macarthur A, Macarthur C, Weeks S. Epidural anesthesia and low back pain after delivery: a prospective cohort study. *BMJ* 1995;**311**:1336–9.

26 Macarthur AJ, Macarthur C, Weeks SK. Is epidural anesthesia in labor associated with chronic low back pain? A prospective cohort study. *Anesth Analg* 1997;**85**:1066–70.

27 Patel M, Fernando R, Gill P, Urquart J, Morgan B. A prospective study on long-term backache after childbirth in primigravidae: the effect of ambulatory epidural analgesia during labor. *Int J Obstet Anesth* 1995;**4**:187.

28 Russell R, Dundas R, Reynolds F. Long-term backache after childbirth: prospective search for causative factors. *BMJ* 1996;**312**:1384–8.

29 Thompson JF, Roberts CL, Currie M, Ellwood DA. Prevalance and persistence of health problems after childbirth: associations with parity and method of birth. *Birth* 2002;**29**:83–94.

30 To WW, Wong MW. Factors associated with back pain symptoms in pregnancy and the persistence of pain 2 years after pregnancy. *Acta Obstet Gynecol Scand* 2003;**82**:1086–91.

31 Howell CJ, Kidd C, Roberts W, *et al.* A randomised controlled trial of epidural compared with non-epidural analgesia in labour. *Br J Obstet Gynaecol* 2001;**108**:27–33.

CHAPTER 18

Analgesia for external cephalic version

William Wight

Introduction

Approximately 3–5% of term, singleton pregnancies are associated with the breech position.[1,2] The international Term Breech Trial provided sufficient evidence to convince obstetricians that planned cesarean section is better than planned vaginal birth for the term fetus in the breech presentation.[1] This study was a multicenter randomized controlled trial in 2088 women with singleton breech at term (≥ 37 weeks' gestation). The perinatal and neonatal morbidity and serious neonatal morbidity was significantly lower in the planned cesarean section group compared with the planned vaginal birth group (relative risk [RR] 0.33; 95% confidence interval [CI], 0.19–0.56). The study involved a large number of participants and was well conducted, giving the potential for broad generalizability to the care of women with a singleton fetus presenting in the breech position at term. This was especially apparent when applied to countries with low perinatal mortality, as demonstrated by subgroup analysis within the study.

Because of the results of the Term Breech Trial, most obstetricians feel obliged to deliver all singleton breech fetuses by cesarean section. External cephalic version (ECV) is an obstetric maneuver used during pregnancy to attempt to turn the breech fetus to a cephalic presentation, so attempting to reduce the need for surgical delivery. Indeed, using ECV at term has been shown to decrease the number of noncephalic presentations at birth and lower the rate of cesarean section associated with breech pregnancy.[3]

There is considerable variation in the reported success rate of ECV. In prospective investigations the success rate ranges from 35% to 86%, with an overall average of 58%.[4] A number of attempts have been made to identify maternal or fetal variables that are influential in the success or failure of ECV. Most studies report a positive association between parity and successful version.[4] Opinion is divided about how well other factors predict success, including amniotic fluid volume, location of placenta and maternal weight.[4] There are several interventions that may improve the success rates for ECV. The use of tocolytic drugs, which relax the uterus, results in fewer failures (RR 0.74; 95% CI, 0.64–0.87).[5] In one small study enhancement of fetal movement through vibroacoustic stimulation in the midline fetal spinal position is also associated with fewer failures.[6]

Maternal discomfort during attempted ECV may lead to involuntary splinting of abdominal musculature that may interfere with version efforts. At times, considerable force directed towards the maternal abdomen[7] can cause enough pain that some patients may request that version be discontinued.[8] Maternal analgesia may obtund any painful stimuli and so decrease maternal anxiety and promote muscle relaxation.

Historically, general anesthesia has been used to increase the success of ECV.[9] These authors noted a success rate of 50% after failure of ECV without anesthesia. Unfortunately, there was a relatively high incidence of fetal demise (1%) in their series. The use of general anesthesia was abandoned after similar results were noted by other investigators.[10]

The purpose of this chapter is to review the available evidence regarding the influence of maternal regional analgesia on the success rate of ECV. There are currently no randomized trials evaluating other forms of analgesia for ECV. The search strategy consisted of the use of electronic databases (MEDLINE®, EMBASE® and Science Citation Index®), manual searches of major obstetric and anesthesia journals and reference listings. The last search was performed in March 2004. The following MeSH terms and text words were used in the search: [analgesia, epidural], [anesthesia, epidural], [anaesthesia, epidural], [analgesia, spinal], [anesthesia, spinal], [anaesthesia, spinal], [analgesia, obstetrical], [anesthesia, obstetrical], [anaesthesia, obstetrical], [breech] and [external cephalic version]. Abstracts and articles in languages other than English were considered. Included in the review are all studies, but critical appraisal is reserved only for studies that are either randomized controlled trials or prospective cohort studies.

Non-randomized trials

There was one retrospective[8] and one prospective[11] clinical trial that studied the incidence of successful version with and without regional anesthesia. In addition, there were three studies that reported the incidence of successful version under regional anesthesia after a failed version without anesthesia.[12–14] The design of these studies are shown in Table 18.1. The main results are shown in Table 18.2.

Retrospective studies

There has been one retrospective cohort study assessing the effect of epidural anesthesia on the success and safety of ECV performed at term.[8] In this study, the records of 61 patients who underwent ECV were reviewed; of these, eight patients had ECV terminated because of pain but later had ECV under epidural analgesia during the same hospitalization. In total there were 69 ECV attempts: 32 with epidural and 37 without epidural. ECV was successful in 59% of the women with epidurals (including seven of the eight having a second attempt with analgesia) and in 24% of women with no epidural ($P < 0.05$). There has been one retrospective cohort study looking at the effect of regional anesthesia on success rates of ECV at term only after a failed ECV attempt with no maternal analgesia.[12] In this study, 52% of ECV attempts with no analgesia were successful in a cohort of 77 patients. Of the 37 failures, 15 consented to further attempts under regional anesthesia. Five of six (83%) of ECV attempts were successful with spinal anesthesia and eight of nine (89%) ECV attempts were successful with epidural anesthesia.

Prospective studies

Birnbach et al.[11] attempted to determine whether analgesia produced by subarachnoid sufentanil would improve the success of ECV at term. Patients who were candidates for term ECV were offered spinal analgesia for the procedure, consisting of 10 μg intrathecal sufentanil following a 500-mL intravenous bolus of Ringer's solution. All patients from both groups received subcutaneous tocolysis before the procedure. Twenty of 35 patients receiving ECV opted for spinal analgesia. The two groups were well matched for parity, gestational age, estimated fetal weight and other demographic parameters. ECV was successful in 80% of the spinal analgesia group and 33% of the no analgesia group ($P = 0.005$). This difference was still statistically significant when the number of attempts was taken into account using logistic regression. There were no episodes of fetal bradycardia or placental abruption in the spinal group, although one patient in the control group required an emergency cesarean section for fetal distress. None of the study patients developed a postdural puncture headache (PDPH). Of note, the pain scores in the control group were much higher (median score 6 out of 10 vs 2 out of 10) than in the spinal anesthesia group. Further, patient satisfaction was significantly better in the study group (median visual analog score [VAS] score of 10 out of 10 vs 5 out of 10). Forty percent of patients in the spinal group complained of pruritus, although none required treatment. In this clinical trial, the success in the control group was lower than the historical success rate under similar circumstances (33% vs 45%). However, the use of spinal anesthesia was still associated with a significantly better incidence of success ($P = 0.03$).

The effect of epidural analgesia on term ECV success rates after a failed ECV attempt with no analgesia has been explored in two prospective studies.[13,14] Neiger et al.[13] studied 83 women undergoing ECV without analgesia. Of these, 33 were unsuccessful and 16 elected to undergo repeat ECV attempts under epidural analgesia. Nine of the 16 previous failures (56%) were successful. Rozenberg et al.[14] studied 73 out of a total of 169 patients having failed ECV with no analgesia, of whom 68 consented to a second attempt under epidural analgesia. An additional 22 (39.7%) of these were successful.

All studies reported a very low incidence of complications which appeared to be unrelated to regional

Table 18.1 Non-randomized trials.

Study	Population	Study design	Control (N)	Study (N)	Intervention	Tocolysis	Comments
Studies of first attempted versions							
Carlan et al. 1994[8]	Mixed, > 36 weeks, some dilated or in labor	Retrospective	37	32	Epidural	According to physician preference	More versions attempted by housestaff in the epidural group. 4/37 (control) vs 11/32 (epidural) patients in labor at the time of version
Birnbach et al. 2001[11]	Mixed, > 36 weeks, not in labor	Prospective	15	20	Spinal sufentanil	Subcutaneous terbutaline	Non-spinal group were offered IV meperidine
Studies of repeat versions							
Neiger et al. 1998[13]	Mixed, > 36 weeks	? Retrospective	83 failed versions		Epidural	Subcutaneous terbutaline	Comparison group of patients who underwent initial version (n = 25) with epidural
Rozenberg et al. 2000[14]	Mixed, about 36 weeks	Prospective	68 failed versions		Epidural	Subcutaneous salbutamol	Cost analysis
Cherayil et al. 2002[12]	Mixed, > 36 weeks, not in labor	Retrospective	15 failed versions		Epidural or spinal	Terbutaline for the first attempt, nitroglycerin during the trial	

IV, intravenous

Table 18.2 Non-randomized trials results.

Study	Success rate (treatment vs control)	Risk difference (and 95% CI)	Cesarean delivery rate	Complications
Studies of first attempted versions				
Carlan *et al.* 1994[8]	Treatment 19/32 (59%) Control 24/37 (24%)	35% (13–57%) in favor of the treatment group	Treatment 15/32 Control 24/37 $P < 0.05$	The incidence of abruptio placentae, fetal bradycardia, low Apgar scores, and low umbilical artery pH was similar External cephalic version in the control group was discontinued in 8 women because of pain – 7 of these were successful after epidural analgesia
Birnbach *et al.* 2001[11]	Treatment 16/20 Control 5/15	47% (17–76%) in favor of the treatment group	NA	One patient in the control group had a placental abruption
Studies of repeat versions				
Neiger *et al.* 1998[13]	50/83 (60%) 16/33 failures underwent repeat version 1 week later with 7/16 success	NA	17/33 failures had an elective cesarean section ? cesarean section rate in successes	Fetal bradycardia in 2 patients with successful version, associated with oligohydramnios and good Apgar scores
Rozenberg *et al.* 2000[14]	27/68 (40%)	NA		Complications in 2 patients Higher cost associated with version than expectant management
Cherayil *et al.* 2002[12]	13/15	NA	3/13 2/2 (after 2nd failed version)	2 patients had fetal bradycardia resulting in emergency cesarean delivery

CI, confidence interval; NA, not applicable.

analgesia (Table 18.2). Only one of the studies clearly reported the cesarean section rate after successful version.[12] From these results it would appear that there may be some value to attempting ECV with epidural analgesia after a failed attempt. This is true now, from a cost–benefit point of view, when most obstetric units follow a policy of planned cesarean section for breech deliveries.[14]

Randomized controlled trials

There are four randomized controlled trials comparing success rates of ECV with and without regional analgesia.[15–18] The design of these studies is shown in Table 18.3. The main results are shown in Table 18.4. Schorr *et al.*[18] randomized 69 patients to receive either epidural analgesia or no analgesia for ECV at term. Sample size was calculated to determine a 30% difference with a power of 80% and alpha of 0.05, although

the baseline success rate is not stated. Inclusion criteria were breech presentation or transverse lie. Exclusion criteria were placenta previa, fetal compromise, intrauterine growth restriction and ruptured membranes. Because of the nature of the intervention, there was no blinding of patients, obstetricians or investigators in this study beyond the randomization process. Those assigned to the epidural group received an intravenous preload of 2000 mL lactated Ringer's solution and then epidural anesthesia consisting of 2% lidocaine with 1 : 200,000 epinephrine administered in a manner to obtain anesthesia at the level of the sixth thoracic dermatome. Tocolysis with terbutaline was performed in all patients, in sequential standardized doses, titrated to effect. ECV was attempted up to a maximum of three attempts, with transvaginal elevation of the fetus performed when deemed necessary by the obstetrician performing the version. All randomized patients were included in the analysis. Patient demographics were

Table 18.3 Study design of randomized trials.

Study	Parity	Quality	Control (N)	Study (N)	Intervention	Tocolysis	Comments
Schorr et al. 1997[18]	Mixed	Concealed randomization Sample size calculation All patients accounted for	35	34	Epidural lidocaine 2% to T6 level	Subcutaneous terbutaline	Performed by 3rd and 4th year residents with perinatal fellow as back-up
Dugoff et al. 1999[16]	Mixed	Concealed randomization Sample size calculation based on a 50% baseline success rate All patients accounted for	52	50	Spinal sufentanil and bupivacaine to T6 level	Subcutaneous terbutaline	Performed by "staff physicians" under supervision of attending physicians Maximum 4 attempts
Mancuso et al. 2000[17]	Mixed	Concealed randomization, adequacy of randomization checked Sample size calculation based on a baseline success rate of 30%	54	54	Epidural lidocaine 2% 13 mL	Subcutaneous terbutaline	Residents performed the versions in the presence of experienced staff
Delisle et al. 2001[15]	Mixed	Sample size calculation based on a baseline success rate of 22%	99	103	Spinal fentanyl and bupivacaine	Nitroglycerin in 60% of controls and 29% of study patients	Abstract + personal communication 4 attempts

Table 18.4 Randomized trials – results.

Study	Success rate (treatment vs control)	Risk difference (95% CI)	Cesarean delivery rate	Complications
Schorr et al. 1997[18]	24/35 with epidural 10/34 control	39% (17–61%)	12/35 with epidural 27/34 control	Unsuccessful epidural (1 patient) No placental abruptions in either group
Dugoff et al. 1999[16]	22/50 with spinal 22/52 control	2% (–18 to 21%)	34/50 with spinal 27/52 control	*Fetal bradycardia* 11/50 with spinal 6/52 control *Hypotension* 4/50 with spinal 0/52 control *Abruption* 0/50 with spinal 1/52 control *Patient discomfort* 0/50 with spinal 4/52 control
Mancuso et al. 2000[17]	32/54 with epidural 18/54 control	26% (8–44%)	25/54 with epidural 37/54 control	*Fetal bradycardia* 2/54 with epidural 3/54 control *Hypotension* 0/54 with epidural 0/54 with control
Delisle et al. 2001[15]	41/99 with spinal 31/103 control	11% (–2 to 24%)	?	1 urgent cesarean section in the spinal group for non-reassuring fetal heart rate tracing

CI, confidence interval.

not significantly different between the groups. Patients with a transverse lie were included in the study, and were evenly distributed between the groups.

There was a significantly higher success rate in the epidural group (69%) compared with the no epidural group (29%). The risk difference (RD) was 39% and the 95% CI was 17–61% (Table 18.4). The number-needed-to-treat (NNT) with epidural analgesia was 2.5 (95% CI, 1.6–5.8) patients to have a successful ECV in one additional patient. The corresponding cesarean section rate was 34% in the epidural group compared with 79% in the no epidural group (Table 18.4). The RD was 45% and the 95% CI was 24–66%. The NNT was 2.2 (95% CI, 1.5–4.1). ECV was abandoned in one patient in the epidural group (failed epidural) and in four patients in the no epidural group because of discomfort. There were no epidural complications reported, and no episodes of maternal hypotension or fetal bradycardias occurred. Only one patient (control group) reverted to breech after ECV. Of interest, patients in the epidural group spent less time in hospital (3.1 vs 4.9 days, $P = 0.05$) than patients in the control group.

Transvaginal elevation of the fetus may be particularly useful in a well-descended breech but may not be tolerated by the control patients because of the absence of maternal analgesia. The success rate in the control group was low when compared with published success rates for ECV, possibly indicating differences between this patient population and other population groups. The epidural group received intravenous preloading with 2000 mL lactated Ringer's solution prior to siting of the epidural and then presumably several minutes to achieve analgesia. This co-intervention may have led to an increase in the volume of amniotic fluid in the epidural group compared with the no epidural group,[19] and therefore may have contributed to the improved ECV success rate in the epidural group.[20]

Mancuso et al.[17] studied the effect of epidural analgesia on ECV success rates. In this study, 108 parturients were randomized to either receive epidural or no epidural prior to ECV. This was based upon a sample size estimation with a power of 80% and an alpha of 0.05, in an attempt to see a twofold increase in ECV success from an institutional baseline success rate of 30%. Inclusion and exclusion criteria were similar to the study by Schorr et al.[18] including the enrollment of parturients with a transverse lie. Also, the baseline

success rate, without analgesia, was similar. Patients in both groups received an intravenous preload of 1500 mL lactated Ringer's solution before version attempts. Those assigned to the epidural group received epidural anesthesia consisting of 2% lidocaine with 1 : 200,000 epinephrine and fentanyl 100 µg administered in a manner to obtain anesthesia at the level of the tenth thoracic dermatome. Tocolysis was given to all patients prior to ECV attempts. ECV was attempted up to a maximum of four attempts, with no employment of the transvaginal elevation technique. Demographics between the two groups were similar and all patients were included in the analysis. There was a significantly higher success rate in the epidural group (59%) compared with the no epidural group (33%). The RD was 26% and the 95% CI was 8–44% (Table 18.4). The NNT with epidural analgesia was 3.8 (95% CI, 2.2–12.5) patients to have a successful ECV in one additional patient. The corresponding cesarean section rate was 46% in the epidural group compared with 68% in the no epidural group (Table 18.4). The RD was 22% and the 95% CI was 4–40%. The NNT was 4.5 (95% CI, 2.5–25). The study does not report the number of ECV procedures that were abandoned because of patient discomfort. None of the fetuses reverted to breech position after successful version, although one of the unsuccessful versions in the control group became a cephalic presentation spontaneously. Four patients (one in the epidural group and three in the control group) had a vaginal delivery of a breech fetus. Two patients in the epidural group and three in the control experienced fetal bradycardia. None developed hypotension.

The results of this study are similar to that of Shorr et al.[18] in a number of important respects. In both studies, the treatment group was epidural analgesia with lidocaine. In both studies, the success rate in the control group was low – approximately 33%. Although both groups received an intravenous preload prior to ECV attempts, the fluid was administered in the epidural group prior to commencing the epidural, whereas the no epidural group received the fluid bolus immediately prior to the ECV. The time needed for the fluid in the no epidural group to affect amniotic fluid volume may have been insufficient compared with the epidural group.

Dugoff et al.[16] studied 102 term parturients who were randomized to receive either spinal anesthesia or no spinal (control) for ECV. Using a baseline success rate of 50% for ECV, the sample size was calculated to determine a clinically significant 20% difference in the two groups on the basis of a power of 80% and an alpha of 0.05. Unlike the previous two studies, patients with a transverse lie were excluded. Those parturients in the spinal group received an intrathecal injection of 10 µg sufentanil and 2.5 mg plain bupivacaine after prehydration with 500 mL lactated Ringer's solution. The level of anesthesia obtained was the sixth thoracic dermatome. Parturients in both groups received tocolysis prior to ECV attempts. ECV was performed by two physicians, up to a total of four attempts. No attempt to elevate the breech by the transvaginal route was performed. The analysis of results was performed on an intent-to-treat basis and all patients were included in the analysis. Patient demographics were similar between the two groups. There was no difference between success rates for the spinal group (44%) and the control group (42%). Sixty eight percent of patients in the spinal group had a cesarean section compared with 52% of control ($P = 0.1$). ECV was terminated before a successful result in four patients in the control group because of discomfort. Transient fetal bradycardia occurred in 22% of the spinal group and 11% of the control group ($P = 0.2$). Four parturients in the spinal group had transient hypotension, three of whom needed pharmacologic intervention. One patient, in the control group, had placental abruption necessitating cesarean delivery despite a successful version. Two of the patients in the spinal group who had a successful version reverted to the breech position before delivery.

The final randomized control trial, conducted by Delisle et al.,[15] has been published in abstract form only; further information has been made available by personal communication with the study's main author (M.F. Delisle, personal communication 2004). Two hundred and two parturients were randomized to receive spinal anesthesia or no spinal (control), based upon detecting a 50% difference in success rate from a baseline of 22% with a power of 80% and an alpha of 0.05. The inclusion and exclusion criteria were similar those of Schorr et al.,[18] including the enrollment of all non-vertex lies. The spinal anesthesia was performed using 2.5 mg plain bupivacaine with 20 µg fentanyl to obtain anesthesia to the sixth thoracic dermatome. The use of fluid preload is not reported. Patients received

tocolysis with intravenous nitroglycerin at the discretion of the physician. ECV attempts were made up to a total of four attempts. It is not reported whether the transvaginal elevation technique was employed.

Demographics data were similar between the two groups, and all patients were included in the analysis. There was no statistical difference between the success rates in the spinal group and the control group (41% vs 30%, $P = 0.09$). However, the use of tocolysis was higher in the control group (60% vs 29%). After controlling for the use of tocolysis there was still no evidence that the success rate differs between the two groups. The cesarean section rate was not reported. There were more complications such as maternal hypotension and fetal heart rate abnormalities in the spinal group compared with the control group (39% vs 15%). One patient in the spinal group needed urgent delivery 55 min after the procedure for a non-reassuring fetal heart rate trace.

Conclusions

The evidence supports the use of ECV in an attempt to reduce the incidence of breech presentation because there was a low incidence of reverting after turning. Further, a large proportion of those that turned eventually went on to vaginal delivery. The complication rate is low and therefore the maneuver is potentially useful in reducing the cesarean section rate.

The current published data give conflicting evidence on the influence of maternal analgesia on the success rate of ECV at term. While the non-randomized trials are positive,[8,11] the randomized controlled trials do not show a clear advantage to regional analgesia before ECV.[15–18] Of interest when examining the randomized controlled trials, epidural analgesia appears to be more useful than spinal anesthesia for the facilitation of ECV. While both techniques provide analgesia, epidural analgesia, using the doses of lidocaine reported in these studies, is more likely to produce muscle relaxation – thus making ECV easier. However, it should be noted that in both studies using epidural analgesia, the success rate in the control group was low. One could postulate that the control rate, rather than the technique used, may be more important in determining the success than the type of analgesia. Alternately, the additional fluid given to patients who received epidural analgesia may have played a part.

Finally, other evidence suggests that the use of tocolytics on all patients may help increase the success rate[5] and therefore selective use[15] may not yield optimal results.

All of the studies show an improvement in success rate when regional analgesia is used after ECV without analgesia fails.[12–14] It may therefore be useful to use regional analgesia in those patients.

It should be noted that regional analgesia adds risk to ECV. Although none of the studies reported significant side-effects, these may become apparent when regional analgesia is used on more patients. Other, less invasive methods of producing analgesia prior to ECV, in conjunction with tocolytics, need to be evaluated.

References

1 Hannah ME, Hannah WJ, Hewson SA, Hodnett ED, Saigal S, Willan AR. Planned caesarean section versus planned vaginal birth for breech presentation at term: a randomised multicentre trial. Term Breech Trial Collaborative Group. *Lancet* 2000;**356**:1375–83.

2 Hickok DE, Gordon DC, Milberg JA, Williams MA, Daling JR. The frequency of breech presentation by gestational age at birth: a large population-based study. *Am J Obstet Gynecol* 1992;**166**:851–2.

3 Hofmeyr GJ, Kulier R. External cephalic version for breech presentation at term (Cochrane Review). *Cochrane Library* January 2004.

4 American College of Obstetricians and Gynecologists. ACOG practice patterns. External cephalic version. *Int J Gynaecol Obstet* 1997;**59**:73–80.

5 Hofmeyr GJ. Interventions to help external cephalic version for breech presentation at term. [Update of *Cochrane Database Syst Rev* 2001;**1**:CD000184; PMID: 11687071. Review. 37 refs.] *Cochrane Database Syst Rev* 2002;CD000184.

6 Annapoorna V, Arulkumaran S, Anandakumar C, Chua S, Montan S, Ratnam SS. External cephalic version at term with tocolysis and vibroacoustic stimulation. *Int J Gynaecol Obstet* 1997;**59**:13–8.

7 Leung TY, Sahota DS, Fok WY, Chan LW, Lau TK. Quantification of contact surface pressure exerted during external cephalic version. *Acta Obstet Gynaecol Scand* 2003;**82**:1017–22.

8 Carlan SJ, Dent JM, Huckaby T, Whittington EC, Shaefer D. The effect of epidural anesthesia on safety and success of external cephalic version at term. *Anesth Analg* 1994;**79**:525–8.

9 Ellis R. External cephalic version under anesthesia. *J Obstet Gynaecol Br Comm* 1968;**75**:865–70.

10 Mushambi M. External cephalic version: new interest and old concerns. *Int J Obstet Anesth* 2001;**10**:263–6.

11 Birnbach DJ, Matut J, Stein DJ, *et al.* The effect of intrathecal analgesia on the success of external cephalic version. *Anesth Analg* 2001;**93**:410–3.

12 Cherayil G, Feinberg B, Robinson J, Tsen LC. Central neuraxial blockade promotes external cephalic version success after a failed attempt. *Anesth Analg* 2002;**94**:1589–92.

13 Neiger R, Hennessy MD, Patel M. Reattempting failed external cephalic version under epidural anesthesia. *Am J Obstet Gynecol* 1998;**179**:1136–9.

14 Rozenberg P, Goffinet F, de Spirlet M, *et al.* External cephalic version with epidural anaesthesia after failure of a first trial with beta-mimetics. *Br J Obstet Gynaecol* 2000;**107**:406–10.

15 Delisle MF, Kamani A, Douglas J, Bebbington M. Antepartum external cephalic version under spinal anesthesia: a randomized controlled trial. *Am J Obstet Gynecol* 2001;**185**:A124.

16 Dugoff L, Stamm CA, Jones OW, III, Mohling SI, Hawkins JL. The effect of spinal anesthesia on the success rate of external cephalic version: a randomized trial. *Obstet Gynecol* 1999;**93**:345–9.

17 Mancuso KM, Yancey MK, Murphy JA, Markenson GR. Epidural analgesia for cephalic version: a randomized trial. *Obstet Gynecol* 2000;**95**:648–51.

18 Schorr SJ, Speights SE, Ross EL, *et al.* A randomized trial of epidural anesthesia to improve external cephalic version success. *Am J Obstet Gynecol* 1997;**177**:1133–7.

19 Hofmeyr GJ. Maternal hydration for increasing amniotic fluid volume in oligohydramnios and normal amniotic fluid volume. In: *Cochrane Update Software*, issue 1. Oxford, 2002.

20 Hellstrom AC, Nilsson B, Stange L, Nylund L. When does external cephalic version succeed? *Acta Obstet Gynaecol Scand* 1990;**69**:281–5.

CHAPTER 19

Is there a difference between the obstetric and non-obstetric airway?

Eric Goldszmidt

Introduction

Failed endotracheal intubation with subsequent inability to ventilate the parturient is an important cause of maternal mortality and morbidity.[1] Many review articles[1-8] and book chapters[9,10] declare that airway management – in particular endotracheal intubation – in the parturient is more difficult than in the non-parturient. Some authors suggest that a significant proportion of pregnant women should be intubated awake to avoid this complication.[11] Common reasons offered to explain the difference between the pregnant and non-pregnant patient include: increased upper airway edema and fat deposition causing decreased soft-tissue mobility and increased tongue size. Most pregnant patients have full dentition, enlarged breasts and may have gained significant amounts of weight. Thoracic lift from a poorly placed hip wedge and overly aggressive cricoid pressure may exacerbate a difficult situation.

General anesthesia for pregnant patients under emergency conditions may be anxiety-provoking for the anesthesiologist, leading to an incomplete assessment of the patient. This further compounds any potential difficulties. Parturients undergoing emergency general anesthesia are seldom fasted and are at increased risk for aspiration pneumonitis. Further, because of a high metabolic rate and decreased functional residual capacity, oxygen desaturation may occur during apnea, increasing the risk of fetal and caregiver distress. Finally, as a consequence of the increased use of regional anesthesia, it is more difficult for trainees to gain experience using general anesthesia in the parturient[1] and possibly more difficult for the more experienced anesthesiologist to maintain expertise.

This chapter discusses whether or not it is more difficult to perform endotracheal intubation in parturients compared with non-pregnant patients. Ideally, this question could be answered in an appropriately designed prospective cohort study. The patients would be matched for identifiable risk factors for difficult intubation and the same anesthesiologists would perform endotracheal intubation using the same techniques for both populations. In addition, the ancillary help and work environment would be controlled. The definition of "difficulty" or "failure to intubate" would be standardized. Finally, because the incidence is small, a large study would be needed. If one considers that the rate of difficult intubation is approximately 2% in parturients, the study would need to include approximately 9000 patients per group to find a difference of 75% (to 0.5% in non-parturients) to demonstrate a difference if one existed. Unfortunately, such a clinical trial does not currently exist. However, considerable data do exist that may help determine:

1 whether endotracheal intubation is more difficult in the population of parturients than in the population of non-parturients; and

2 which parturients are at risk for difficult airway management.

Population-based studies

The data for this systematic review are derived from all studies that report and estimate the incidence of difficult intubation in the parturient. These studies were located using MEDLINE® and EMBASE® from 1966 and 1980, respectively, until the end of December 2002. These studies were either comparative (obstetric and non-obstetric populations in the same study) or derived an incidence of difficult intubation from the collected data. Additional comparative data were derived from large prospective studies (N > 5000) in non-pregnant patients. Case reports, case series and case–controlled studies were not included because an incidence from this type of data cannot be calculated.

The primary outcome was the incidence of failure to intubate as defined by the authors. Secondary outcomes were the incidence of difficult intubation (as defined by the authors) and the total of grade 3 and 4 laryngoscopic views as defined by Cormack and Lehane.[2] Grade 3 laryngoscopies yield only a view of the epiglottis, whereas grade 4 views do not even reveal the epiglottis.

Eleven studies reported the incidence of difficult intubation or failed intubation in parturients. Two of these were abstracts,[11,12] the rest were full manuscripts.[13–21] One paper included the data from a previous paper[16] so those data are only considered once.[15] Four of these studies include an obstetric and non-obstetric comparison group.[12,18,20,21] The study characteristics are shown in Table 19.1.

For comparison, five large studies of the non-obstetric airway were found.[22–26] Their characteristics, along with the four studies with both an obstetric and non-obstetric group, are shown in Table 19.2.

Quality of studies

Obstetric patients

Many studies that determine the incidence of difficult or failed endotracheal intubation in the obstetric patient do not provide reliable data. The two comparative prospective studies that are published as full manuscripts are too small to determine the accurate incidence of difficult intubation, as defined by grade 3 or 4 laryngoscopic view.[20,21] A third study, available only as an abstract, does not describe the laryngoscopic view seen by the anesthesiologist, rather it reports quality assurance markers for difficult intubation such as trauma to the airway, documented esophageal intubation or the need to change from the planned method endotracheal intubation.[12] The fourth – and largest – study is retrospective.[18] The data were obtained from a registry of difficult intubation, but it is not possible to tell how complete the data collection was. In addition, the authors classified endotracheal intubation as difficult subjectively.

There are six large studies designed to determine the incidence of difficult or failed endotracheal intubation in the parturient. One prospective cohort study (N = 1500) defined difficult endotrachal intubation as a grade 3 or 4 laryngoscopic view.[17] A second prospective study, from the same institution (N = 523), reported a higher incidence of difficult endotracheal intubation using the same criteria.[13] Unfortunately, data on 90 of the patients who received general anesthesia during the time of the study are not available, reducing the reliability of the estimated incidence. A second retrospective study (N = 536) reported a high incidence of difficult endotracheal intubation. In this study, the definition of "difficult" was not reported and therefore a comparison cannot be made with other studies.[19]

One study, reported as an abstract,[27] suggests that fiberoptic endotracheal intubation on selected obstetric patients may reduce the incidence of failed intubation. Because only an abstract is available, many of the details concerning patient assessment and operator training are missing, making the results of the study difficult to interpret. However, the investigators reported that the incidence of failed endotracheal intubation was reduced by changing their policy for the use of fiberoptic intubation in the parturient. The two remaining studies are audits.[14,16] While these are the largest studies, it is impossible to determine the completeness of data collection. Further, the definition of difficult endotracheal intubation is lacking.

Non-obstetric patients

Five large studies reported the incidence of difficult endotracheal intubation in non-obstetric patients.[22–26] All were prospective cohort studies, although one was a self-report questionnaire.[24] One study excluded emergency surgeries.[26] The primary purpose of all studies was to correlate physical examination criteria with the laryngoscopic view and therefore the data on this parameter are complete. However, the incidence of failed endotracheal intubation was dependent on the protocol. For example, in one study[23] all patients with a grade 4 view of the glottis on rigid laryngoscopy were intubated using a fiberoptic scope, reducing the incidence of failed intubation to 0%. One study excluded difficult endotracheal intubations performed by trainees with less than 6 months' experience.[24]

Table 19.1 Characteristics of obstetric airway studies. For comparative studies N is the number of pregnant patients.

Reference	Study period	Patient population	N	Airway assessment (Yes/No)	Operator experience	Definition of difficult airway or failed intubation	Quality	Comments
Comparative studies								
Wong & Hung 1999[20]	1998	Ethnic Chinese Elective cesarean section	151	Yes Assessor did not take part in intubation	Consultant or trainees with more than 3 years experience	Difficult – grade 3 or 4 view on direct laryngoscopy	Prospective comparative study, elective gynecology control group No sample size calculation	Excluded patients if an alternative method of intubation was chosen preoperatively or if delivered in previous 2 weeks (control group); only 1 failure (the only one with a group 4 view) Demonstrated poor positive predictive value for Mallampati score, thyromental distance, atlanto-occipital extension and for combinations of these Suggest that Chinese airways are no more difficult than others
Yeo & Chang 1992[21]	1991	All obstetric patients (including postpartum sterilization) vs gynecological patients	277	Yes	Registrars, senior registrars and consultants	Not formally defined	Comparative, prospective cohort study	Study designed to compare the predictive ability of a preoperative Mallampati score in obstetric and non-obstetric patients Patients were Chinese, Malay or Indian
Dhaliwal et al. 1996[12]	1991–1994	All obstetric general anesthetics vs all non-obstetric general anesthetics (n = 15,150)	466	Unknown	Unknown	A list of difficulties, both subjective (e.g. "difficult intubation") and objective (e.g. chipped tooth, alternate method of intubation used)	Abstract Audit	Differences between main operating room and obstetric difficult intubation (1.16% vs 0.86%), esophageal intubation (0.40% vs 1.29%), inability to intubate by the planned route (0.28% vs 0%) and failed rapid sequence induction (0.10% vs 1.50%) 3.64% difficulties in obstetrics vs 1.95% in main operating room Most of the difference accounted for by the number of failed rapid sequence inductions
Samsoon & Young 1987[18]	1982–1985	All obstetric patients	1980	Unknown	Unknown	Difficult – inadequate visualization of the glottis Failure – inability to insert a tracheal tube	Comparative retrospective cohort Patients were selected from a registry	Unable to assess whether all cases were found All of the obstetric patients with failed intubation had class 4 airway views except for 1 who had tracheal stenosis All of the non-obstetric patients had class 4 airway views

Continued

Table 19.1 (*continued*)

Reference	Study period	Patient population	N	Airway assessment (Yes/No)	Operator experience	Definition of difficult airway or failed intubation	Quality	Comments
Cohort studies without control group								
Barnardo & Jenkins 2000[14]	1993–1998	All obstetric patients receiving care in the South Thames region of the UK	8970	26 charts reviewed evidence of an assessment found in only 11 of these	7/26 senior house officer 14/26 registrar 5/26 staff grade or clinical assistant 1/26 consultant	Failure – intubation not accomplished with a single dose of succinylcholine	Audit 36 known failures 26 reviewed	Quality of data is unknown 23 were cesarean sections, only 4 were elective 10 general anesthetics for maternal request 16 cases occurred between 17:30 and 08:30 (outside normal working hours) Most views at laryngoscopy were grade 3–4
Ramadhani et al. 1996[13]	1994–1995	All cesarean sections	523	Yes	Consultants and trainees with more than 2 years experience	Difficult – grade 3 or 4 view on direct laryngoscopy Failure – not defined	Prospective cohort study Collected data on 523/613 patients	13/17 Grade III easily intubated 2/17 Grade III intubated blindly 2/17 Grade III failed – laryngeal mask airway 1/1 Grade IV failed – regional
Tsen et al. 1998[19]	1990–1995	All cesarean sections	536	Unknown	Unknown	Not defined	Retrospective cohort	1 failure (parturient died, general anesthesia after failure to place a spinal for elective cesarean section) It is not known if this patient was the index case which prompted the study Her preoperative airway assessment and history were unremarkable 4.5% of cesarean sections under general anesthesia with incidence decreasing over period secondary to increased use of epidurals 86% of general anesthetics because of contraindication to regional or perceived lack of time 41% of general anesthetics were given during daytime hours

Study	Years	Population	N	Airway assessment	Operator	Definitions	Study type	Comments
Hawthorne et al. 1996[15] Lyons 1985[16]	1978–1994	All cesarean sections	5802	Yes but assessments not formally recorded	78% of incidents involved a senior house officer or registrar 13% involved a senior registrar or consultant	Failure – intubation not accomplished with a single dose of succinylcholine requiring initiation of a failed intubation drill	Prospective audit	23 failures (5 Asian, 5 Afro Caribbean) 78% during evening or night 87% considered emergency 1/3 were predicted to be difficult All had at least one airway abnormality and 13 had more than one abnormality on postoperative examination 14 of the patients were easily intubated prior to or subsequent to the event 1 was intubated in the lateral position During the failed intubation drill: 6 patients were said to have laryngeal edema, at least 2 were known difficult airways and 2 others were subsequently shown to have Klippel–Feil syndrome, 1 had masseter spasm and her mouth could not be opened
Rocke et al. 1992[17]	1990–1991	Elective and emergency cesarean sections	1500	Yes	Unknown but if two anesthesiologists present, intubation by the most junior	Difficult – required some adjustment of laryngoscope or head Very difficult – required removal of laryngoscope, mask ventilation and intubation using additional equipment or senior assistance Failure – several attempts or unrecognized esophageal intubation	Prospective cohort	All airway assessments by the most senior anesthesiologist but intubations by the most junior Only 2 failures, 1 of which was easily intubated by the consultant Multivariate analysis of risk factors
Glassenberg et al. 1990[27]	1980–1989	All obstetric patients with liveborn singletons vaginal delivery of liveborn singletons	1349 (1980–1984) 744 (1985–1989)	Unknown	Unknown	Difficult – intubation on 1st attempt with difficulty or multiple attempts required Failure – could not be intubated by direct laryngoscopy	Abstract Retrospective chart review	Review performed to determine whether or not fiberoptic intubation should be carried out on anticipated difficult intubations in obstetrics

Table 19.2 Characteristics of non-obstetric airway studies with more than 5000 patients in the operating room with a comparison between obstetric and non-obstetric patients. N is the number of non-obstetric patients in comparative studies.

Reference	Study period	Patient population	N	Airway assessment (Yes/No)	Operator experience	Definition of difficult airway or failed intubation	Quality	Comments
Comparative studies								
Wong & Hung 1999[20]	1998	Ethnic Chinese women undergoing elective gynecological operations	260	Yes assessor did not take part in intubation	Consultant or trainees with more than 3 years experience	Difficult – grade 3 or 4 view on direct laryngoscopy	Prospective cohort study	See Table 19.1
Yeo et al. 1992[21]	1991	Gynecologic elective	283	Yes	Registrars, senior registrars and consultants	Not formally defined	Prospective, comparative cohort	See Table 19.1
Dhaliwal et al. 1996[12]	1991–1994	All patients	15,150	Unknown	Unknown	See Table 19.1	See Table 19.1	See Table 19.1
Samsoon & Young 1987[18]	1982–1985	Failed intubation registry	13,380	Unknown	Unknown	Difficult – inadequate visualization of the glottis Failure – inability to insert a tracheal tube from the oropharynx	Comparative retrospective cohort Patients were selected from a registry	See Table 19.1

Cohort studies without control group

Study	Year	N	Control group	Population	Operator	Difficulty definition	Study type	Comments
Yamamoto et al. 1997[26]	1996	6184	Yes	Japanese study Elective surgery, adult patients	Consultants	Difficult – grade 3 or 4 view on direct laryngoscopy	Prospective	17/19 patients with grade 4 views at laryngoscopy had anatomic abnormalities such as micrognathia, trismus or cervical spine abnormalities unanticipated grade 4 view = 0.03% of all patients
el Ganzouri et al. 1996[23]	1996	10,507	Yes	Consecutive adults	Anesthesiologists with more than 2 years experience	Difficult – grade 3 or 4 view on direct laryngoscopy	Prospective	Excluded patients with obvious airway malformations scheduled for awake intubation. Attempt to optimize intubating conditions 91% of all grade 4 views intubated fiberoptically but none of these reported as failures
Koay 1998[24]	1994–1995	5379	Yes	All patients	More than 6 months training in anesthesia	Difficult – failure to visualize the larynx during laryngoscopy after using neck flexion and cricoid pressure	Prospective cohort study Self-report	Excluded 'clinically obvious' difficult airways and difficult intubations by operators with less than 6 months experience. 40.5% of the difficult intubations were unexpected
Rose & Cohen 1994[25]	1991–1993	18,500	Yes	All patients	Not specified	Difficult – grade 3 or 4 view on direct laryngoscopy. Failure – abandonment of direct laryngoscopy	Prospective	1.9% had initial intubation attempt with alternative methods to direct laryngoscopy. No cases of failure to intubate and ventilate. 1/3 had incomplete documentation of airway assessment
Deller et al. 1990[22]	1989	8538	Yes	Consecutive surgical patients	Consultants and trainees	Difficult defined as failure by trainee and difficult for consultant	Abstract Prospective	

Table 19.3 Results of obstetric airway studies.

Study	Grade 3 % (95% CI)	Grade 4 % (95% CI)	Grade 3 + 4 % (95% CI)	Difficult intubation % (95% CI)	Failures % (95% CI)
Wong & Hung 1999[20]	1.3% (0.02–5%)	0.7% (0.01–3.6%)	1.99% (0.04–5.7%)	1.99% (0.04–5.7%)	0.7% (0.01–3.6%)
Barnardo & Jenkins 2000[14]	–	–	–	–	0.4% (0.2–0.5%)
Ramadhani et al. 1996[13]	3.3% (1.9–5.1%)	0.2% (0.02–1.0%)	3.5 (2.1–5.4%)	–	0.6% (0.1–1.6%)
Tsen et al. 1998[19]	–	–	–	5.8% (3.9–8.1%)	0.19% (0.047–1.1%)
Hawthorne et al. 1996[15]	–	–	–	–	0.4% (0.2–0.6%)
Dhaliwal et al. 1996[12]*	–	–	–	3.6% (2.1–5.6%)	–
Yeo et al. 1992[21]	–	–	2.2% (0.2–3.0%)	–	0% (0–1.1%)
Rocke et al. 1992[17]	1.7% (1.1–2.5%)	0.1% (0.02–0.5%)	1.8% (1.2–2.6%)	2% (1.3–2.8%)	0.13% (0.016–0.48%)
Samsoon & Young 1987[18]	–	–	–	–	0.35% (0.14–0.72%)
Glassenberg et al. 1990[27]†	–	–	–	2.2% (1.5–3.2%)	0.37% (0.12–0.86%)
Glassenberg et al. 1990[27]‡	–	–	–	2.6% (1.5–4.0%)	0.2% (0.34–0.74%)

CI, confidence interval.

* For this set of data, difficult defined by authors of this review as total incidence of difficult intubation, esophageal intubation, inability to intubate by the planned route and failed rapid sequence induction.

† This set of data spans 1980–1984 where no awake intubations were performed.

‡ This set of data spans 1985–1989 where 14% of anticipated difficult airways received awake intubations.

Incidence of difficult endotracheal intubation

Obstetric patients

The incidence of difficult endotracheal intubation is shown in Table 19.3. Four studies reported the incidence of grade 3 and 4 laryngoscopic view.[13,17,20,21] The incidence ranged from 1.8% to 3.5% and the 95% confidence interval range is 0.04–5.7%. This large range is because of the relatively small sample sizes of most of the studies. Two studies, using different criteria, reported the incidence of difficult intubation as 3.6%[12,21] and 5.8%,[19,21] respectively.

Inability to perform endotracheal intubation in the parturient was uncommon. The point estimate of the incidence range is 0–0.7%. The 95% confidence interval for the estimate was as high as 3.6%.[20] This study was small, resulting in a very low event rate (one).

Non-obstetric patients

The incidence of difficult endotracheal intubation in non-obstetric studies is similar (Table 19.4). Four studies reported the incidence of grade 3 and 4 laryngoscopic views.[20,21,23,24,26] The incidence ranged from 0.66% to 6.1% and the 95% confidence interval is 0.47–6.6%. The studies that report difficult intubation using other criteria[12,22,25] report an incidence between 1.2% and 1.95%. The incidence of failure of endotracheal intubations is extremely low. Of the five studies that reported the incidence, three had no failures.[20,21,23]

Table 19.4 Results of non-obstetric airway studies with more than 5000 patients in the operating room with a comparison of obstetric and non-obstetric patients.

Study	Grade 3 % (95% CI)	Grade 4 % (95% CI)	Grade 3 + 4 % (95% CI)	Difficult intubation % (95% CI)	Failures % (95% CI)
Wong & Hung 1999[20]	1.54% (0.4–3.9%)	0 (0–1.1%)	1.54% (0.4–3.9%)	1.54% (0.4–3.9%)	0% (0–1.1%)
Yamamoto et al. 1997[26]	1% (0.7–1.2%)	0.3% (0.18–0.48%)	1.3% (1.0–1.6%)	1.3% (1.0–1.6%)	–
El-Ganzouri et al. 1996[23]	5.1% (4.6–5.5%)	1.0% (0.81–1.2%)	6.1% (5.6–6.6%)	6.1% (5.6–6.6%)	0% (0–0.02%)
Koay 1998[24]	0.64% (0.44–0.88%)	0.02% (0.005–0.10%)	0.66% (0.47–0.92%)	0.7% (0.50–0.97%)	–
Dhaliwal 1996[12]*	–	–	–	1.95% (1.7–2.2%)	–
Rose & Cohen 1994[25]	–	–	–	1.8% (1.6–2.0%)	0.3% (0.23–0.39%)
Yeo et al. 1992[21]	–	–	1.8% (0.057–4.1%)	–	0% (0–1.0%)
Deller et al. 1990[22]	–	–	–	1.2% (0.05–0.2%)	–
Samsoon & Young 1987[18]	–	–	–	–	0.045% (0.03–0.06%)

CI, confidence interval.
* For this set of data, difficult was defined by authors of this review as total incidence of difficult intubation, esophageal intubation, inability to intubate by the planned route and failed rapid sequence induction.

Two of these were small studies[20,21] and the third specifically avoided attempted endotracheal intubation with a rigid laryngoscope in high-risk patients.[23]

Discussion

Data from separate clinical trials that report the incidence of difficult or failed endotracheal intubation do not confirm the impression that pregnant patients are more difficult to manage than non-pregnant patients. However, there are a number of factors that must be considered before applying these results to individual patients. In particular, it is most important to reduce the incidence of unanticipated difficult intubations.

Airway changes related to pregnancy

Although airway changes induced by pregnancy are thought to be at least partially responsible for the added difficulty in intubation, this has not been well studied. Hawthorne et al.[15] found 14/23 failures had been successfully intubated prior to or subsequent to the failure and that 6/23 failures were reported as being caused by laryngeal edema, implying that the airway changes of pregnancy were responsible for these cases. However, six other patients had anatomic or physiologic abnormalities unrelated to pregnancy. Two were documented as difficult before pregnancy, two had Klippel–Feil syndrome, one had masseter muscle spasm and one was easily intubated in the lateral position after the initial failure. Similarly, Fahy et al.[28] noted that 5/8 parturients in whom endotracheal intubation failed had persistent X-ray findings, consistent with difficult endotracheal intubation, 4–7 years later.

Rocke et al.,[17] using multivariate analysis of risk factors for difficult intubation, found that facial and tongue edema, the only factors related to pregnancy, failed to appear as independent risk factors. This may have occurred because these contributed to other assessments such as the Mallampati score.

Two recent abstracts attempted to document airway changes with labor. In the first, the investigators photographed the oropharynx of 61 healthy primigravidas in early active labor, after delivery and at 36–48 h postpartum.[29] Those who reviewed the photographs were unaware of the stage of labor at which the photographs were taken. Patients with Mallampati class 4 airways on admission were excluded. Thirty-eight percent of the included parturients had an increase of one grade (e.g. grade 1–2) at the end of labor and 5% increased by two grades. The airway reverted to the admission grade in 82% of patients by 48 h. No correlation was found between airway changes and age, height, prepregnant weight, weight gain during pregnancy, duration of stages of labor, intravenous fluid administration during labor and type of labor analgesia. The second abstract, using acoustic reflectometry during and after labor, confirmed that mean pharyngeal volumes decreased during labor in a sample of five patients.[30] Two of the five had an increase of one grade in Mallampati score. These abstracts suggest that labor and delivery may induce airway changes but their significance with respect to ease of intubation was not determined.

Pilkington et al.,[31] using standardized photography, documented an increase in the incidence of Mallampati grades 3 and 4 in term parturients compared with the first trimester. In a sample of 242 patients at 12 weeks' gestation, they documented an incidence of Mallampati class 3 of 36% and class 4 of 42%. At 38 weeks', the rates were 29% and 56%. The authors concluded that "pharyngeal edema causes some hindrance to tracheal intubation but not enough to explain the high failure rate reported." It is interesting to note such a high rate of Mallampati class 3 and 4 patients. In the original study in non-pregnant patients, Mallampati et al.[32] only reported a 7% incidence in this class. Whether or not this striking difference is because of early pregnancy requires confirmation.

Airway assessment

Because the incidence of difficult or failed endotracheal intubation is rare, tests that evaluate the airway will have a poor positive predictive value when applied to a population of patients.[20,21] However, negative tests, such as a Mallampati score[32] of 1 or 2 are comforting. Ramadhani et al.[13] demonstrated a significant correlation between sternomental distance, age,

weight and laryngoscopic view. Rocke et al.[17] performed a multivariate analysis looking at the relationship between airway abnormalities and difficult intubation in obstetric patients. Mallampati score, short neck, retrognathia and overbite were the only factors that correlated positively. Their model also predicted that the probability of a difficult intubation increases dramatically with increasing numbers of these abnormalities in an individual patient. It should be noted that the factors identified are not related to pregnancy.

The lack of appropriate airway assessment may lead to unanticipated difficult endotracheal intubation. Barnardo and Jenkins[14] identified 26 patients with failed intubations out of 8970, but were only able to find evidence of an airway assessment in 11 of these cases. Hawthorne et al.[15] noted that one-third of the failed endotracheal intubations were predicted to be difficult and 2/23 had medical records that noted previous difficulties.

Whether or not physical examination of the airway reduces the incidence of unanticipated difficult endotracheal intubation is controversial. Samsoon and Young[18] concluded that six of the seven failed intubations in their series of obstetric patients could be anticipated based on the Mallampati score (the seventh had occult tracheal stenosis).

Glassenberg and Freiberger[11] attempted to reduce the incidence of unanticipated difficult intubation by performing awake fiberoptic intubation in an unreported proportion of predicted difficult intubations in pregnant patients. The author noted that 50% of the failed intubations occurred in patients with no risk factors.

Unanticipated difficulties also occur in the nonpregnant surgical population. Two large studies estimated the incidence at between 37%[25] and 40%[24] of all difficult intubations. Of interest, when patients who had experienced difficult endotracheal intubation were re-examined, only 5% had no identifiable risk factors.[24]

A possible reason for a lack of thorough anatomic assessment of the upper airway leading to unanticipated problems in securing the airway, is that many of these cases are carried out under emergency conditions. Three studies assessed the time of day and indications for cesarean section in patients in whom endotracheal intubation was difficult or failed.[14,15,19] There was no consistent pattern in the time of day at which these problems occurred. However, 70–90% of the cases were considered to be an emergency.

Who are the operators?

Most of the prospective studies that had an airway assessment protocol specified the experience of the operators, usually at least 2 years of anesthesia training. Several studies do not define the experience of the operator.[11,12,17–19] Three studies, in particular, make special note of this issue.

Barnardo and Jenkins[14] noted that, of the patients classified as "failed intubation," over 80% of the cases were carried out by the most junior anesthesia trainees. Similarly, Hawthorne *et al.*[15] reported an incidence of 78%. These trainees provided most of the general anesthetics during the time period and therefore highlight the risk of remote supervision of junior staff.

In the study by Rocke *et al.*,[17] the most senior anesthesiologist performed the airway assessment but the most junior performed the endotracheal intubation. They recorded only two failures out of 1500 patients, one of these was easily intubated by the consultant.

Conclusions

From the available population data, there does not appear to be a difference between the obstetric and non-obstetric airways with respect to the incidence of difficult intubation or grade 3 or 4 laryngoscopy, both of which seem to occur at a frequency of approximately 1–6%. There also appears to be no difference in the incidence of failed intubation, which is approximately 10% of the incidence of difficult intubation.

Changes in upper airway anatomy related to pregnancy may contribute to difficulties in the airway management of individual patients. There is no doubt that some patients have abnormalities that are unrelated to pregnancy. It is possible that these are more pronounced during pregnancy and increased further during labor and delivery. As in the non-pregnant population, a thorough airway examination helps the anesthesiologist anticipate many of the problems. While this is helpful, unanticipated problems with endotracheal intubation do occur. It is therefore important to have a plan to deal with the situation if it arises. This plan should include a means of obtaining skilled help and additional equipment such as aids to laryngoscopy. Other techniques of airway management should be considered. Finally, it may be necessary to consider alternate modes of anesthesia.[3]

Many of the obstetric airway problems occur under emergency conditions and involve junior staff. Recommendations from the 1997–1999 Confidential Inquiries into Maternal Deaths in the UK include the need for a multidiscipinary approach to the parturient and better communication between the obstetric and anesthetic staff to allow time for appropriate assessments and preparation. Further, the Inquiry stresses the need for appropriate supervision of junior staff.[33]

In summary, only a small proportion of parturients will present difficulties in airway management. Many of these difficulties can be anticipated using a thorough clinical examination of the upper airway. Time to assess the parturient in an unhurried manner and the presence of an experienced anesthesiologist should decrease the incidence of difficult or failed intubation in the parturient.

Failure of endotracheal intubation will occur in the parturient with approximately the same frequency as in the non-pregnant population. It is therefore extremely important to be familiar with an alternative plan, using ancillary airway equipment when difficult or failed intubation occurs.

References

1 Hawkins JL. Anesthesia-related maternal mortality. *Clin Obstet Gynecol* 2003;**46**:679–87.
2 Cormack RS, Lehane J. Difficult tracheal intubation in obstetrics. *Anaesthesia* 1984;**39**:1105–11.
3 Crosby ET, Cooper RM, Douglas MJ, *et al.* The unanticipated difficult airway with recommendations for management. *Can J Anaesth* 1998;**45**:757–76.
4 Davies JM, Weeks S, Crone LA, Pavlin E. Difficult intubation in the parturient. *Can J Anaesth* 1989;**36**:668–74.
5 Ezri T, Szmuk P, Evron S, Geva D, Hagay Z, Katz J. Difficult airway in obstetric anesthesia: a review. *Obstet Gynecol Surv* 2001;**56**:631–41.
6 Halpern S, Preston R, Davies S. The airway in obstetrics. *Anesthesiol Clin North America* 1995;**13**:665–82.
7 King TA, Adams AP. Failed tracheal intubation. *Br J Anaesth* 1990;**65**:400–14.
8 Wilson WC, Benumof JL. Pathophysiology, evaluation and treatment of the difficult airway. *Anesthesiol Clin North America* 1998;**16**:29–75.
9 Barash PG, Cullen BF, Stoelting RK. *Clinical Anesthesia*. Philadelphia: Lippincott-Raven, 1997.
10 Chestnut DH. *Obstetric Anesthesia Principles and Practice*. St. Louis: Mosby, 1994.
11 Glassenberg R, Freiberger D. Beating the odds of a failed intubation: number needed to treat or the trick of turning to binomial tables. *Anesthesiology* 2002;**96**:A1022.

12 Dhaliwal AS, Tinnell CA, Palmer SK. Difficulties encountered in airway management: a review of 15,616 general anesthetics at a university medical center. *Anesth Analg* 1996;**82**:S92.

13 Al Ramadhani S, Mohamed LA, Rocke DA, Gouws E. Sternomental distance as the sole predictor of difficult laryngoscopy in obstetric anaesthesia. *Br J Anaesth* 1996;**77**:312–6.

14 Barnardo PD, Jenkins JG. Failed tracheal intubation in obstetrics: a 6-year review in a UK region. *Anaesthesia* 2000;**55**:690–4.

15 Hawthorne L, Wilson R, Lyons G, Dresner M. Failed intubation revisited: 17-year experience in a teaching maternity unit. *Br J Anaesth* 1996;**76**:680–4.

16 Lyons G. Failed intubation: six years' experience in a teaching maternity unit. *Anaesthesia* 1985;**40**:759–62.

17 Rocke DA, Murray WB, Rout CC, Gouws E. Relative risk analysis of factors associated with difficult intubation in obstetric anesthesia. *Anesthesiology* 1992;**77**:67–73.

18 Samsoon GL, Young JR. Difficult tracheal intubation: a retrospective study. *Anaesthesia* 1987;**42**:487–90.

19 Tsen LC, Pitner R, Camann WR. General anesthesia for cesarean section at a tertiary care hospital 1990–1995: indications and implications. *Int J Obstet Anesth* 1998;**7**:147–52.

20 Wong SH, Hung CT. Prevalence and prediction of difficult intubation in Chinese women. *Anaesth Intens Care* 1999;**27**: 49–52.

21 Yeo SW, Chong JL, Thomas E. Difficult intubation: a prospective study. *Singapore Med J* 1992;**33**:362–4.

22 Deller A, Schreiber MN, Gramer J, Ahnefeld FW. Difficult intubation: incidence and predictability – a prospective study of 8248 adult patients. *Anesthesiology* 1990;**73**:A1054.

23 el Ganzouri AR, McCarthy RJ, Tuman KJ, Tanck EN, Ivankovich AD. Preoperative airway assessment: predictive value of a multivariate risk index. *Anesth Analg* 1996;**82**:1197–204.

24 Koay CK. Difficult tracheal intubation: analysis and management in 37 cases. *Singapore Med J* 1998;**39**:112–4.

25 Rose DK, Cohen MM. The airway: problems and predictions in 18,500 patients. *Can J Anaesth* 1994;**41**:372–83.

26 Yamamoto K, Tsubokawa T, Shibata K, Ohmura S, Nitta S, Kobayashi T. Predicting difficult intubation with indirect laryngoscopy. *Anesthesiology* 1997;**86**:316–21.

27 Glassenberg R, Vaisrub N, Albright G. The incidence of failed intubation in obstetrics: is there an irreducible minimum? *Anesthesiology* 1990;**73**:A1062.

28 Fahy L, Horton WA, Charters P. Factor analysis in patients with a history of failed tracheal intubation during pregnancy. *Br J Anaesth* 1990;**65**:813–5.

29 Bhavani-Shankar K, Bulich LS, Kafiluddi R, Kral M, Datta S. Does labor and delivery induce airway chages? *Anesthesiology* 2000;**93**:A1072.

30 Chandrasekhar S, Topulus G, Bhavani-Shankar K. Upper airway study in pregnancy using acoustic reflectometry. *Anesthesiology* 2001;**95**:A1035.

31 Pilkington S, Carli F, Dakin MJ, *et al.* Increase in Mallampati score during pregnancy. *Br J Anaesth* 1995;**74**:638–42.

32 Mallampati SR, Gatt SP, Gugino LD, *et al.* A clinical sign to predict difficult tracheal intubation: a prospective study. *Can Anaesth Soc J* 1985;**32**:429–34.

33 Why mothers die 1997–99. Midwifery Summary and Key Recommendations. *The Confidential Inquiries into Maternal Deaths in the United Kingdom*. RCOG Press, 2002.

Jadad scale for reporting randomized controlled trials

Many of the chapters in this book have reported the quality of the randomized trials using elements from one scale.[1] The main advantages of this scale are that:

1 it is easy to use;

2 it contains many of the important elements that have empirically been shown to correlate with bias; and

3 it has known reliability and external validity.

In order to avoid duplication, the elements of scale are presented in full here (Table A1).

It should be noted that there are other factors that are important in describing the quality of reporting and these have been formally incorporated into the CONSORT (**Con**solidated **S**tandards **o**f **R**eporting **T**rials) checklist.[2] For example, some of the chapters make reference to blinding of allocation, *a priori* sample size calculation and statistical adjustment for multiple testing.

Some quality issues are unique to a particular problem. For example, it impossible to blind the patient or caregivers to treatment group when epidural analgesia is given to one group (and not the other) for labor pain. Therefore another method, such as a written protocol, is necessary to minimize bias for that particular set of randomized controlled trials. Clinical trials that involve administration of a specialized test

Table A1 Jadad scale for reporting randomized controlled trials.

Item	Maximum points	Description	Examples
Randomization	2	1 point if randomization is mentioned	"The patients were randomly assigned into two groups"
		1 additional point if the method of randomization is appropriate	The randomization was accomplished using a computer-generated random number list, coin toss or well-shuffled envelopes
		Deduct 1 point if the method of randomization is inappropriate (minimum 0)	The group assignment was accomplished by alternate assignment, by birthday, hospital number or day of the week
Blinding	2	1 point if blinding is mentioned	"The trial was conducted in a double-blind fashion"
		1 additional point if the method of blinding is appropriate	Use of identical tablets or injectables, identical vials Use of tablets with similar looks but different taste
		Deduct 1 point if the method of blinding is inappropriate (minimum 0)	Incomplete masking
An account of all patients	1	The fate of all patients in the trial is known. If there are no data the reason is stated	"There were 40 patients randomized but the data from 1 patient in the treatment group and 2 in the control were eliminated because of a break in protocol"

or procedure should report the training of the individuals in the procedure.

It should also be noted that there is no scale in common use to assess non-randomized (cohort and case-controlled) trials.

References

1 Jadad AR, Moore RA, Carroll D, *et al.* Assessing the quality of reports of randomized clinical trials: is blinding necessary? *Control Clin Trials* 1996;**17**:1–12.

2 Altman DG, Schulz KF, Moher D, *et al.* The revised CONSORT statement for reporting randomized trials: explanation and elaboration. *Ann Intern Med* 2001;**134**:663–94.

Index